NATIONAL ACADEMIES *Sciences Engineering Medicine*

NATIONAL ACADEMIES PRESS
Washington, DC

Regulatory Processes for Rare Disease Drugs in the United States and European Union

Flexibilities and Collaborative Opportunities

Jeffrey P. Kahn, Carson W. Smith, Tequam L. Worku, and Carolyn K. Shore, *Editors*

Committee on Processes to Evaluate the Safety and Efficacy of Drugs for Rare Diseases or Conditions in the United States and the European Union

Board on Health Sciences Policy

Health and Medicine Division

Consensus Study Report

NATIONAL ACADEMIES PRESS 500 Fifth Street, NW Washington, DC 20001

This activity was supported by a contract between the National Academy of Sciences and the U.S. Food and Drug Administration (75F40123C00077). Any opinions, findings, conclusions, or recommendations expressed in this publication do not necessarily reflect the views of any organization or agency that provided support for the project.

International Standard Book Number-13: 978-0-309-72655-9
International Standard Book Number-10: 0-309-72655-7
Digital Object Identifier: https://doi.org/10.17226/27968

This publication is available from the National Academies Press, 500 Fifth Street, NW, Keck 360, Washington, DC 20001; (800) 624-6242 or (202) 334-3313; http://www.nap.edu.

Copyright 2024 by the National Academy of Sciences. National Academies of Sciences, Engineering, and Medicine and National Academies Press and the graphical logos for each are all trademarks of the National Academy of Sciences. All rights reserved.

Printed in the United States of America.

Suggested citation: National Academies of Sciences, Engineering, and Medicine. 2024. *Regulatory processes for rare disease drugs in the United States and European Union: Flexibilities and collaborative opportunities*. Washington, DC: The National Academies Press. https://doi.org/10.17226/27968.

The **National Academy of Sciences** was established in 1863 by an Act of Congress, signed by President Lincoln, as a private, nongovernmental institution to advise the nation on issues related to science and technology. Members are elected by their peers for outstanding contributions to research. Dr. Marcia McNutt is president.

The **National Academy of Engineering** was established in 1964 under the charter of the National Academy of Sciences to bring the practices of engineering to advising the nation. Members are elected by their peers for extraordinary contributions to engineering. Dr. John L. Anderson is president.

The **National Academy of Medicine** (formerly the Institute of Medicine) was established in 1970 under the charter of the National Academy of Sciences to advise the nation on medical and health issues. Members are elected by their peers for distinguished contributions to medicine and health. Dr. Victor J. Dzau is president.

The three Academies work together as the **National Academies of Sciences, Engineering, and Medicine** to provide independent, objective analysis and advice to the nation and conduct other activities to solve complex problems and inform public policy decisions. The National Academies also encourage education and research, recognize outstanding contributions to knowledge, and increase public understanding in matters of science, engineering, and medicine.

Learn more about the National Academies of Sciences, Engineering, and Medicine at **www.nationalacademies.org**.

Consensus Study Reports published by the National Academies of Sciences, Engineering, and Medicine document the evidence-based consensus on the study's statement of task by an authoring committee of experts. Reports typically include findings, conclusions, and recommendations based on information gathered by the committee and on the committee's deliberations. Each report has been subjected to a rigorous and independent peer-review process, and it represents the position of the National Academies on the statement of task.

Proceedings published by the National Academies of Sciences, Engineering, and Medicine chronicle the presentations and discussions at a workshop, symposium, or other event convened by the National Academies. The statements and opinions contained in proceedings are those of the participants and are not endorsed by other participants, the planning committee, or the National Academies.

Rapid Expert Consultations published by the National Academies of Sciences, Engineering, and Medicine are authored by subject-matter experts on narrowly focused topics that can be supported by a body of evidence. The discussions contained in rapid expert consultations are considered those of the authors and do not contain policy recommendations. Rapid expert consultations are reviewed by the institution before release.

For information about other products and activities of the National Academies, please visit www.nationalacademies.org/about/whatwedo.

COMMITTEE ON PROCESSES TO EVALUATE THE SAFETY AND EFFICACY OF DRUGS FOR RARE DISEASES OR CONDITIONS IN THE UNITED STATES AND THE EUROPEAN UNION[1]

JEFFREY P. KAHN (*Chair*), Andreas C. Dracopoulos Director and Levi Professor of Bioethics and Public Policy, Johns Hopkins Berman Institute of Bioethics
RONALD J. BARTEK, President, Director, and Co-Founder, Friedreich's Ataxia Research Alliance
TERRY JO BICHELL, Founder and Director, COMBINEDBrain
EDWARD A. BOTCHWEY, Professor, Georgia Tech and Emory University
SHEIN-CHUNG CHOW, Professor of Biostatistics and Bioinformatics, Duke University School of Medicine
HANS-GEORG EICHLER, Consulting Physician, Austrian Association of Social Insurance Bodies
PAT FURLONG, Founding President and Chief Executive Officer, Parent Project Muscular Dystrophy
STEVEN K. GALSON, Senior Advisor, Boston Consulting Group
GAVIN HUNTLEY-FENNER, Principal Consultant, Huntley-Fenner Advisors
ANAEZE C. OFFODILE II, Chief Strategy Officer, Memorial Sloan Kettering Cancer Center
ANNE R. PARISER, Physician, Indian Health Service, Crow/Northern Cheyenne Hospital
JONATHAN H. WATANABE, Professor of Clinical Pharmacy, Associate Dean of Assessment and Quality, University of California, Irvine, School of Pharmacy and Pharmaceutical Sciences

National Academies of Medicine Fellow

SANKET DHRUVA, University of California, San Francisco

Study Staff

CAROLYN K. SHORE, Study Co-Director and Senior Program Officer
TEQUAM L. WORKU, Study Co-Director and Program Officer (*as of March 2024*)
EESHAN KHANDEKAR, Study Co-Director and Program Officer (*until March 2024*)

---

[1] See Appendix A: Disclosure of Unavoidable Conflicts of Interest

CARSON SMITH, Research Associate
MELVIN JOPPY, Senior Program Assistant
NOAH ONTJES, Associate Program Officer
KYLE CAVAGNINI, Associate Program Officer (*from April to June 2024*)
CLARE STROUD, Senior Board Director, Board on Health Sciences Policy

Consultants

ERIN HAMMERS FORSTAG, Science Writer
MAGDA BUJAR, Centre for Innovation in Regulatory Science
ADEM KERMAD, Centre for Innovation in Regulatory Science
JUAN LARA, Centre for Innovation in Regulatory Science
NEIL McAUSLANE, Centre for Innovation in Regulatory Science
ANNA SOMUYIWA, Centre for Innovation in Regulatory Science

Reviewers

This Consensus Study Report was reviewed in draft form by individuals chosen for their diverse perspectives and technical expertise. The purpose of this independent review is to provide candid and critical comments that will assist the National Academies of Sciences, Engineering, and Medicine in making each published report as sound as possible and to ensure that it meets the institutional standards for quality, objectivity, evidence, and responsiveness to the study charge. The review comments and draft manuscript remain confidential to protect the integrity of the deliberative process.

We thank the following individuals for their review of this report:

ERIKA FULLWOOD AUGUSTINE, Kennedy Krieger Institute
BARBARA BIERER, Harvard Medical School
CHERIÉ BUTTS, Biogen
KARIN HOELZER, National Organization for Rare Disorders
MWANGO A. KASHOKI, Parexel International
CHAITAN KHOSLA, Stanford University
ESTHER KROFAH, Milken Institute Health
LISA M. LAVANGE, University of North Carolina
BRENDAN LEE, Baylor College of Medicine
DONALD C. LO, European Infrastructure for Translational Medicine (EATRIS)
CHARLENE SON RIGBY, Global Genes, STXBP1 Foundation
JOSH SHARFSTEIN, Johns Hopkins University
FERGUS SWEENEY, Clinical Trail Expert (retired)

MARK TAISEY, Amgen, Inc.
SHARON F. TERRY, Genetic Alliance
JANET WOODCOCK, U.S. Food and Drug Administration (retired)

Although the reviewers listed above provided many constructive comments and suggestions, they were not asked to endorse the conclusions or recommendations of this report, nor did they see the final draft before its release. The review of this report was overseen by **ELI Y. ADASHI,** Brown University, and **DAN G. BLAZER,** Duke University. They were responsible for making certain that an independent examination of this report was carried out in accordance with the standards of the National Academies and that all review comments were carefully considered. Responsibility for the final content rests entirely with the authoring committee and the National Academies.

Acknowledgments

To begin, the committee would like to thank the sponsor of this study. This report would not be possible without the U.S. Food and Drug Administration (FDA), whose affiliates were instrumental in conceptualizing the study's statement of task. Numerous individuals and organizations made important contributions to the study process and this report. In particular, the committee wishes to thank the staff teams at FDA, particularly Rachael Anatol, Jacqueline Corrigan-Curay, Martha Donoghue, Lewis Fermaglich, Emily Freilich, Kerry Jo Lee, Akua Mfum-Gyau, James Myers, Miranda Raggio, Sandra Retzky, Quyen B. Tran, Katherine Tyner, Julienne Vaillancourt, Celia Witten, Sarah Zaidi, Samantha Zenlea, and Hao Zhu; and the European Medicines Agency, particularly Steffen Thirstrup, for lending their time and expertise, sharing information and data with the committee, and providing technical review of draft manuscript sections.

The committee thanks representatives from the following companies for taking the time to participate in a series of semi-structured qualitative interviews that helped inform the committee's deliberations: AMO Pharma; AbbVie; Affinia Therapeutics; Agios; Bayer; BioMarin Pharmaceuticals; Biogen; BridgeBio; Dyne Therapeutics; GlaxoSmithKline; Glycomine; Janssen Pharmaceutical Companies of Johnson & Johnson; Mahzi Therapeutics; Prilenia Therapeutics; Reata; Recordati; Roche; Sanofi; Stealth BioTherapeutics; Takeda; Ultragenyx Pharmaceutical Inc. The committee would also like to acknowledge the many individuals who took the time to share information, perspectives, and insights during open sessions of committee meetings. Their names and affiliations can be found in the committee meeting agendas in Appendix B.

The committee wish to express special thanks to the Centre for Innovation in Regulatory Science (CIRS) for its commissioned and pro bono contribution to this report. At CIRS, the committee thanks Magda Bujar, Adem Kermad, Juan Lara, Neil McAuslane, and Anna Somuyiwa, and for their collaboration and for carrying out the data analyses that helped inform this report (Appendix D).

The committee would also like to thank National Academy of Medicine fellow, Sanket Dhruva, for his thoughtful contributions throughout the study process; Erin Hammers Forstag for her writing contributions; and additional National Academies' staff, without whom this report would not have been possible: Christie Bell, Lori Brenig, Samantha Chao, Robert Day, Amber McLaughlin, Marguerite Romatelli, Leslie Sim, Clare Stroud, Taryn Young, Megan Lowry, Will Andersen, Christopher Lao-Scott, and Rebecca Morgan.

Above all, the committee would like to express its gratitude to the many patient groups, and people living with rare diseases—including caregivers and their families—for taking time to share their invaluable insights, experiences, and perspectives, which helped shape this report and inform the committee's recommendations.

Contents

ACRONYMS AND ABBREVIATIONS	xix
PREFACE	xvii
SUMMARY	1
Regulatory Flexibilities, Authorities, and Mechanisms, 3	
Use of Alternative and Confirmatory Data, 9	
FDA and EMA Collaboration, 13	
1 INTRODUCTION	19
Clinical Trials for Rare Diseases and Conditions, 22	
Context for this Study, 30	
Study Approach, 36	
References, 39	
2 FDA FLEXIBILITIES, AUTHORITIES, AND MECHANISMS	45
Drug Review and Approval, 46	
Designation for Rare Disease Products, 53	
Expedited Regulatory Programs, 62	
Inclusion of Pediatric Populations, 80	
Stakeholder Engagement, 86	
Select Rare Disease Programs, 97	
Transparency, 103	
Summary of Conclusions and Recommendations, 104	
References, 107	

3	**EMA FLEXIBILITIES, AUTHORITIES, AND MECHANISMS**	115

Drug Review and Approval, 116
Orphan Medicine Designation, 120
Expedited Regulatory Programs, 124
Stakeholder Engagement, 132
Rare Disease Initiatives, 135
Transparency, 136
References, 138

4	**ALTERNATIVE AND CONFIRMATORY DATA**	143

Guidance on Alternative and Confirmatory Data, 144
Sources of Alternative and Confirmatory Data, 146
Trends in Regulatory Use, 163
Novel Approaches for Data Analysis, 169
Biomarkers, 179
Opportunities to Enhance Innovation, 182
Summary of Conclusions and Recommendations, 184
References, 186

5	**FDA AND EMA COLLABORATION**	195

Similarities and Differences Between FDA and EMA, 197
Collaboration Between Regulatory Agencies, 214
Opportunities for Enhanced Collaboration, 230
Summary of Conclusions and Recommendations, 231
References, 235

APPENDIXES

A	Biographical Sketches of Committee Members And Staff	241
B	Disclosures of Unavoidable Conflicts of Interest	253
C	Public Meeting Agendas	257
D	Centre for Innovation in Regulatory Science Data Analysis Methodology	271
E	Qualitative Interview Summary and Methodology	283
F	Non-Exhaustive List of Patient Focused Drug Development Meetings and Patient Listening Sessions for Rare Diseases Between 2013 and 2023	303
G	List of Orphan Approvals by FDA or EMA Between 2018 and 2022	309
H	Select Examples of Rare Disease Drug Products	321
I	FDA and EMA Resources, Policies, and Programs Relevant for Drug Development for Rare Diseases and Conditions	337

Boxes, Figures, and Tables

BOXES

1-1 Orphan Designation, 20
1-2 Types of Clinical Trials, 24
1-3 Select Publications on Regulatory Processes for Evaluating the Safety and Efficacy of Drugs to Treat Rare Diseases and Conditions, 30
1-4 Statement of Task, 32
1-5 Key Terms and Definitions, 34

2-1 Benefit–Risk Assessment, 50
2-2 Reforms and Future Direction of Accelerated Approval, 67
2-3 Pilot Program: Collaboration on Gene Therapies Global Pilot, 75
2-4 Best Pharmaceuticals for Children Act (BPCA) and Pediatric Research Equity Act (PREA), 82
2-5 What is Patient-Focused Drug Development?, 88
2-6 Select Eastern Research Group Report Findings and Recommendations, 92

4-1 Use Case: SkyClarys (Friedreich's Ataxia), 149
4-2 Diseases Studied by Ongoing and Past FDA Office of Orphan Products Development Natural History Grants from 2016 to 2023, 151
4-3 Diseases Covered by Critical Path Institute's Rare Disease Cures Accelerator–Data and Analytics Platform, 152

xiii

4-4   Use Case: Relyvrio (Amyotrophic Lateral Sclerosis), 159
4-5   Application of Bayesian Method: Hypoxic Ischaemic Encephalopathy, 172
4-6   Use Case: Nexviazyme® (Pompe Disease), 177
4-7   Regulatory Guidance and Guidelines on Biomarkers, 180

5-1   FDA Demonstration of Discretion about Disclosure: COVID-19 Pandemic, 213
5-2   Gaucher Disease: A Strategic Collaborative Approach from EMA and FDA, 221
5-3   Select Examples of Drug Products to Treat Rare Diseases and Conditions that Received Parallel Scientific Advice, 228

FIGURES

S-1   Number of orphan drugs approved by FDA and EMA from 2018 to 2022, 4

2-1   FDA drug review process, 48
2-2   Proportion of CDER novel drug approvals that were orphan from 2010 to 2022, 56
2-3   Proportion of CBER novel biologic approvals that were orphan from 2010 to 2022, 58
2-4   Novel approval rates for non-orphan and orphan new drug applications submitted to CDER from 2015 to 2020 by office, 59
2-5   FDA approval of orphan and non-orphan drugs by therapeutic area from 2013 to 2022, 60
2-6   Entry points of expedited approval programs by clinical development stage, 63
2-7   FDA approval rates for orphan and non-orphan drugs using expedited approval pathways from 2013 to 2022, 64
2-8   Number of orphan and non-orphan drug products that received accelerated approval designation by FDA between 2013 and 2022, 66
2-9   Number of orphan and non-orphan drug products that received fast track designation approved by FDA between 2013 and 2022, 69
2-10 Number of orphan and non-orphan drug products that received breakthrough therapy designation approved by FDA between 2013 and 2022, 71
2-11 Number of orphan and non-orphan drug products that received priority review designation approved by FDA between 2013 and 2022, 72

2-12   Number of orphan and non-orphan drug products using the real-time oncology review program approved by FDA between 2013 and 2022, 77
2-13   Approval time of orphan and non-orphan drug products approved by FDA from 2018 to 2022 by regulatory pathway, 78
2-14   Use of expedited development programs in CDER and CBER from 2013 to 2022, 79
2-15   Expedited program approvals for new molecular entities and novel biologics in CDER and CBER from 2013 to 2022, 80

3-1   EMA committees in human medicines regulatory process, 117
3-2   Orphan product designation and maintenance along drug life cycle, 122
3-3   Designation and authorization of orphan medicines in the EU from 2001 to 2022, 123
3-4   EMA approval rates for orphan and non-orphan drugs using expedited approval pathways from 2015 to 2020, 125
3-5   Approval rates for non-orphan and orphan NAS applications submitted to EMA from 2015 to 2020 per therapeutic area, 126
3-6   Evolution of the number of orphan medicinal products that have received a non-standard marketing authorization, are non-small molecules, and have benefited from accelerated assessment, 129
3-7   Patient involvement along the medicines lifecycle at EMA, 134

4-1   Distribution of types of alternative and confirmatory data referenced by EMA and FDA for orphan drug products between 2013 and 2022, 147
4-2   The Rare Disease Cures Accelerator–Data and Analytics Platform process, 154
4-3   Use of alternative and confirmatory data by FDA and EMA in marketing authorization approvals for orphan drug products from 2013 to 2022, 165
4-4   Accepted alternative and confirmatory data for orphan drug products approved by FDA and EMA from 2013 to 2022 by therapeutic area, 166
4-5   Comparison between Bayesian and frequentist approaches, 171
4-6   The number of annual QSP publications deposited to PubMed vs. QSP-based regulatory submissions reported by FDA from 2008 to 2022, 178

5-1   Number of orphan drugs approved by FDA and EMA from 2018 to 2022, 199

5-2   Discordance on the approval of orphan new active substances approved by FDA and EMA from 2018 to 2022, 200
5-3   Approval rates for new active substance applications submitted to FDA and EMA between 2015 and 2020, 203
5-4   Novel approval rates for non-orphan and orphan new drug applications submitted to the Center for Drug Evaluation and Research from 2015 to 2020 by office, 204
5-5   Approval rates for non-orphan and orphan new active substance applications submitted to the European Medicines Agency from 2015 to 2020 per therapeutic area, 205
5-6   FDA and EMA expedited programs, 206
5-7   20 years of EU/U.S. collaboration on medicines regulation, 215
5-8   Top topic areas discussed in clusters, 217
5-9   Accepted Parallel Scientific Advice requests (N=26) by product category from 2017 to 2021, 225
5-10 Parallel Scientific Advice submissions by year from 2017 to 2021, 226

D-1   Project timelines and steps, 272
D-2   Overall methods and data sources used based on the contract agreement with the National Academies, 273

TABLES

1-1   Clinical Trial Options for Rare Disease Drug Development, 26

2-1   Components of an Action Package for an NDA or BLA, 49
2-2   CDER Decisions to Grant or Deny Breakthrough Therapy Designation Requests for Non-Oncology Drugs and Biological Products from 2017 to 2019, 70
2-3   FDA Guidance on Pediatric Drug Development, 81

3-1   Components of European Public Assessment Reports, 118
3-2   EMA Guidelines on Collection of Data, 119

4-1   Examples of Types of Confirmatory Evidence from FDA Guidance, 145
4-2   EMA Resources on Trial Design, Statistical Methods, and Alternative and Confirmatory Data, 146

5-1   Examples of Clusters Relevant for Rare Diseases, 218
5-2   Timeline for Parallel Scientific Advice, 224

D-1   Variables and Data Points Collected for Each New Active Substance, 279

Preface

The challenges for people living with rare diseases and conditions are numerous and often daunting. The Orphan Drug Act, passed some 40 years ago, was an attempt to remove policy roadblocks and create market incentives to increase research and development and bring new therapies for rare diseases to market. The impact was real, with nearly 900 new drugs for rare diseases since the Act was passed, but it was insufficient as that number barely scratches the surface in terms of the need. Of the rare diseases so far identified, fewer than 5 percent have available therapies.

This committee was tasked with examining regulatory processes in both the United States and the European Union for evaluating the safety and efficacy of drugs for rare diseases, and with identifying flexibilities and mechanisms available to regulators, all in service of increasing the number of available therapies.

Our conclusions and recommendations were informed by data available to us from both FDA and EMA, from information about policies and practices shared by colleagues from both agencies, by oral and written feedback from rare disease advocates, and by the experiences and expertise of our diverse committee members. This report represents the work of true consensus—a committee that was focused on its charge, careful in its analyses, informed by each other's expertise, and committed to going wherever the facts would take us, free of personal or self-interested agenda. The result is a clear-eyed assessment of the status quo, conclusions that point to needed change, and actionable recommendations for doing so.

We were aided by an incredibly committed, hardworking, and expert National Academies staff: Carolyn Shore, Eeshan Khandekar, Carson Smith, Tequam Worku, Melvin Joppy, Noah Ontjes, Kyle Cavagnini, and Clare Stroud. This report truly would not have been possible without them. Lastly, my personal thanks to my committee colleagues, for their careful attention and parsing of often complex data, for their patience and willingness to learn from each other, and mostly for their incredible commitment to improving the lives of those with rare diseases. It was truly a privilege to work with you all.

Jeffrey P. Kahn, *Chair*
Committee on Processes to Evaluate the Safety
and Efficacy of Drugs for Rare Diseases or Conditions
in the United States and the European Union

Acronyms and Abbreviations

AACC	Accelerated Approval Coordinating Council
AAV	adeno-associated virus
ACD	alternative and confirmatory data
AIDS	acquired immunodeficiency syndrome
ARC	Accelerating Rare Disease Cures program
ATMP	Advanced Therapy Medical Products
BLA	biologics license application
BPCA	Best Pharmaceuticals for Children Act
CBER	Center for Biologics Evaluation and Research
CDER	Center for Drug Evaluation and Research
CDRH	Center for Devices and Radiological Health
CHMP	Committee for Medicinal Products for Human Use
CID	Complex Innovative Trial Design
CIRS	Centre for Innovation in Regulatory Science
CMS	congenital myasthenic syndrome
CoGenT	Collaboration on Gene Therapies Global Pilot
COMP	Committee for Orphan Medicinal Products
CTIS	Clinical Trial Information System
CTTI	Clinical Trials Transformation Initiative
DMD	Duchenne muscular dystrophy

EC	European Commission
ECD	Erdheim-Chester disease
eCTD	electronic common technical document
EMA	European Medicines Agency
EPAR	European public assessment report
ERG	Eastern Research Group
EU	European Union
EUA	emergency use authorization
EU-IN	EU Innovation Network
FA	Friedreich's ataxia
FD&C Act	Federal Food, Drug and Cosmetic Act
FDA	U.S. Food and Drug Administration
FDARA	Food and Drug Administration Reauthorization Act
FDASIA	Food and Drug Administration Safety and Innovation Act
FDORA	Food and Drug Omnibus Reform Act
GAO	U.S. Government Accountability Office
GD1	Gaucher disease type 1
HC	Health Canada
HHS	U.S. Department of Health and Human Services
HIPAA	Health Insurance Portability and Accountability Act
HIV	human immunodeficiency virus
ICD	International Classification of Diseases
ICH	International Council for Harmonisation of Technical Requirements for Pharmaceuticals for Human Use
IND	investigational new drug
iPSP	initial pediatric study plan
IRB	institutional review board
ITF	Innovation Task Force
LADDER	Linking Angelman and Dup15q Data for Expanded Research
LEADER 3D	Learning and Education to Advance and Empower Rare Disease Drug Developers
MAA	Marketing Authorization Application
MDRI	multi-domain responder index
MHLW	Ministry of Health, Labour and Welfare of Japan
MIDD	Model-Informed Drug Development Paired Meeting Program

NAS	new active substance
NCATS	National Center for Advancing Translational Sciences
NDA	new drug application
NIH	National Institutes of Health
NMA	network meta-analysis
NME	new molecular entity
NORD	National Organization for Rare Disorders
OBRR	Office of Blood Research and Review
OCE	Oncology Center of Excellence
ODD	orphan drug designation
OMP	orphan medicinal product
OND	Office of New Drugs
OOPD	Office of Orphan Products Development
OTP	Office of Therapeutic Products
OVRR	Office of Vaccines Research and Review
PCWP	Patients' and Consumers' Working Party
PDCO	Paediatric Committee
PDUFA	Prescription Drug User Fee Act
PEC	Patient Engagement Collaborative
PED	patient experience data
PFDD	patient-focused drug development
PIP	paediatric investigational plan
PMDA	Pharmaceuticals and Medical Devices Agency
PREA	Pediatric Research Equity Act
PRIME	Priority Medicines program
PRO	patient-reported outcome
PRV	priority review voucher
PSA	Parallel Scientific Advice
QSP	quantitative systems pharmacology
RACE Act	Research to Accelerate Cures and Equity for children Act
RBI	randomization-based inference
RCT	randomized controlled trial
RDCA-DAP®	Rare Disease Cures Accelerator-Data and Analytics Platform
RDEA	Rare Disease Endpoint Advancement Pilot Program
RMAT	regenerative medicine advanced therapy
RPM	regulatory project manager
RTOR	real-time oncology review
RWD	real-world data
RWE	real-world evidence

SMA	spinal muscular atrophy
SME	small or medium-sized enterprise
SMN	survival motor neuron 1 (gene)
START	Support for clinical Trials Advancing Rare disease Therapeutics
TGA	Therapeutic Goods Administration

Summary[1]

There are an estimated 7,000 to 10,000 life-threatening and chronically debilitating rare diseases. While each disease affects only a small number of people, together rare diseases affect up to 30 million individuals in the United States, 36 million in the European Union, and at least 300 million across the globe. The impact of rare diseases extends well beyond the affected individual to include family members and caregivers, imposing a significant burden on an estimated 1 billion people globally, when accounting for both people living with a rare disease or condition and their caregivers.

The U.S. Food and Drug Administration (FDA) and the European Medicines Agency (EMA) play a critical role in protecting public health by ensuring that drugs to treat rare diseases and conditions are safe and effective. Additionally, the agencies help advance the public health by actively promoting scientific and technological innovation for advancing drug development. Before the Orphan Drug Act[2] was passed in 1983 the development of drugs to treat rare diseases[3] was largely neglected by the pharmaceutical industry. Following passage of the Orphan Drug Act and subsequent policy measures implemented around the world, including the European Union (EU) regulation on orphan medicinal products, which was adopted

---

[1] This summary does not include references. Citations for the discussion presented in the Summary appear in the subsequent report chapters.
[2] P.L. 97-414
[3] The Orphan Drug Act defines a rare disease as one that affects fewer than 200,000 people in the United States.

in 1999, there has been a marked increase in the investment and successful development of drugs to treat rare diseases and conditions. And yet today, less than 5 percent of rare diseases have approved products on the market.

For people living with rare disease and conditions, there is an urgent need to increase the pace and volume of drug development and of regulatory approval processes. Patient groups have expressed frustration with regulatory agencies, raising legitimate questions about how agencies analyze data gathered from small trials and consider patient and caregiver input in regulatory decision-making, noting seeming inconsistencies around drug products that are approved by one agency and not the other, and asking how and when FDA applies regulatory flexibilities across its centers and divisions.

The U.S. Congress called on FDA to contract with the National Academies of Sciences, Engineering, and Medicine (the National Academies) to conduct a study on processes for evaluating the safety and efficacy of drugs for rare diseases in the United States and the European Union. The statement of task includes: (1) flexibilities and mechanisms available to regulators, (2) the consideration and use of "supplemental data" submitted during the review process, and (3) an assessment of collaborative efforts between FDA and EMA.

The committee was specifically asked to focus on the regulatory processes for the review and approval of new molecular entities (NMEs) and biologics. As requested by the sponsor, drug repositioning or repurposing, new indications for drugs already approved, N-of-1 or single-participant clinical trials, devices, new modalities, and platform technologies were considered outside the scope of this report. While the committee looked at areas for collaboration between the United States and the European Union, recommendations are focused primarily on the United States.

The committee gathered information through open presentations from topic experts, public comments from interested parties, literature review, and semi-structured interviews. To supplement information gathered from the peer reviewed literature and during open sessions of committee meetings, the committee commissioned work to analyze: (1) success rates of orphan product authorization submissions and approvals by FDA and EMA; (2) distribution of products approved by FDA and EMA by therapeutic area; (3) use of expedited pathways by products approved by FDA and EMA; (4) use of "supplemental data" in applications for products approved by FDA and EMA.

Recommendations in this report seek to enhance strategic engagement of FDA with people living with a rare disease or condition, their caregivers, and patient representatives, especially patient groups that are small and under-resourced, throughout the full continuum of the drug development process; advance regulatory science, including the use of innovative study designs and methods and application of alternative and confirmatory data to inform regulatory decision-making for rare disease drug products; and improve collaboration between FDA and EMA.

It is important to note that at the time of this report's writing, there were several activities underway that could affect the landscape for the approval of treatments for rare diseases, including the Consolidated Appropriations Act of 2023 (PL 117-328) and the Food and Drug Omnibus Reform Act of 2022, which contain multiple provisions intended to improve rare disease drug development.

REGULATORY FLEXIBILITIES, AUTHORITIES, AND MECHANISMS

In the United States, FDA has authority under the Federal Food, Drug, and Cosmetic Act to regulate medical products and devices to ensure that they are safe and effective for the intended use. EMA is a decentralized agency of the European Union that is responsible for evaluating the safety and efficacy of drugs in Europe. To gain access to the U.S. and European markets, drug sponsors must submit marketing applications to both the agencies, which have different organizational structures, applicable laws, risk management procedures, and regulations.

Both FDA and EMA have regulatory flexibilities and mechanisms designed to facilitate the development and approval of drug products to treat rare diseases. These include programs to expedite the review and approval of certain types of drug products; mechanisms for engaging patients, caregivers, and patient groups; incentives for orphan drug designated[4] products (FDA) or orphan medicines[5] (EMA); and guidance (FDA) and guidelines (EMA) on study design, methodologies, and the use of alternative and confirmatory data. Together, these efforts help the agencies execute their missions to protect and advance the public's health with the goal of ensuring that patients have access to safe and effective treatments for rare diseases in a timely manner.

FDA and EMA Alignment on Evidence-Based Approaches and Programs

While FDA and EMA generally align on evidence-based approaches and have similar programs in place to expedite the review and approval of

---

[4] FDA has authority to grant orphan drug designation to a drug or biological product to prevent, diagnose or treat a rare disease or condition.
[5] EMA may designate an orphan medicine for certain products intended to treat a rare disease or condition.

drugs to treat rare diseases and conditions, there is no required process for regulators to jointly discuss drug products under review. That said, the two agencies often reach the same regulatory decisions when it comes to submitted applications for marketing approval for drugs to treat rare diseases and conditions (see Figure S-1).

Inclusion of Pediatric Populations

The majority of rare diseases affect the pediatric population. Evidence has shown there can be substantial differences in the way that children respond to drug treatment compared to adults. Thus, the inclusion of pediatric populations in clinical trials should be a core component for rare disease drug development.

Over the past several decades, a combination of legislation, regulatory action and the accumulation of scientific evidence has enabled what some have considered to be a "revolutionary change" in pediatric drug development—a shift from considering pediatric populations as "therapeutic orphans" to a current state in which the number of drug products

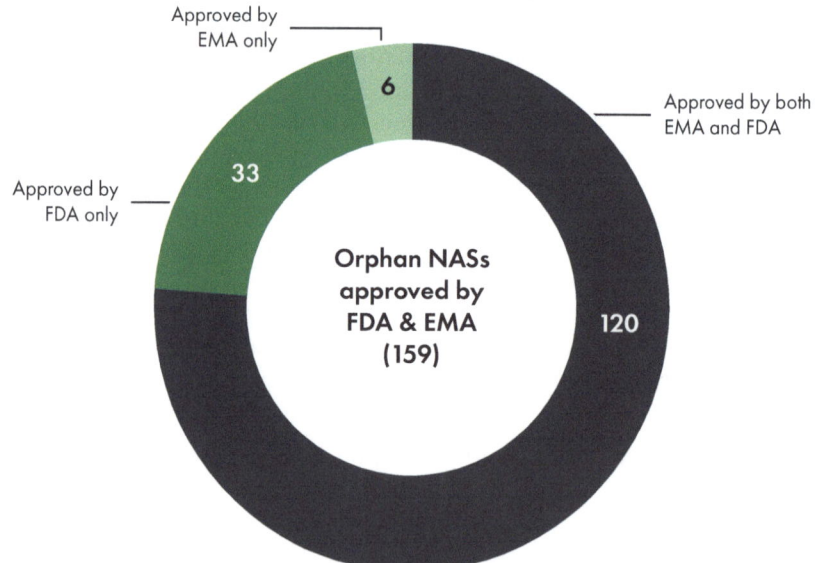

FIGURE S-1 Number of orphan drugs approved by FDA and EMA from 2018 to 2022.
NOTE: NASs = new active substances.
SOURCE: CIRS Data Analysis, 2024.

approved for use in children continues to increase. Two laws—the Pediatric Research Equity Act (PREA) of 2003, the Best Pharmaceuticals for Children Act (BPCA) of 2002—work together to address the need for pediatric drug development. In particular, PREA authorizes FDA to require pediatric studies for certain drugs and biological products. Despite these efforts, off-label drug use remains an issue for pediatric populations, particularly those living with rare diseases and conditions for whom there is no available treatment on the market. Notably, orphan designated drug products are generally exempted from PREA requirements.

In addition to measures taken by Congress to incentivize the inclusion of pediatric populations in rare disease drug development, FDA and the National Institutes of Health (NIH), in partnership with nongovernmental organizations—including patient and disease advocacy groups, academic clinical investigators, and biopharmaceutical companies—have an opportunity to better collaborate on approaches to include pediatric populations as early as possible in clinical trials and meet the needs of children living with rare diseases and conditions.

> RECOMMENDATION 2-1: Congressional action is needed to encourage and incentivize more studies that provide information about the use of rare disease drug products in pediatric populations. To that end, Congress should remove the Pediatric Research Equity Act orphan exemption and require an assessment of additional incentives needed to spur the development of drugs to treat rare diseases or conditions.[6]
>
> Additionally, the U.S. Food and Drug Administration (FDA) and the National Institutes of Health in partnership with nongovernmental organizations, including patient groups, clinical investigators, and biopharmaceutical companies, should work to provide clarity regarding the evolving regulatory policies and practices for the inclusion of pediatric populations as early as possible in rare disease clinical trials. Actions should include, but are not limited to the following:
> - FDA should convene a series of meetings with relevant stakeholders and participate in relevant meetings convened by others to clarify what data are required to support the early inclusion of pediatric populations in clinical trials for rare diseases as well as other key considerations.
> - Publish or revise guidance for industry on pediatric study plans for rare disease drug development programs.

---

[6] This sentence was edited after release of the prepublication version of the report to clarify the intent of the recommendation.

Enhancing Mechanisms for Patient Input

FDA has made important strides through guidance and policy to engage people with lived experience—people who are living with a rare disease or condition and their caregivers—throughout the regulatory review process. FDA advisory committees offer independent expert advice and recommendations on scientific, technical, and policy matters related to FDA-regulated products. In addition to including a patient representative who provides lived experience with a particular disease, condition, or medical product, all advisory committee meetings include an open public hearing session during which patients and their caregivers have an opportunity to share relevant information about a given drug and disease or condition. In principle, open public hearing sessions should inform the advisory committee on the drug product under consideration.

Conclusion 2-2: FDA is using available mechanisms to gather patient input. However, there are opportunities to better ensure that patient input informs the development of treatments for rare diseases as well as the design and conduct of clinical trials for rare diseases. More clarity is needed on the part of patient groups and people with lived experience on how the agency is using patient input to inform regulatory decision-making and what types of patient input are most relevant.

Patients and caregivers are experts in their own experience of living with or caring for someone with a disease or condition and their perspectives and insights should be valued alongside those of regulators, sponsors, and researchers when it comes to informing the development of drugs to meet their needs.

RECOMMENDATION 2-2: The U.S. Food and Drug Administration (FDA) should strengthen mechanisms to integrate input from people living with a rare disease or condition, their caregivers, and patient representatives, especially patient groups that are small and under-resourced, throughout the full continuum of the drug development process. To that end, FDA should take the steps necessary to fully implement Section 1137 of the Food and Drug Administration Safety and Innovation Act (Public Law 112-144), which directs the Secretary of Health and Human Services to develop and implement strategies to solicit the views of rare disease patients during the full range of regulatory review discussions. This should include but not be limited to:
- Implementing strategies to meaningfully engage people living with a rare disease or condition, their caregivers, and patient

representatives throughout the review process, from initial review discussions to final regulatory decisions.
- Ensuring equitable representation of people living with a rare disease or condition, their caregivers, and patient representatives throughout the review process by actively recruiting and supporting participation from underrepresented and under-resourced patient groups, providing necessary support and accommodations to enable their full participation.
- Developing a structured approach to directly engage people with lived experience (those living with or caring for someone living with a rare disease or condition), including in all open public hearing sessions of advisory committee meetings by establishing a mechanism to prioritize and provide speaking opportunities for people with lived experience, particularly patients and caregivers, to inform advisory committees on how primary or secondary outcome measures relate to functional status and quality of life.
- Developing in-person and hybrid education and training programs to assist rare disease patient groups in creating and maintaining tools (e.g., patient registry, natural history data, translational tools) that can contribute to research and development.

Enhancing Mechanisms for Sponsor Engagement

Sponsors developing new drugs must navigate a range of complex challenges when designing and conducting studies for regulatory submission. These challenges are heightened when it comes to rare diseases and conditions, particularly given that many companies developing rare disease drugs are small and medium-sized enterprises, which may have fewer resources and less in-house expertise than large pharmaceutical companies.

Conclusion 2-4: FDA engagement with rare disease drug development sponsors is of particular importance because compared to common diseases, rare diseases are less well understood, more often do not have regulatory precedent, more commonly lack validated endpoints and outcome measures, and involve small patient populations limit the size and number of clinical trials that can be conducted.

RECOMMENDATION 2-3: The U.S. Food and Drug Administration and the National Institutes of Health in collaboration with the European Medicines Agency, nongovernmental organizations, patient groups, and biopharmaceutical sponsors should implement a sponsor, investigator, and patient group navigation service to support the development of drugs to treat rare diseases and conditions (1) by advising on the range of available regulatory pathways and flexibilities and (2)

by providing clarity on how to comply with regulatory policies, apply guidances, and meet requirements in rare disease drug development. Actions should include:
- Facilitation including, but not limited to, consultation, referral to other organizations, services to identify and overcome regulatory barriers, needs assessment, and regular follow-up; and
- The development of educational materials and tools.

In addition to programs intended to facilitate and expedite development and review of new drugs, FDA has several newer programs relevant to rare diseases, including the Rare Disease Endpoint Advancement (RDEA) pilot program, the Model-Informed Drug Development (MIDD) Paired Meeting Program, Support for clinical Trials Advancing Rare disease Therapeutics (START) Pilot Program, the Complex Innovative Trial Design (CID) meeting program, the FDA-NIH Bespoke Gene Therapy Consortium, programs and pilots led by the Oncology Center of Excellence (e.g., real-time oncology review [RTOR], Project Orbis), and notably a newly announced Rare Disease Innovation Hub. These programs are welcome developments, but most are limited in scope and scale compared to the scale of unmet need in rare disease drug development. Several of these programs are early on in implementation, making it difficult to assess their impact on drug development for rare diseases and conditions.

RECOMMENDATION 2-4: The U.S. Food and Drug Administration (FDA) should assess the impact of new and ongoing programs and approaches that support drug development for rare diseases and conditions to improve the regulatory decision-making process; publicly share the results of these assessments in a timely manner; take steps to ensure that lessons learned across different programs are disseminated throughout FDA centers and divisions, including a summary of regulatory flexibilities and novel innovative approaches that were considered acceptable; scale-up and expand successful programs across therapeutic areas; and modify or sunset programs that are not improving the regulatory decision-making process. Programs and regulatory approaches should include, but not be limited to:
- Rare Disease Endpoint Advancement Pilot Program
- Support for clinical Trials Advancing Rare Disease Therapeutics pilot program
- Complex Innovative Trial Design meeting program
- FDA-NIH Bespoke Gene Therapy Consortium
- Programs and pilots led by the Oncology Center of Excellence (e.g., real-time oncology review, Project Orbis);
- Flexibility and leadership in the review and oversight of genetically-targeted advanced therapeutics (e.g., genetic therapies), especially for very low-prevalence patient populations;

- Adoption and support of master protocols, particularly basket trials, to support mutationally defined product approvals;
- Guidance development on cutting-edge topics to support drug research and development, such as the use of accelerated approval in tissue-agnostic drug development (i.e., drugs that target specific molecular alterations) and master protocols, among others.

USE OF ALTERNATIVE AND CONFIRMATORY DATA

For the purposes of this report, the committee uses the term "alternative and confirmatory data" (ACD) to mean data that are collected outside the setting of a randomized controlled clinical trial and used as supplementary, alternative and/or confirmatory evidence in support of regulatory submission and review of a drug product. These data include natural history data, registry data, data from expanded access or compassionate use, data from open-label extension studies, data from studies using external control groups, patient reported outcomes, and real-world evidence.

The statutory requirements for drug review and approval for rare diseases and conditions are the same as for non-rare diseases or conditions. However, when a disease is life-threatening or severely debilitating with unmet need, both FDA and EMA have flexibility to consider the use of ACD along with a single adequate and well-controlled clinical trial. The agencies have published guidance on how these data sources can support a marketing application. However, in the United States, there is little publicly available information about whether and how these data are taken into account during regulatory decision-making.

Natural history data are particularly important to rare disease drug development. The use of biomarkers or a panel of biomarkers can help alleviate diagnostic challenges and facilitate clinical trials based on smaller sample sizes and shorter duration. However, limited populations and the heterogeneity in clinical presentation combined with a lack of information about disease emergence and progression makes it difficult to validate biomarkers for regulatory decision-making. Natural history studies can provide information about potential endpoints and the relationship between disease severity/progression and biomarker changes as well as clinical outcome assessments—measures that describe or reflect how a patient feels, functions, or survives. While natural history registries have been established for a growing number of rare diseases and conditions, they have not been established for the majority of rare diseases and conditions.

FDA supports programs aimed at developing alternative data sources, notably the Rare Disease Cures Accelerator-Data and Analytics Platform (RDCA-DAP®), which is funded by FDA and operated by the Critical Path

Institute in collaboration with the National Organization of Rare Disorders (NORD). This platform is a centralized database and analytics hub that contains standardized data on a growing number of rare diseases and allows secure sharing of data collected across multiple sources, including natural history studies and patient registries, control arms of clinical trials, longitudinal observational studies, and real-world data. Drug developers and other data users can access the platform to better understand disease progression and heterogeneity, better target therapeutics, and inform trial design and other aspects of rare disease drug development. The European Reference Networks contribute work on registries.

> **RECOMMENDATION 4-1: The U.S. Food and Drug Administration (FDA) should enable the collection and curation of regulatory-grade natural history data to enhance the quality and accessibility of data for all rare diseases.** This should include, but not be limited to:
> - Continuation and expansion of support for current rare disease natural history design and data collection programs, such as FDA's Office of Orphan Products Development awarding clinical trial and natural history study grants
> - Continuation and expansion of data aggregation, standardization, and analysis programs, including, but not limited to Critical Path Institute's Rare Disease Cures Accelerator-Data and Analytics Platform
> - Support, education, training, and access to resources/infrastructure for nascent rare disease advocacy groups to enable the standardization and integration of patient-level data for future regulatory use.
> - Continuation and expansion of collaboration with other agencies (e.g., National Institutes of Health Rare Disease Clinical Research Network) to expand natural history design and data collection resources for all rare diseases.
> - Periodic assessment regarding the impact and opportunities for improvement of ongoing programs for the collection, curation, and use of natural history data in regulatory decision-making for rare disease drug development programs.

Given proven examples of success, the evolution in regulatory thinking, and advances in new trial designs and methods for data analysis, there is a growing impetus to apply and expand available opportunities for collecting, analyzing, and using ACD to inform researchers, sponsors, regulators, and patient groups on when and how alternative and confirmatory data have informed regulatory decision-making to ensure the integration of lessons learned from past successes and failures.

EMA and FDA can facilitate the use of these types of data in marketing submission applications by standardizing, documenting, and publicly sharing information to enable stakeholders to track over time how alternative and confirmatory data have successfully and unsuccessfully informed regulatory decision-making for rare disease drug products. A publicly available and easily accessible (indexed and searchable) listing of products coupled with standardized information on the types and sources of alternative and confirmatory data that were considered as part of a marketing authorization application, would enable drug sponsors, patient and disease advocates, researchers, and regulators to improve the collection and use of these data for rare disease drug development going forward.

An understanding of the opportunities as well as the gaps and inadequacies in alternative and confirmatory data would help guide data collection strategies on the part of patients, caregivers, sponsors, and researchers, and ensure that the data gathered are both relevant and robust enough to support regulatory needs.

RECOMMENDATION 4-2: The U.S. Food and Drug Administration (FDA) should invite the European Medicines Agency (EMA) to jointly conduct systematic reviews of submitted and approved marketing authorization applications to treat rare diseases and conditions that document cases for which alternative and confirmatory data have contributed to regulatory decision-making. The systematic reviews should include relevant information on the context for whether these data were:
- found to be adequate, and why they were found to be adequate
- found to be inadequate, and why they were found to be inadequate
- found to be useful in supporting decision making and to what extent

Findings from the systematic reviews should be made publicly available and accessible for sponsors, researchers, patients, and their caregivers through public reporting or publication of the results. EMA and FDA should establish a public database for these findings that is continuously updated to ensure that progress over time is captured, opportunities to clarify agency thinking over time are identified, and information on the use of alternative and confirmatory data to inform regulatory decision-making is publicly shared to inform the rare disease drug development community.

Several novel approaches for analyzing relevant data on drug safety and efficacy that can make it possible to generate useful information for regulatory decision-making based on limited data. Further acceptance of these methods on the part of regulatory agencies and sponsors would better enable the use of alternative and confirmatory data as well as data collected through traditional randomized clinical trials for rare diseases and conditions. While this report focuses on rare diseases and conditions, the committee notes that it is not uncommon for innovations in rare disease drug development to be a vanguard for applications across therapeutic areas, so lessons learned in the rare disease space could be considered by the agencies on a broader scale.

Conclusion 4-3: Given the variable and often longtime horizons for rare disease progression, gaps in the knowledge of disease etiology, ethical concerns, severity of disease, small sample sizes, and unmet medical need, rare diseases require additional methods of demonstrating substantial evidence of effectiveness. New approaches in study design and data analysis need not require lower regulatory standards, but rather they enable the consideration of alternative and confirmatory data and a nuanced interpretation of the benefit–risk assessments that take into account the limited availability of data, limited treatment availability and the risk acceptance threshold in these unique patient populations.

RECOMMENDATION 4-3: The U.S. Food and Drug Administration (FDA) should collect and disseminate information on how state-of-the art regulatory science; innovative study designs and methods; tools, including biomarkers and surrogate endpoints; and effective applications of alternative and confirmatory data inform regulatory decision-making for rare disease drug products by:

- Annually convening the European Medicines Agency, National Institutes of Health (NIH) National Center for Advancing Translational Sciences, industry, patient groups, and the broad stakeholder community to review new advances in regulatory science (preclinical, clinical, and platform technologies), iterate on innovative study design and methods, and consider other uses of alternative and confirmatory data for regulatory decision-making. Following each meeting, FDA and NIH should publish a publicly accessible summary of key themes and issues discussed;
- Publishing innovative methods for data analysis that have been used to support regulatory approval of drugs for a rare disease or condition, including information about how the methods were used or considered by the agency;
- Collaborating on the validation of clinical and pre-clinical drug development tools for drugs to treat rare diseases and conditions.

FDA AND EMA COLLABORATION

The complex regulatory landscape and the differences between regulatory agencies can have an outsized impact on patients with rare diseases and conditions. Due to the nature of rare disease drug development (e.g., small patient populations, high rates of morbidity and mortality), early collaboration and information exchange between the agencies to coordinate on study design and align on data requirements could help reduce duplication of clinical testing and streamline the regulatory process for sponsors submitting marketing authorization applications to both agencies.

Conclusion 5-1: Despite some key differences, FDA and EMA have similar approaches to the evaluation and approval of drugs for rare diseases. Given these parallel approaches, there are existing mechanisms for close collaboration between the two agencies, as well as opportunities for enhanced collaboration in the future, that would allow each agency to retain sovereign authority and accountability in regulatory decision-making.

Enhancing Information Sharing

Under EU regulations, transparency is an important feature of EMA's operations. Starting in 2016, EMA has published clinical data submitted by sponsors in support of marketing applications for human medicines. EU law mandates that EMA make clinical trial data publicly available while also protecting personal data and commercially confidential information. In addition to the European public assessment report (EPAR) and clinical trial data, EMA makes other information available to improve transparency, including dates, agendas, minutes, and outcomes of its scientific committee meetings; information about staff and experts' conflicts of interest; information about manufacturing inspections; pediatric investigation plans; and orphan designations.

Conclusion 5-2: To meet the needs of rare disease patients and their caregivers, there is an ethical obligation on the part of regulatory agencies to share relevant information on the review and approval of drugs to treat rare diseases and conditions. If researchers and sponsors working on rare disease drug development had a better understanding of the reasons for successes and failures of marketing authorization applications, they could better innovate new therapeutics that have a higher likelihood of reaching patients. Additionally, more transparency would enhance public understanding and confidence in the important work carried out by regulatory agencies.

RECOMMENDATION 5-1: The U.S. Food and Drug Administration (FDA) should take steps to make relevant information on marketing authorization submissions, review milestones, approval and negative review decisions (refusal to file, clinical hold, and complete response letters), and the use of regulatory flexibilities for rare disease drug products publicly available and easily accessible to inform sponsors, patients, researchers, and reviewers on decision-making rationales and when and how available policies are applied. While the committee acknowledges the legal challenges surrounding disclosure of information, actions should include, but not be limited to:
- Mirroring the level of information disclosed by the European Medicines Agency (EMA) presented on submissions, review milestones, and review decisions, such that there is parity between what FDA and EMA share publicly;
- Building on the work of the 2010 FDA Transparency Task Force, to implement Phase II product application's disclosure requirements:[7] considerations for product applications (including investigational applications);
- Organizing and structuring the information made public in such a way that the public can identify trends (e.g., increases or decreases in the use of regulatory flexibility by product type or therapeutic area over time and expedited and designation program use);
- Link clinical trials to FDA disclosures by using national clinical trial identifiers[8] to allow the public to better understand the connection between clinical trials and the regulatory process.

The committee recognizes there are multiple barriers to achieving greater transparency on the part of FDA, including laws that govern how the agency can or cannot share information. Some have argued that FDA has broad discretion on what is considered confidential. FDA has the ability to incentivize and facilitate pathways for enhancing information sharing, but there are practical and legal considerations, which may require modification of some of the laws that restrict the agency from sharing certain types of information. For these reasons, the committee recognizes the need

---

[7] On May 19, 2010, the Transparency Task Force released a report containing 21 draft proposals about expanding the disclosure of information by FDA while maintaining confidentiality for trade secrets and individually identifiable patient information. FDA accepted public comment on the proposals, as well as on which draft proposals should be given priority, on this website from May 19, 2010, through July 20, 2010. https://wayback.archiveit.org/7993/20171105152021/https://www.fda.gov/AboutFDA/Transparency/PublicDisclosure/DraftProposalbyTopicArea/ucm211691.htm (accessed May 14, 2024).

[8] A national clinical trial number is an 8-digit unique identifier assigned to a clinical study when it is registered on ClinicalTrials.gov.

Clusters

One of the primary formal mechanisms for collaboration between EMA and FDA is holding so-called "clusters"—regular virtual meetings between EMA and FDA staff, that are focused on specific topics and therapeutic areas that would benefit from an "intensified exchange of information and collaboration." Documents exchanged within clusters may include draft guidelines; assessment reports, review memos; and minutes from investigational new drug (IND), pre-IND, and pre-biologics-license-application meetings. While clusters help inform drug development and approval processes and provide a valuable forum for collaboration between the regulatory agencies, there is substantial unfulfilled potential. The impact of the clusters on the drug development ecosystem may be limited by the fact that cluster discussions are largely focused on specific issues such as an existing development plan or safety concern. The existing cluster structure could instead more prospectively address common challenges for rare disease drug development, thereby harmonizing and streamlining the orphan designation and drug evaluation process.[9]

An expansion and shift in focus on the part of the clusters to include prospective issues facing rare disease drug development would align with current objectives and build on existing collaborative efforts and help inform regulatory decision-making. There may be concerns on the part of the agencies or sponsors that such an approach could constrain discussions if information were to be made publicly available. However, the agencies have in place mechanisms to share non-binding documents that lay out common thinking on how the agencies weigh urgency and pragmatic limitations against the need for data to support marketing authorization applications for rare diseases and conditions and considerations for how FDA and EMA might address areas of misalignment on clinical trial endpoints, the determination of non-inferiority (or similarity) margins, use and acceptance of statistical methodologies, and totality of evidence determinations.

RECOMMENDATION 5-2: To facilitate the efficient global development of orphan drugs, the U.S. Food and Drug Administration (FDA) and the European Medicines Agency (EMA) should build upon the existing clusters relevant for rare diseases by undertaking the following:

---

[9] This section was edited after release of the prepublication version of the report to more precisely describe cluster discussions.

- Create a forum, which includes key decision makers within the agencies, for forward-looking discussion of issues and common challenges for rare disease drug development that EMA and FDA could use to achieve a more harmonized approach to rare disease development.
- Devote resources to discuss and resolve misalignment related to rare disease drug development.
- Publicly issue findings on key scientific or regulatory topics related to rare disease drug development.
- Conduct and publicly share an annual review of all orphan drug applications for the agencies to facilitate more immediate sharing of lessons learned and surface issues that cut across rare disease drug development programs.

Increasing the Use of Parallel Scientific Advice

Another formal mechanism for collaboration between FDA and EMA is the Parallel Scientific Advice (PSA) program. PSA is a voluntary mechanism through which the two agencies can concurrently provide scientific advice to sponsors during the development of new drugs, biologics, vaccines, or advanced therapies. The program does not guarantee EMA and FDA alignment but can offer potential benefits for sponsors, including agency convergence on approaches for drug development, a better understanding of each agency's concerns and requirements, and opportunity for sponsors and agencies to ask and answer questions. Despite the potential benefits of the PSA program, only a handful of sponsors apply each year. Reasons for the lack of uptake may include real and perceived concerns on the part of drug sponsors about the value of the program, practical limitations in participating in PSA, and a lack of incentives for using the program.

Conclusion 5-3: Despite the underuse of the PSA program and lack of available evidence related to its impact, the committee acknowledges and expects that, in principle, concurrent scientific discourse through PSA should better enable more streamlined clinical trials, regulatory review, and approval of drugs to treat rare diseases and conditions.

RECOMMENDATION 5-3: The U.S. Food and Drug Administration (FDA), along with the European Medicines Agency (EMA) and other key stakeholders, should assess the impact of the Parallel Scientific Advice (PSA) program over the past decade on drug development for rare diseases and conditions, publicly share the results of this assessment, seek sponsor input on approaches to improve and enhance the use and utility of the program, and take action to increase access, use,

and impact of the PSA program going forward. This assessment and plan for improvement should include:
- Reasons (real and perceived) for continued underuse of the PSA program and address the issues identified;
- Information-gathering on sponsor experience with PSA regarding the practical considerations (e.g., resources, location) for large and small companies to participate in PSA;
- Incentives that encourage use of the PSA program earlier in development (i.e., prior to enrolling patients in trials);
- Metrics for assessing the impact of the PSA program; and
- Criteria and goals for demonstrating improvement of the PSA program with established timeframes over a 5-year period.

If the actions taken do not lead to an increased use and greater impact of the PSA program within a 5-year period after the assessment and improvement plan has taken place, FDA should implement other mechanisms for parallel advice between FDA and EMA on drug development programs for rare diseases and conditions.

This report evaluates and makes recommendations for one part of a multifaceted ecosystem that determines which diseases are studied, what types of drug research and development are prioritized, how the safety and efficacy of drug products are reviewed and approved, which products are brought to market, and how approved and marketed therapies are made available (or not) to patients. While the adoption of the recommendations in this report will serve to foster transparency, streamline regulatory processes, and facilitate more collaboration between FDA and EMA, regulators review what is submitted to them. The gap between the needs of patients living with rare diseases and conditions and the therapies available for treating them cannot be closed by focusing solely on regulatory processes. Increasing the number of available therapies for rare diseases and conditions will require additional attention upstream of regulatory decision-making—investment in basic research to understand the underlying biology of rare diseases and conditions, approaches to ensure patient input is incorporated early on and throughout the research process—as well as downstream from the regulatory process—policies, incentives, and business models to address issues with drug pricing and payer decisions that have outsized impacts on the accessibility and affordability of treatments for rare disease patients. The committee believes this framing is critical for understanding the report recommendations and considerations for implementation.

1

Introduction

Rare diseases are a heterogenous group of between 7,000 and 10,000 life-threatening and chronically debilitating conditions (Haendel et al., 2019; NIH, 2023). Each condition may only affect a small percentage of the population, but they collectively affect up to 30 million people in the United States, 36 million in the European Union, and at least 300 million across the globe (EMA, n.d.; GAO, 2021; Gopal-Srivastava and Kaufmann, 2017; Haendel et al., 2019; NIH, 2023; Wakap et al., 2020). The majority of rare diseases have genetic precursors and over half manifest during childhood (Chung et al., 2022b; FDA, 2023c; Wakap et al., 2020). The impact of rare diseases extends well beyond the affected individual to include family members and caregivers, imposing a significant burden on an estimated 1 billion people globally, when accounting for both patients and their caregivers (Groft and Posada de la Paz, 2017).

The U.S. Food and Drug Administration (FDA) and the European Medicines Agency (EMA) play a critical role in ensuring that drugs to treat rare diseases and conditions are safe and effective. Additionally, regulatory agencies help advance public health by actively promoting scientific and technological innovation for advancing drug development. Before the Orphan Drug Act[1] was passed in 1983 (see Box 1-1), the development of drugs to treat rare diseases was largely neglected by the pharmaceutical industry (IOM, 2009). Following passage of the Orphan Drug Act and the subsequent policy measures implemented around the world, including the European Union (EU) regulation on orphan medicinal products, which was

---

[1] P.L. 97-414. *Orphan Drug Act* (January 4, 1983).

BOX 1-1
Orphan Designation

U.S. Food and Drug Administration

The Orphan Drug Designation program at the U.S. Food and Drug Administration was launched following enactment of the Orphan Drug Act in 1983 with the goal of stimulating development of drugs and biologics for rare diseases. A drug may qualify for orphan drug designation if it is intended to treat a condition affecting fewer than 200,000 individuals in the United States, or if it affects more than 200,000 individuals but there is "no reasonable expectation that the cost of developing a drug for the condition would be recovered by sales of the drug." Once designated as an orphan drug, sponsors receive the following incentives:

- Tax credits worth 25 percent of costs for qualified clinical trials;
- Waiver of the prescription drug user fee ($4 million for fiscal year 2024); and
- Potential 7 years of market exclusivity after approval.

European Medicines Agency

To qualify for orphan designation by the European Medicines Agency, a medicine must meet a number of criteria:

- "It must be intended for the treatment, prevention or diagnosis of a disease that is life-threatening or chronically debilitating;
- "The prevalence of the condition in the EU must not be more than 5 in 10,000 or it must be unlikely that marketing of the medicine would generate sufficient returns to justify the investment needed for its development; and
- "No satisfactory method of diagnosis, prevention or treatment of the condition concerned can be authorised, or, if such a method exists, the medicine must be of significant benefit to those affected by the condition" (EMA, n.d.)

NOTES: See Chapter 2 for more details on FDA's Orphan Drug Designation Program. See Chapter 3 for more details on EMA's Orphan Designation.
SOURCES: EMA, n.d.; FDA, 2022c, 2024b; Michaeli et al. 2023.

adopted in 1999, there has been a marked increase in the investment and successful development of drugs to treat rare diseases and conditions. Prior to 1983, only 38 drugs were available to treat rare diseases in the United States; by the end of 2022, FDA had cumulatively approved 882 drugs for 392 rare diseases (Saltonstall et al., 2024).

Over the past 40 years, patient groups, policy makers, research funders, drug sponsors, researchers, and regulatory agencies have worked to address the devastating impact of rare diseases on millions of patients and their families by facilitating and accelerating the development and approval of new therapies. There has been tremendous progress made in research and innovation as well as in regulatory policy, and yet today, only around 5 percent of rare diseases and conditions have FDA approved products on the market (Fermaglich and Miller, 2023).

The path to diagnosis for a patient living with a rare disease or condition is often long and arduous (GAO, 2021). Studies have shown that many patients visit multiple doctors and receive multiple misdiagnoses before receiving an accurate diagnosis; others remain undiagnosed (EURODIS, 2017; Shire, 2013; The Lancet Diabetes & Endocrinology, 2019). All hospitals and health care providers covered by the Health Insurance Portability and Accountability Act (HIPAA)[2] in the United States and most hospital systems in the European Union record patient diagnoses using the World Health Organization's International Classification of Diseases (ICD). Only around 500 hundred rare diseases were listed in the 10th ICD version (ICD-10) and only half of these had a specific code (Rath et al., 2012). A retrospective analysis of 2019 claims data showed that most (92 percent) of the assigned ICD-10 diagnosis codes associated with a rare disease were broadly defined and only 16 percent were diagnosed using a specific code (Kuester et al., 2022). In the 11th ICD version (ICD-11) published in 2022, there is an estimated 5,500 rare diseases included—around 11 times more than ICD-10 (WHO, n.d.). Prior to this increase, it was difficult for clinicians to appropriately document the care and treatment of patients with rare diseases and conditions. Additionally, the lack of ICD-10 codes made it hard for researchers to identify and track patients with rare diseases or conditions and study the epidemiology. Even still with a diagnosis in hand, patients face additional hurdles to receiving appropriate care and treatment, including the fact that very few approved therapies are on the market.

As is the case for other therapeutic areas, limited access to appropriate diagnosis and treatment of rare diseases and conditions for minority populations—African Americans, Native Americans, Hispanics, and several Asian subgroups—is further exacerbated by preexisting inequities in access to clinical care and social determinants of health. Inequities are further

---

[2] P.L. 104-191. Health Insurance Portability and Accountability Act (August 21, 1996).

embedded in the context of an appreciable geographic dispersion in rare disease presentation and prevalence across the United States and European Union (Adachi et al., 2023). Such inequities are particularly problematic for certain rare diseases (Everylife Foundation for Rare Diseases, 2024), including sickle cell disease (Pokhrel et al., 2023) and thalassemia (Lorey et al., 1996), which have higher prevalence and mortality rates for ethnic and racial minorities in the United States. These realities reinforce the importance of identifying and addressing barriers to research, development, and approval of new therapies for rare diseases and conditions to help ensure that products are made readily accessible to the full breadth of patients and communities who most need them.

While beyond the scope of this report, it is important to recognize that the economic burden and impact of rare diseases should be acknowledged. In the United States alone, the annual economic burden of rare disease, including direct and indirect health care costs, has been estimated to be in the range of $1.0 trillion to $8.6 trillion (Andreu et al., 2022; Yang et al., 2022). On an individual level, the average health care cost per year for people with a rare disease may be 2.8 to 4.8 times higher than for people without a rare disease (Tisdale et al., 2021). Rare disease drug products are also associated with higher costs compared to other therapeutic areas (EvaluatePharma, 2019). Some of the most expensive drugs on the market are for the treatment of rare diseases and conditions, which creates disproportionate barriers for patient access and a strain on public and private health care payers (Tozzi, 2019). These barriers are particularly severe for underserved communities, for which inequities in access to clinical care and underlying community health risks further complicate access to diagnosis and treatment. While payer programs should be designed to protect patients from high orphan drug prices, in practice this protection is not equally distributed or enforced among patients with rare diseases (Hyde and Dobrovolny, 2010). Ensuring equitable access to rare disease treatments will require vigilance on the economic burden and cost structure of diagnosing and treating rare diseases (Adachi et al., 2023), particularly given increased applications for more complex medical therapies.

CLINICAL TRIALS FOR RARE DISEASES AND CONDITIONS

Clinical trials are the primary method by which drug sponsors can demonstrate whether a new form of drug treatment or prevention is likely to be safe and effective in people (see Box 1-2). When it comes to rare diseases and conditions, there are several barriers that make it particularly difficult to design and implement clinical trials, a few of which are described below.

Small Patient Populations

By definition, rare disease populations are small and often geographically dispersed, which can limit the ability of researchers to enroll adequate numbers of trial participants in an interventional study. In general, trials that involve small numbers of participants raise methodologic concerns, given that results are more prone to variability and may lack statistical power and generalizability. The following concerns with small trials have been identified: low-power leaving too much to chance, lower probability that an observed effect reaches statistical significance, multiple variables making it hard to determine cause and effect to a meaningful degree, safety issues not being adequately studied, and subgroups cannot be analyzed (IOM, 2001). With small sample sizes, p-values (the probability that an observed effect would have occurred by chance if the test drug had no effect) are vulnerable to small deviations in observed effect and may inaccurately convey the statistical significance of results (Mitani and Haneuse, 2020). If an intervention has a large effect on clinical trial participants, the effect can be detected even with a relatively small sample size. Conversely, if the effect size is small, the trial needs a larger sample size to detect the effect with statistical significance (Serdar et al., 2021). Given that trials for rare diseases have small sample sizes, it may be difficult or impossible to detect an effect based on a traditional randomized clinical trial design; a product that has a real but small impact on patient outcomes may not show statistically significant efficacy and thus not be approved for marketing.

While randomized controlled clinical trials are the gold standard for establishing the safety and efficacy of a test drug, this approach may not be feasible for certain rare disease populations. In addition to the lack of patients who may be eligible to participate in a clinical trial, there may be ethical or logistical considerations that make it difficult to enroll people in a given study (Pizzamiglio et al., 2022). For many rare diseases and conditions, including an untreated or placebo control group can raise ethical concerns due to a greater risk of harm for participants who do not receive the active treatment. In such cases, different trial designs, such as crossover, adaptive, master protocol, and decentralized trial designs, may offer additional options for testing new drugs for the treatment of rare diseases or conditions (see Table 1-1).

As described in Chapter 4, alternative and confirmatory data—data that are collected outside the setting of a randomized controlled clinical trial—can be used to support regulatory submission and review of a drug product. Additionally, advanced statistical methods can be applied to address some of the analytic challenges with rare disease trials.

> **BOX 1-2**
> **Types of Clinical Trials**
>
> *"Clinical trials are research studies in which researchers assign participants to get one or more interventions to test what happens in people. Because of this, clinical trials are also called interventional studies. Often, the intervention is investigational, which means it is not approved for doctors to prescribe to people. In some clinical trials, researchers assign participants to interventions randomly. This means that researchers assign the participants by chance. Usually, participants (or their doctors) don't choose what intervention they will get when they join a clinical trial"* (NIH, 2023)
>
> **Types of Clinical Trials**
> - Phase 1 trials initiate the study of candidate drugs in humans. Such trials assess the safety and tolerability of a drug, routes of administration and safe dose ranges, and the way the body processes the drug (e.g., how it is absorbed, distributed, metabolized, and excreted). Phase 1 trials are often conducted in healthy volunteers, typically 20–100 participants. However, for some products, such as gene therapies or certain types of oncology drugs, phase 1 trials may not be feasible due to a lack of eligible participants or a toxicity risk and may be conducted in the patient population for a disease instead. Given the small number of patients with a rare disease, phase 1 trials may involve small numbers of patients or may be combined with a phase 2 trial (often referred to as a phase 1-2 trial), and in some cases, may often involve only around 10–20 patients.
> - Phase 2 trials continue the assessment of a drug's safety and dosing, but also begin to test efficacy in people with the target disease. These studies may include a range of controls on potential bias, including the

Preexisting Health Inequities

Widespread demographic disparities in health care access and outcomes in Europe and the United States are well documented. Studies have consistently shown that racial and ethnic minorities, low-income populations, and other disadvantaged groups experience higher rates of chronic disease, worse health outcomes, and more limited access to quality health care than more privileged populations (Clark et al., 2019; Docteur and Berenson, 2014; Ndugga and Artiga, 2023; Satcher et al., 2005; Williams et al., 2010). These disparities are compounded by the unequal geographic distribution of health care resources and disease burden, both within countries and globally (Docteur and Berenson, 2014). Although the primary

> use of a control group that receives a standard treatment or a placebo, the random assignment of research participants to the experimental and control groups, and the concealment (blinding or masking) from participants and researchers of a participant's assignment. For cases in which it may be unfeasible for a patient to receive a placebo or for randomization to occur (e.g., diseases with very low prevalence, ethical considerations with the use of a placebo control), as may be the case for some rare disease trials, all trial volunteers may receive the treatment, or phase 2 and 3 trials may be combined to answer research questions with fewer patients, or both. In these instances, trials may often only include tens of patients.
> - Phase 3 trials are expanded investigations of safety and efficacy that are intended to allow a fuller assessment of a drug's benefits and harms and to provide information sufficient to prepare labeling or instructions for the use of the drug. For common diseases, these studies may involve thousands of research participants and multiple sites and often include more than one trial. For rare diseases, especially for very low prevalence disorders, Phase 3 is often limited to a single clinical trial and may include fewer than 100 patients, where feasible.
> - Post-marketing studies are conducted after a product is approved for marketing and are highly variable in their design. FDA may require post-marketing studies to gather additional information about the risks, benefits, and use of a given drug, such as outcomes in clinical practice or to assess safety in a larger patient population. Results from these studies can be useful for understanding how a drug performs in broader populations or over longer periods than studied in the trials used to support FDA approval.
>
> SOURCES: FDA, 2018b; IOM, 2010; NIH, 2023.

contributing causes are structural and may even be subject to legal sanction today, current approaches to drug research and development continue to reflect and contribute to preexisting disparities. Clinical trials often lack adequate representation from minority groups (Turner et al., 2022), leading to limited data on the safety and efficacy of treatments in diverse populations. This lack of representation may be due to several factors associated with health inequities: differential screening and diagnosis as well as increased prevalence of exclusion criteria in underserved populations (e.g., smoking cessation and mental illness) (NASEM, 2022). Medical devices and diagnostic tools may be designed based on data from predominantly White populations, resulting in worse performance for patients of color

TABLE 1-1 Clinical Trial Options for Rare Disease Drug Development

Trial Design	Description	Relevance for Rare Diseases	FDA Resources
Adaptive	Enables prospectively planned modifications to a trial based on accumulated data from trial participants	Can help reduce the number of trial participants needed and increase the likelihood that trial participants receive the most effective investigational drug	FDA (2019a)
Crossover	Trial participants may receive a sequence of investigational drugs over time and serve as their own comparison control	Can help reduce the number of trial participants needed by allowing all trial participants to receive an investigational drug	21 CFR §320.27
Decentralized	Some or all trial activities take place at locations other than a traditional trial site; can range from hybrid (some activities involve in-person visits to traditional trial sites) to fully decentralized (all activities take place outside of a traditional clinical trial site)	Can help lower geographic barriers to trial participation and increase retention (e.g., trial participants may participate in trial activities at home or other convenient locations)	FDA (2023a)
Master Protocol	Allows multiple sub-studies, which can evaluate one or more investigational drug or one or more diseases or conditions	Can help expedite drug development and increase the likelihood a participant receives the experimental treatment	FDA (2022a)
Real-World Evidence	Clinical evidence about the use and potential benefits or risks of a drug product for disease/condition based on analysis of real-world data—data related to patient health status and/or delivery of health care that are routinely collected from various sources (e.g. electronic health records and patient registries)	Can help bridge evidence gaps not addressed by a traditional randomized clinical trial (e.g., serving as an external control, providing insights on the natural history of disease or condition)	FDA (2023e)

SOURCES: Chodankar, 2021; Park et al., 2024; Pizzamiglio et al., 2022; Zhou and Chow, 2023.

(Kadambi, 2021). Inequitable access to cutting-edge treatments and technologies can further widen gaps in health outcomes between advantaged and disadvantaged communities. Addressing these ongoing issues will require concerted and sustained efforts to increase diversity in medical research, ensure equitable design of health technologies, and promote policies that dismantle structural barriers to accessing high-quality care for all.

The committee observed that current approaches to drug research and development for rare diseases may inadvertently perpetuate existing inequities for already marginalized populations. For example, in the current environment, patient groups, which include patient advocacy organizations, disease-advocacy organizations, and nonprofit organizations, play a critical role in raising awareness, driving research and innovation, and informing drug development. Therefore, the patient groups with the most economic and social means are more likely to succeed in effectively advocating for much-needed resources and therapeutic advances. Conversely, patient groups that represent marginalized populations with fewer resources and less social capital are more likely to be left behind (Halley et al., 2022). This further exacerbates the scarcity of rare disease advocates with a lived experience of a specific disease. Given this context, the current advocacy-based model primarily serves a small select population of rare disease patients and has the potential to worsen current health disparities for marginalized subpopulations.

Additional resources are needed to ensure that research and development for new drugs to treat rare diseases and conditions are predicated on current epidemiology, health services usage, public health impact, and patient-centered outcomes and that it helps close the health disparities gaps for the underserved, minorities, and other marginalized populations. Preexisting health inequities also present additional challenges in the regulation of treatments for rare diseases. Understanding of efficacy of a treatment depends on an understanding of the disease and its progression. A lack of research and information on a rare disease that affects predominately marginalized populations could result in inaccurate understandings of the efficacy of the treatment.

Pediatric Considerations

Rare diseases commonly present during childhood, and, for some diseases, irreparable harm or death may occur before a child reaches adulthood (Chung et al., 2022a). When this is the case, clinical trials aimed at a rare disease should enroll pediatric patients as early as possible. FDA encourages sponsors to study a product in all relevant pediatric populations, from birth through 17 years of age, and to consider the relevance and comparability of endpoints for patients of different ages (FDA, 2023b). Conducting trials that include pediatric patients requires a number of special considerations, such as balancing of risks and benefits, obtaining informed consent of parents and agreement from children when possible, and ensuring the protection of child participants (IOM, 2004). The added layers of complexity for studying a treatment intended for a pediatric population makes regulation of these treatments more difficult.

Informed consent and privacy are fundamental principles of research; participants or their legal proxies need adequate information about the risks and benefits, the ability to make an informed choice whether to participate, and an assurance that data they provide will be kept private. In the context of rare disease research, informed consent and privacy are complicated by several issues. First, obtaining consent from parents while respecting the autonomy of the child can be a difficult balance. Second, due to the small numbers of available research participants, data sharing among researchers may be necessary, raising privacy concerns. Third, rare disease research may require the collection and sharing of genetic data as well as phenotypic data such as images or videos. Research participants may be able to be identified based on these data, particularly if they are one of only a few patients with a disease. These types of challenges require that researchers be thoughtful about how to conduct research while respecting the autonomy and privacy of rare disease patients (Nguyen et al., 2019). At the same time, people living with rare diseases may be highly motivated to participate in clinical trials and contribute to the research process, which further supports the need for informed consent that is person-centered and tailored to the needs and interests of the patient population (Gainotti et al., 2016)

As discussed in Chapter 2, there are several laws and regulatory policies in place to address barriers to pediatric drug development, but more is needed to address the unmet medical need for children living with rare diseases and conditions.

Complex and Heterogenous Clinical Manifestation of Disease

Successful drug development is built on a foundation of scientific insights, including an understanding of the natural history of disease—the progression of a disease or condition in a person over time. High-quality natural history data play a critical role in rare disease drug development as this information helps sponsors establish inclusion or exclusion criteria for interventional studies, determine clinical outcomes that are meaningful for patients, and identify relevant biomarkers and it can serve as or augment control arms in a clinical trial and serve as an external control to provide confirmatory evidence of a single adequate and well-controlled trial (FDA, 2023d). While natural history registries have been established for some rare diseases and conditions, for most rare diseases, the natural history is poorly understood (Liu et al., 2022).

The same condition can present differently across individuals and over time; this heterogeneity in clinical manifestation is more acute in the case of rare diseases, which further complicates the design and implementation of clinical trials (Murray et al., 2023). Clinical trials are generally designed to study the effect of an intervention on one or more outcomes, but for conditions with heterogenous clinical manifestations, the targeted measure(s) may not be relevant for all trial participants (Murray et al., 2023). Poor understanding of disease symptoms or progression can further impede the selection of relevant outcome(s) (Murray et al., 2023). There are several approaches for addressing the challenge of heterogeneity, including using multicomponent or composite endpoints that combine several outcomes into one measure (Chow and Huang, 2019; Chow et al., 2020; Murray et al., 2023).

For most rare diseases, there are often few, if any, validated endpoints—reliable measurements of a clinical trial outcome (Busner et al., 2021). The endpoints chosen for a particular trial depend on the design of the trial as well as the nature of the condition or the expected effect of the drug or both (NIH, n.d.). Endpoints (including surrogate endpoints) can be developed and selected in a number of ways—through natural history data, using measures developed for other conditions, or based on measures used in clinical practice. However, there are challenges in applying each of these approaches for rare diseases. Natural history data are often lacking, measures for other conditions may not capture all relevant symptoms, and there may be few clinical measures, depending on the rarity of the condition.

While there are many challenges common to drug development for all rare diseases, some are particularly pronounced for diseases for which information may be extremely limited or nonexistent. Due to this lack of information, the benefit–risk assessment that is integral to the drug approval process can be more difficult to conduct. If a drug is approved based on the limited information available, post-marketing surveillance, post-marketing studies, and registries can be effective tools for collecting additional information about benefits and risks (Sardella and Belcher, 2018).

Due to the complexity and heterogeneity of rare diseases, it is often the case that drug development programs must be tailored to address particular challenges. FDA encourages sponsors seeking to develop new drug products for the treatment of rare diseases or conditions to engage with the agency early and often and to review relevant guidance documents. There is no one-size-fits-all regulatory process for rare disease products, which can increase the time, effort, and difficulty for sponsors pursuing rare disease development programs.

CONTEXT FOR THIS STUDY

For people living with rare disease and conditions, there is an urgent need to increase the pace and volume of drug development and of regulatory approval processes. Patient groups have expressed frustration with regulatory agencies, raising legitimate questions about how agencies analyze data gathered from small trials and consider patient and caregiver input in regulatory decision-making, noting seeming inconsistencies around drug products that are approved by one agency and not the other, and asking how and when FDA applies regulatory flexibilities across its centers and divisions (EveryLife Foundation for Rare Diseases, 2023; Haystack Project, 2023).

Given the challenges associated with rare disease research and development and the need for new drug products to treat rare diseases and conditions, policy makers have attempted to understand the underlying issues and find potential solutions.

BOX 1-3
Select Publications on Regulatory Processes for Evaluating the Safety and Efficacy of Drugs to Treat Rare Diseases and Conditions

- 2001: The U.S. Department of Health and Human Services (HHS) Office of Inspector General published a report that assessed the implementation and impact of the Orphan Drug Act of 1983. The report found that the Orphan Drug Act was successful in motivating pharmaceutical companies to develop orphan products, which were generally accessible to patients. The report also found that the Office of Orphan Products Development provides a valuable service to companies and patients (HHS, 2001).
- 2010: The Institute of Medicine published a consensus study report, *Rare Diseases and Orphan Products: Accelerating Research and Development*, which made recommendations for the U.S. Food and Drug Administration (FDA) to (1) "develop guidelines for CDER [Center for Drug Evaluation and Research] reviewers to promote consistency and reasoned flexibility in the review of orphan drugs" and "use the analysis and the review guidelines to inform the advice and formal guidance given to sponsors about the evidence needed to support orphan drug approvals"; (2) examine the use of small clinical trials and adjust educational programs and guidance to align with advances in the science of small clinical trials and associated analytical methods; and the National Institutes of Health (NIH) and FDA to support NIH-funded studies involving rare disease research and development that are designed to fulfill requirements for FDA approval (IOM, 2010).

INTRODUCTION

The U.S. Congress requested that the National Academies of Sciences, Engineering, and Medicine (the National Academies) convene a committee to conduct a study on the processes for evaluating the safety and efficacy of drugs for rare diseases. The statement of task (see Box 1-4) asked the committee to examine processes in both the United States and the European Union, and specifically tasked the committee with identifying flexibilities and mechanisms available to regulators, considering the use of "supplemental data" during review (see Box 1-5 for key terminology), and assessing existing and potential collaborative efforts between the United States and the European Union. Several other publications on similar topics have been produced in the previous decades (see Box 1-3).

It is important to note that at the time of this report's writing, there were several activities underway that could positively affect the landscape for the approval of treatments for rare diseases. As part of the Consolidated

- 2018: The U.S. Government Accountability Office (GAO) was tasked with examining the process by which FDA reviews applications for orphan designation and published a report that looked at (1) FDA actions to address the demand for orphan designations, (2) the extent to which FDA has used consistent criteria to review orphan designation applications, and (3) steps FDA has taken to address barriers to rare disease drug development. GAO recommended that FDA ensure that information from orphan drug applications is consistently recorded and evaluated by reviewers (GAO, 2018).
- 2019: The European Commission (EU) published a study that evaluated the extent to which the EU Orphan Regulation, which was introduced in 2000, has been effective, efficient, and relevant. The study found that the incentives for development of medicines for rare diseases that were put in place through the regulation helped improve drug development. The report also stated that "the needs and problems to which the EU Orphan Regulation responded still exist, and, as such, the objectives of the Regulation remain as important today as they were nearly two decades ago" (European Commission, 2019).
- 2024: The National Academies published a consensus study report, *Living with ALS*, which made recommendations for actions the NIH, the Centers for Disease Control and Prevention (CDC), and public–private partnerships funded under the Accelerating Access to Critical Therapies Act should take to improve research and development for drugs to treat ALS (NASEM, 2024).

> **BOX 1-4**
> **Statement of Task**
>
> In response to a congressional request, an ad hoc committee of the National Academies of Sciences, Engineering, and Medicine will conduct a study on processes for evaluating the safety and efficacy of drugs for rare diseases or conditions in the United States and the European Union, including:
>
> - flexibilities, authorities, or mechanisms available to regulators in the United States and the European Union applicable to rare diseases or conditions;
> - the consideration and use of supplemental data submitted during review processes in the United States and the European Union, including data associated with open label extension studies and expanded access programs specific to rare diseases or conditions;
> - an assessment of collaborative efforts between United States and European Union regulators related to:
>   - product development programs under review;
>   - policies under development and those recently issued; and
>   - scientific information related to product development or regulation.
>
> Based on its information gathering and internal deliberations, the committee will develop a report with its findings, conclusions, and recommendations for actions that Congress, federal agencies, the pharmaceutical industry, and nongovernmental organizations can take to support collaborative efforts.

Appropriations Act of 2023,[3] the Food and Drug Omnibus Reform Act of 2022 (FDORA) contains several provisions directed at improving the number of rare disease treatments. Among other provisions, FDORA:

- Requires FDA to publish a report summarizing its activities related to designating and approving or licensing drugs and biologics for rare diseases (Sec. 3202);
- Creates a Rare Disease Endpoint Advancement Pilot Program (Sec. 3208);

---

[3] P.L. 117-328. Consolidated Appropriations Act (December 29, 2023).

- Reauthorizes orphan drug grants (Sec. 3107); and
- Requires the drafting of a U.S. Government Accountability Office (GAO) report assessing FDA's policies, practices, and programs regarding treatments for rare diseases (Sec. 3202).

In 2024, FDA announced a plan to establish a Rare Disease Innovation Hub (the Hub) to establish a new model for the agency to leverage cross-agency expertise and enhance shared learnings to spur drug development for rare diseases and conditions (FDA, 2024a). As outlined in this chapter and in the details of this report, there are numerous challenges for rare disease drug development—challenges that must be overcome to increase the likelihood of success for drug development across rare diseases and conditions and ensure that these therapies are accessible to patients to address their unmet medical needs.

Historically marginalized communities in the United States have faced heightened challenges in the realm of rare diseases and conditions. These challenges include inadequate federal and foundation funding, exclusionary research practices, and inequitable access to emerging therapies (Docteur and Berenson, 2014). As solutions are developed to address the needs of those affected by rare diseases, it will be imperative that the unique needs and perspectives of marginalized groups are centered in the process. Failure to do so will perpetuate health disparities and limit the overall impact of efforts to improve access to rare disease therapies. Inclusive funding, research, and treatment access strategies will be essential to comprehensively address the needs of all individuals affected by rare diseases and conditions in the United States.

This report evaluates and makes recommendations for one part of a multifaceted ecosystem that determines which diseases are studied, what types of drug research and development are prioritized, how the safety and efficacy of drug products are reviewed and approved, which products are brought to market, and how approved and marketed therapies are made available (or not) to patients. While the adoption of the recommendations in this report will serve to foster transparency, streamline regulatory processes, and facilitate more collaboration between FDA and EMA, regulators review what is submitted to them. The gap between the needs of patients living with rare diseases and conditions and the therapies available for treating them cannot be closed by focusing solely on regulatory processes. Filling the gap will require additional attention upstream of regulatory decision-making—investment in basic research to understand the underlying biology of rare diseases and conditions, approaches to ensure patient input is incorporated early on and throughout the research process—as well as downstream from the regulatory process—policies, incentives, and business models to address issues with drug pricing and

BOX 1-5
Key Terms and Definitions

- **Adequate and Well-Controlled Trial:** A clinical trial or clinical investigation that includes the characteristics defined in regulation:[a] a clear statement of objective, comparison with a valid control (types of valid control defined in regulation), adequate method of participant selection, method of patient assignment to treatment group (e.g., randomization), method to reduce bias (e.g., blinding), well-defined and reliable method of assessing participants' response, and adequate analysis of the results to assess effect of the treatment (FDA, 2019b).
- **Alternative and Confirmatory Data:** For the purposes of this report, the committee uses the term *alternative and confirmatory data* to mean data that are collected outside the setting of a randomized controlled clinical trial and used as supplementary, alternative, or confirmatory evidence in support of regulatory submission and review of a drug product. See Chapter 4 for additional context.
- **Benefit–Risk Assessment:** A comprehensive evaluation of the benefits and risks (along with uncertainties in managing the risks) for a drug product that is part of the drug review and approval process. Regulatory agencies use benefit–risk assessments to help ensure that approved drugs offer therapeutic benefit while minimizing risk to patients.
- **Biologics License Application:** "A request for permission to introduce, or deliver for introduction, a biologic product into interstate commerce (21 CFR 601.2). The BLA is regulated under 21 CFR 600 – 680" (FDA, 2021b).
- **Biomarker:** A drug development tool used to measure a biological or pathogenic process, a response to an exposure or intervention, including therapeutic interventions (e.g., molecular, histologic, radiographic, or physiologic measurements) (FDA, 2021a). Biomarkers are used in clinical trials to help diagnose, monitor, or stratify patients and to predict clinical outcomes and can also serve as surrogate endpoints.
- **Clinical Trials:** This report generally uses the term *clinical trials* to mean "voluntary research studies conducted in people and designed to answer specific questions about the safety or effectiveness of drugs, vaccines, other therapies, or new ways of using existing treatments." (FDA, 2018a)
- **Diseases and Conditions:** This report generally uses the term *disease* to mean a disruption of normal functions of the body that can be diagnosed by a health care provider. A *disease* or *condition* is an affliction that causes harm to an organ, part, structure, or system of the body that results in improper functioning, or a state of health that causes such dysfunction, with the exception of diseases caused by essential nutrient deficiencies.
- **Drug Effectiveness**: How well a drug provides the expected therapeutic effect on a disease or symptom in clinical practice in the real world (NCATS, n.d.-a).

- **Drug Efficacy:** How well a drug provides the expected therapeutic effect on a disease or symptom under controlled conditions, such as a clinical trial (NCATS, n.d.-b).
- **Drug Product:** The finished dosage form containing a drug substance (may include other active or inactive ingredients), which is intended for the diagnosis, treatment, or prevention of a disease (FDA, 2017). Biological products are included within this definition.
- **Drug Safety and Effectiveness:** For a drug product to receive the U.S. Food and Drug Administration (FDA) approval or European marketing authorization, it must first undergo a rigorous evaluation process in which evidence is reviewed by regulatory personnel to evaluate the likelihood of adverse effects and ability of the drug to produce the desired result (IOM, 2010).
- **Drug Research and Development:** Broadly defined term that includes laboratory studies (e.g., investigation to understand the biological mechanisms and processes that underpin a disease or condition; testing of molecular compounds to find beneficial effects against a disease or condition), pre-clinical studies to answer basic questions about drug safety (e.g., gathering information on dosing and toxicity levels), and clinical trials to test a drug on people to make sure the drug is safe and effective.
- **New Active Substance:** "A chemical, biological, biotechnology or radiopharmaceutical substance that has not been previously available for therapeutic use in humans and is destined to be made available as a 'prescription-only medicine,' to be used for the cure, alleviation, treatment, prevention or in vivo diagnosis of diseases in humans." (Centre for Innovation in Regulatory Science, 2020)
- **New Drug Application:** Mechanism through which a drug sponsor formally proposes that FDA approve a new drug product for sale and marketing in the United States. Includes relevant data and information (e.g., ingredients of the drug, results from animal studies, how the drug behaves in the body, and how it is manufactured, processed and packaged) that has been collected during research and development (FDA, 2022b).
- **Orphan-Drug Designation:**[b] A status given to drug products that show promise in diagnosing, treating, or preventing rare diseases or conditions. FDA and the European Medicines Agency (EMA) have similar, but not identical criteria for orphan designation. See Chapters 2 and 3 for additional information.
- **People with Lived Experience:** Individuals who have firsthand experience with a diagnosis or health condition. This may include individuals who have a rare disease or condition and individuals who are caregivers and/or family members of those who have a rare disease or condition.
- **Sponsor:** An applicant, such as pharmaceutical company, foundation, medical institution, patient group, or federal agency, that assumes responsibility for a marketing authorization application to a regulatory agency.

---

[a] 21 CFR § 314.126(b).
[b] 21 U.S.C. § 360bb.

payer decisions that have outsized impacts on the accessibility and affordability of treatments for rare disease patients. The committee believes this framing is critical for understanding the report recommendations and considerations for implementation.

To carry out this study, the National Academies convened the Committee on Evaluating the Safety and Efficacy of Drugs for Rare Diseases or Conditions in the United States and the European Union (see Appendix A for biographical sketches of committee members). The project was supported by funding from the U.S. Department of Health and Human Services. This report presents the committee's conclusions and recommendations and identifies the diverse set of stakeholders best positioned to address and implement its recommendations.

Committee's Charge

Given the broad scope of the statement of task, and the limited time it had to carry out the study, the committee focused on certain types of drug products to treat rare diseases and conditions. Specifically, the committee was asked by the sponsor to focus on examining the regulatory processes for the review and approval of new molecular entities (NMEs) and biologics, rather than applications to repurpose or reposition drug products. As requested by the sponsor, drug repositioning or repurposing, new indications for drugs already approved, N-of-1 or single-participant clinical trials, devices, new modalities, and platform technologies were considered to be outside the scope of this report. Finally, while the committee looked at areas for collaboration between the United States and the European Union, recommendations are focused primarily on the U.S. regulatory landscape.

STUDY APPROACH

Committee Composition

To carry out the statement of task, a committee was convened that included experts from a broad array of fields, including bioethics, biomedical engineering, biostatistics, clinical trials, pharmaceutical research and development, patient advocacy, regulatory policy at FDA and EMA, risk analysis, translational science, and technology transfer.

Information Gathering

The committee gathered information through open presentations from topic experts, public comments from interested parties, literature review, commissioned data analysis, and semi-structured interviews. The committee held three open sessions during the course of the study: November 6–7, 2023; December 4–5, 2023; and February 6–7, 2024 (see Appendix C for open session agendas). During these open sessions, the committee received presentations from FDA, EMA, patient advocates, industry drug developers, industry trade organizations, and experts on alternative and confirmatory data and trial design. Stakeholders that were interested in providing a public comment were able to speak as part of the open session meetings with the committee. Interested parties also had opportunities to submit written public comments for the committee's consideration. At the beginning of the project, National Academies staff conducted a literature review to curate research materials for the committee's consideration. The committee was provided with literature in preparation for each committee meeting that was tailored to the planned topics of the open session.

The commissioned analysis and semi-structured interviews were conducted at the request of the committee. Both were designed by the committee. The committee commissioned the Centre for Innovation in Regulatory Science (CIRS) to analyze: (1) the success rates of orphan product approval and authorization submissions at FDA and EMA, respectively; (2) the distribution of products approved by FDA and EMA by therapeutic area; (3) the use of expedited pathways by products approved by FDA and EMA; and (4) the use of "supplemental data" in applications for products approved by FDA and EMA (see Appendix D for a detailed description of CIRS' methodology). At the request of the committee, National Academies staff conducted semi-structured interviews with industry stakeholders who led the clinical development or regulatory submission of rare disease drug products (see Appendix E for a detailed description of the approach, including a recruitment strategy and a summary of the stakeholders interviewed).

Concepts, Definitions, and Conceptual Framework

Orphan designation in the United States is available for drugs aimed at rare diseases that affect fewer than 200,000 people *or* drugs that are aimed at diseases that affect more than 200,000 people in the United States and "for which there is no reasonable expectation that the cost of developing and making available in the United States a drug for such disease or condition will be recovered from sales in the United States of such drug."[4]

EU legislation defines a rare disease or condition as one for which the prevalence is no more than 5 in 10,000 people across the European Union.[5] EMA orphan designation is available for drugs that meet *all* of the following criteria:

---

[4] Federal Food, Drug, and Cosmetic Act, SEC. 526(a)(2), 2023.
[5] EU Pharmaceutical Legislation on Orphan Medicinal Products (Regulation (EC) 141/2000, 1999.

- "it must be intended for the treatment, prevention or diagnosis of a disease that is life-threatening or chronically debilitating;
- "the prevalence of the condition in the EU must not be more than 5 in 10,000 or it must be unlikely that marketing of the medicine would generate sufficient returns to justify the investment needed for its development;
- "no satisfactory method of diagnosis, prevention or treatment of the condition concerned can be authorized, or, if such a method exists, the medicine must be of significant benefit to those affected by the condition." (EMA, n.d.)

While the definitions of a rare disease differ somewhat between FDA and EMA, the numbers are roughly similar. The population in the European Union in January 2023 was 448.4 million (European Commission, 2023); a rare disease or condition as defined by EMA would be one that affects less than 224,200 people (compared to the FDA definition of less than 200,000 people). The population in the United States in 2023 was estimated to be 334.9 million people (USAFacts, n.d.); a rare disease or condition as defined by FDA would be approximately 6 in 10,000 (compared to the EMA requirement of no more than 5 in 10,000 people). For consistency, this report will use the same definition for recurring key terms (see Box 1-5).

Organization of the Report

This report is organized into five chapters. The first chapter provides the context for the study and the committee's approach and gives a brief overview of the topic. The second chapter describes the regulatory functions of FDA and its flexibilities, authorities, and mechanisms related to rare disease drug development, review, and approval. The third chapter reviews the same areas for EMA. In the fourth chapter, the committee explores the various approaches for generating and using alternative and confirmatory data and examines how these data are received by FDA and EMA for the purposes of drug approval. Chapter 5 provides a comparison between the regulatory approaches of FDA and EMA and identifies existing and potential areas for collaboration between the two agencies. The committee's recommendations are presented throughout the report.

REFERENCES

Adachi, T., A. W. El-Hattab, R. Jain, K. A. Nogales Crespo, C. I. Quirland Lazo, M. Scarpa, M. Summar, and D. Wattanasirichaigoon. 2023. Enhancing equitable access to rare disease diagnosis and treatment around the world: A review of evidence, policies, and challenges. *International Journal of Environment Research and Public Health* 20(6).

Andreu, P., J. Karam, C. Child, G. Chiesi, and G. Cioffi. 2022. *The burden of rare diseases: An economic evaluation.* https://chiesirarediseases.com/assets/pdf/chiesiglobalrarediseases. whitepaper-feb.-2022_production-proof.pdf (accessed August 1, 2024).

Busner, J., G. Pandina, S. Domingo, A. K. Berger, M. T. Acosta, N. Fisseha, J. Horrigan, J. Ivkovic, W. Jacobson, D. Revicki, and V. Villalta-Gil. 2021. Clinician and patient-reported endpoints in CNS orphan drug clinical trials: ISCTM position paper on best practices for endpoint selection, validation, training, and standardization. *Innovations in Clinical Neuroscience* 18(10-12):15-22.

Centre for Innovation in Regulatory Science. 2020. *R&D briefing 81: New drug approvals in six major authorities 2011–2020: Focus on facilitated regulatory pathways and worksharing.* London, UK: Centre for Innovation in Regulatory Science (CIRS).

Chodankar, D. 2021. Introduction to real-world evidence studies. *Perspectives in Clinical Research* 12(3):171-174.

Chow, S. C., and Z. Huang. 2019. Innovative thinking on endpoint selection in clinical trials. *Journal of Biopharmaceutical Statistics* 29(5):941-951.

Chow, S.-C., P. J. Lee, J. Gao, R. J. Lee, J. J. Lee, and Z. Soferman. 2020. Statistical method for development of composite index in clinical research. *American Journal of Biomedical Science & Research* 10(4):388-393.

Chung, C. C. Y., A. T. W. Chu, and B. H. Y. Chung. 2022a. Rare disease emerging as a global public health priority. *Frontiers in Public Health* 10:1028545.

Chung, C. C. Y., Hong Kong Genome Project, A. T. W. Chu, and B. H. Y. Chung. 2022b. Rare disease emerging as a global public health priority. *Frontiers in Public Health* 10.

Clark, L. T., L. Watkins, I. L. Piña, M. Elmer, O. Akinboboye, M. Gorham, B. Jamerson, C. McCullough, C. Pierre, A. B. Polis, G. Puckrein, and J. M. Regnante. 2019. Increasing diversity in clinical trials: Overcoming critical barriers. *Current Problems in Cardiology* 44(5):148-172.

Docteur, E., and R. A. Berenson. 2014. In pursuit of health equity: Comparing U.S. and EU approaches to eliminating disparities. *SSRN Electronic Journal.* http://dx.doi.org/10.2139/ssrn.2462922.

EMA (European Medicines Agency). n.d. *Orphan designation: Overview.* https://www.ema.europa.eu/en/human-regulatory-overview/orphan-designation-overview (accessed June 25, 2024).

EURODIS (European Organisation for Rare Diseases). 2017. *Survey of the delay in diagnosis for 8 rare diseases in Europe ('Eurordiscare 2').* https://www.healthworkscollective.com/wp-content/uploads/2013/10/Fact_Sheet_Eurordiscare2.pdf (accessed August 1, 2024).

European Commission. 2019. *Study to support the evaluation of the EU orphan regulation.* https://health.ec.europa.eu/system/files/2020-08/orphan-regulation_study_final-report_en_0.pdf (accessed August 1, 2024).

European Comission. 2023. *Population and population change statistics.* https://ec.europa.eu/eurostat/statistics-explained/index.php?title=Population_and_population_change_statistics (accessed July 9, 2024).

EvaluatePharma. 2019. *Orphan drug report 2019.* 6th Edition. https://info.evaluate.com/rs/607-YGS-364/images/EvaluatePharma%20Orphan%20Drug%20Report%202019.pdf (accessed May 22, 2024).

EveryLife Foundation for Rare Diseases. 2023. *EveryLife Foundation applauds bipartisan congressional letter urging FDA to strengthen rare disease activities.* https://everylifefoundation.org/everylife-foundation-applauds-bipartisan-congressional-letter-urging-fda-to-strengthen-rare-disease-activities/ (accessed June 25, 2024).

Everylife Foundation for Rare Diseases. 2024. *Challenges to diversity in rare diseases.* https://everylifefoundation.org/rare-advocates/rare-diversity-hub/disparities-in-public-health/#toggle-id-1 (accessed June 25, 2024).

FDA (U.S. Food and Drug Administration). 2017. *Drugs@FDA glossary of terms.* https://www.fda.gov/drugs/drug-approvals-and-databases/drugsfda-glossary-terms (accessed August 1, 2024).

FDA. 2018a. *Clinical trials: What patients need to know.* https://www.fda.gov/patients/clinical-trials-what-patients-need-know (accessed June 25, 2024).

FDA. 2018b. *What are the different types of clinical research?* https://www.fda.gov/patients/clinical-trials-what-patients-need-know/what-are-different-types-clinical-research (accessed June 25, 2024).

FDA. 2019a. *Adaptive designs for clinical trials of drugs and biologics: Guidance for industry.* https://www.fda.gov/media/78495/download (accessed August 1, 2024).

FDA. 2019b. *Demonstrating substantial evidence of effectiveness for human drug and biological products: Guidance for industry.* https://www.fda.gov/media/133660/download (accessed August 1, 2024).

FDA. 2021a. *About biomarkers and qualification.* https://www.fda.gov/drugs/biomarker-qualification-program/about-biomarkers-and-qualification#what-is (accessed June 25, 2024).

FDA. 2021b. *Biologics license applications (BLA) process (CBER).* https://www.fda.gov/vaccines-blood-biologics/development-approval-process-cber/biologics-license-applications-bla-process-cber#:~:text=The%20Biologics%20License%20Application%20(BLA,under%2021%20CFR%20600%20E2%80%93%20680 (accessed August 1, 2024).

FDA. 2022a. *Master protocols: Efficient clinical trial design strategies to expedite development of oncology drugs and biologics: Guidance for industry.* https://www.fda.gov/media/120721/download (accessed August 1, 2024).

FDA. 2022b. *New drug application (NDA).* https://www.fda.gov/drugs/types-applications/new-drug-application-nda (accessed June 25, 2024).

FDA. 2022c. *Rare diseases at FDA.* https://www.fda.gov/patients/rare-diseases-fda (accessed June 25, 2024).

FDA. 2023a. *Decentralized clinical trials for drugs, biological products, and devices: Guidance for industry, investigators, and other stakeholders.* https://www.fda.gov/media/167696/download (accessed August 1, 2024).

FDA. 2023b. *Pediatric drug development: Regulatory considerations — complying with the Pediatric Research Equity Act and qualifying for pediatric exclusivity under the Best Pharmaceuticals for Children Act.* https://www.fda.gov/media/168201/download (accessed August 1, 2024).

FDA. 2023c. *Rare diseases: Considerations for the development of drugs and biological products: Guidance for industry.* https://www.fda.gov/media/119757/download (accessed August 1, 2024).

FDA. 2023d. *Real-world data: Assessing registries to support regulatory decision-making for drug and biological products: Guidance for industry.* https://www.fda.gov/media/154449/download (accessed August 1, 2024).

FDA. 2023e. *Real-world evidence.* https://www.fda.gov/science-research/science-and-research-special-topics/real-world-evidence (accessed June 25, 2024).

FDA. 2024a. *FDA Rare Disease Innovation Hub to enhance and advance outcomes for patients.* https://www.fda.gov/news-events/fda-voices/fda-rare-disease-innovation-hub-enhance-and-advance-outcomes-patients (accessed August 15, 2024).

FDA. 2024b. *Prescription Drug User Free Ammendments.* https://www.fda.gov/industry/fda-user-fee-programs/prescription-drug-user-fee-amendments (accessed June 25, 2024).

Fermaglich, L. J., and K. L. Miller. 2023. A comprehensive study of the rare diseases and conditions targeted by orphan drug designations and approvals over the forty years of the Orphan Drug Act. *Orphanet Journal of Rare Diseases* 18(1):163.

Gainotti, S., C. Turner, S. Woods, A. Kole, P. McCormack, H. Lochmüller, O. Riess, V. Straub, M. Posada, D. Taruscio, and D. Mascalzoni. 2016. Improving the informed consent process in international collaborative rare disease research: Effective consent for effective research. *European Journal of Human Genetics* 24(9):1248-1254.

GAO (U.S. Government Accountability Office). 2018. *Orphan drugs: FDA could improve designation review consistency; rare disease drug development challenges continue.* https://www.gao.gov/products/gao-19-83 (accessed June 25, 2024).

GAO. 2021. *Rare diseases: Although limited, available evidence suggests medical and other costs can be substantial.* https://www.gao.gov/products/gao-22-104235 (accessed June 25, 2024).

Gopal-Srivastava, R., and P. Kaufmann. 2017. Facilitating clinical studies in rare diseases. *Advances in Experimental Medicine and Biology* 1031.

Groft, S. C., and M. Posada de la Paz. 2017. Rare diseases: Joining mainstream research and treatment based on reliable epidemiological data. *Advances in Experimental Medicine and Biology* 1031.

Haendel, M., N. Vasilevsky, D. Unni, C. Bologa, N. Harris, H. Rehm, A. Hamosh, G. Baynam, T. Groza, J. McMurry, H. Dawkins, A. Rath, C. Thaxton, G. Bocci, M. P. Joachimiak, S. Köhler, P. N. Robinson, C. Mungall, T. I. Oprea, M. Haendel, N. Vasilevsky, D. Unni, C. Bologa, N. Harris, H. Rehm, A. Hamosh, G. Baynam, T. Groza, J. McMurry, H. Dawkins, A. Rath, C. Thaxton, G. Bocci, M. P. Joachimiak, S. Köhler, P. N. Robinson, C. Mungall, and T. I. Oprea. 2019. How many rare diseases are there? *Nature Reviews Drug Discovery* 19(2).

Halley, M. C., H. S. Smith, E. A. Ashley, A. J. Goldenberg, and H. K. Tabor. 2022. A call for an integrated approach to improve efficiency, equity and sustainability in rare disease research in the United States. *Nature Genetics* 54(3):219-222.

Haystack Project. 2023. *Letter to Dr. Victor Dzau.* https://static1.squarespace.com/static/5966cc2220099e91326caaec/t/646fe0a4ad973d3c9320dcc3/1685053604966/Letter+to+NASEM+Requesting+Meeting+re+HEART+Act.pdf (accessed August 1, 2024).

HHS (U.S. Department of Health and Human Services). 2001. *The Orphan Drug Act: Implementation and impact.* https://oig.hhs.gov/oei/reports/oei-09-00-00380.pdf (accessed July 31, 2024).

Hyde, R., and D. Dobrovolny. 2010. Orphan drug pricing and payer management in the United States: Are we approaching the tipping point? *American Health & Drug Benefits* 3(1):15-23.

IOM (Institute of Medicine). 2001. *Small clinical trials: Issues and challenges.* Edited by C. H. Evans, Jr. and S. T. Ildstad. Washington, DC: The National Academies Press.

IOM. 2004. *Ethical conduct of clinical research involving children.* Washington, DC: The National Academies Press.

IOM. 2009. *Drug development for rare and neglected diseases and individualized therapies.* Washington, DC: The National Academies Press.

IOM. 2010. *Rare diseases and orphan products: Accelerating research and development.* Washington, DC: The National Academies Press.

Kadambi, A. 2021. Achieving fairness in medical devices. *Science* 372(6537):30-31.

Kuester, M. K., J. M. Naber, and C. E. Smith. 2022. *Prevalence of rare disease in a commercial population using ICD-10 diagnosis codes: Milliman Report.* https://www.milliman.com/en/insight/prevalence-of-rare-disease-in-a-commercial-population-icd10-diagnosis (accessed August 1, 2024).

Liu, J., J. S. Barrett, E. T. Leonardi, L. Lee, S. Roychoudhury, Y. Chen, and P. Trifillis. 2022. Natural history and real-world data in rare diseases: Applications, limitations, and future perspectives. *Journal of Clinical Pharmacology* 62(Suppl 2):S38-S55.

Lorey, F. W., J. Arnopp, and G. C. Cunningham. 1996. Distribution of hemoglobinopathy variants by ethnicity in a mulltiethnic state. *Genetics Epidemiology* 13(5):501-512.

Michaeli, T., H. Jürges, and D. T. Michaeli. 2023. FDA approval, clinical trial evidence, efficacy, epidemiology, and price for non-orphan and ultra-rare, rare, and common orphan cancer drug indications: Cross sectional analysis. *BMJ* 381.

Mitani, A. A., and S. Haneuse. 2020. Small data challenges of studying rare diseases. *JAMA Network Open* 3(3).

Murray, L. T., T. A. Howell, L. S. Matza, S. Eremenco, H. R. Adams, D. Trundell, S. J. Coons, and Rare Disease Subcommittee of the Patient-Reported Outcome Consortium. 2023. Approaches to the assessment of clinical benefit of treatments for conditions that have heterogeneous symptoms and impacts: Potential applications in rare disease. *Value Health* 26(4):547-553.

NASEM (National Academies of Sciences, Engineering, and Medicine). 2022. *Improving representation in clinical trials and research: Building research equity for women and underrepresented groups*. Edited by K. Bibbins-Domingo and A. Helman. Washington, DC: The National Academies Press.

NASEM. 2024. *Living with ALS*. Edited by A. I. Leshner, R. A. English and J. Alper. Washington, DC: The National Academies Press.

NCATS (National Center for Advancing Translational Sciences). n.d.-a. *Effectivness: Toolkit for patient-focused therapy development*. https://toolkit.ncats.nih.gov/glossary/effectiveness (accessed June 25, 2024).

NCATS. n.d.-b. *Efficacy: Toolkit for patient-focused therapy development*. https://toolkit.ncats.nih.gov/glossary/efficacy/ (accessed June 25, 2024).

Ndugga, N., and S. Artiga. 2023. *Disparities in health and health care: 5 key questions and answers*. https://files.kff.org/attachment/Issue-Brief-Disparities-in-Health-and-Health-Care-Five-Key-Questions-and-Answer (accessed August 1, 2024).

Nguyen, M. T., J. Goldblatt, R. Isasi, M. Jagut, A. H. Jonker, P. Kaufmann, L. Ouillade, F. Molnar-Gabor, M. Shabani, E. Sid, A. M. Tassé, D. Wong-Rieger, B. M. Knoppers, and IRDiRC-GA4GH Model Consent Clauses Task Force. 2019. Model consent clauses for rare disease research. *BMC Medical Ethics* 20(1):55.

NIH (National Institutes of Health). 2023. *Learn about studies*. https://clinicaltrials.gov/study-basics/learn-about-studies (accessed June 25, 2024).

NIH. 2023. *Genetic and rare diseases information center*. https://rarediseases.info.nih.gov/ (accessed June 25, 2024).

NIH. n.d. *Endpoint*. https://toolkit.ncats.nih.gov/glossary/endpoint/ (accessed June 25, 2024).

Park, J., K. Y. Huh, W. K. Chung, and K. S. Yu. 2024. The landscape of decentralized clinical trials (DCTs): Focusing on the FDA and EMA guidance. *Translational and Clinical Pharmacology* 32(1):41-51.

Pizzamiglio, C., H. J. Vernon, M. G. Hanna, and R. D. S. Pitceathly. 2022. Designing clinical trials for rare diseases: Unique challenges and opportunities. *Nature Reviews Methods Primers* 2(1):13.

Pokhrel, A., A. Olayemi, S. Ogbonda, K. Nair, and J. C. Wang. 2023. Racial and ethnic differences in sickle cell disease within the United States: From demographics to outcomes. *European Journal of Hematology* 110(5).

Rath, A., A. Olry, F. Dhombres, M. M. Brandt, B. Urbero, and S. Ayme. 2012. Representation of rare diseases in health information systems: The Orphanet approach to serve a wide range of end users. *Human Mutation* 33(5):803-808.

Saltonstall, P., H. Ross, and P. T. Kim. 2024. The Orphan Drug Act at 40: Legislative triumph and the challenges of success. *The Milbank Quarterly* 102(1).

Sardella, M., and G. Belcher. 2018. Pharmacovigilance of medicines for rare and ultrarare diseases. *Therapeutic Advances in Drug Safety* 9(11):631-638.

Satcher, D., G. E. Fryer, J. McCann, A. Troutman, S. H. Woolf, and G. Rust. 2005. What if we were equal? A comparison of the black-white mortality gap in 1960 and 2000. *Health Affairs* 24(2):459-464.

Serdar, C. C., M. Cihan, D. Yücel, and M. A. Serdar. 2021. Sample size, power and effect size revisited: Simplified and practical approaches in pre-clinical, clinical and laboratory studies. *Biochemia Medica (Zabreb)* 31(1):010502.

Shire. 2013. *Rare disease impact report: Insights from patients and the medical community.* https://globalgenes.org/wp-content/uploads/2013/04/ShireReport-1.pdf (accessed June 25, 2024).

The Lancet Diabetes & Endocrinology. 2019. Spotlight on rare diseases. *The Lancet Diabetes & Endocrinology* 7(2).

Tisdale, A., C. M. Cutillo, R. Nathan, P. Russo, B. Laraway, M. Haendel, D. Nowak, C. Hasche, C. H. Chan, E. Griese, H. Dawkins, O. Shukla, D. A. Pearce, J. L. Rutter, and A. R. Pariser. 2021. The IDeaS initiative: pilot study to assess the impact of rare diseases on patients and healthcare systems. *Orphanet Journal of Rare Diseases* 16(1):429.

Tozzi, J. 2019. *Gene therapy drugs that cost millions have employers and health plans worried.* https://www.insurancejournal.com/news/national/2019/09/13/539591.htm (accessed August 15, 2024).

Turner, B. E., J. R. Steinberg, B. T. Weeks, F. Rodriguez, and M. R. Cullen. 2022. Race/ethnicity reporting and representation in US clinical trials: A cohort study. *The Lancet Regional Health – Americas* 11.

USAFacts. n.d. *How is the population changing and growing?* https://usafacts.org/state-of-the-union/population/ (accessed July 9, 2024).

Wakap, S. N., D. M. Lambert, A. Olry, C. Rodwell, C. Gueydan, V. Lanneau, D. Murphy, Y. L. Cam, and A. Rath. 2020. Estimating cumulative point prevalence of rare diseases: Analysis of the Orphanet database. *European Journal of Human Genetics: EJHG* 28(2).

WHO (World Health Organization). n.d. *Rare diseases.* https://www.who.int/standards/classifications/frequently-asked-questions/rare-diseases (accessed July 29, 2024).

Williams, D. R., S. A. Mohammed, J. Leavell, and C. Collins. 2010. Race, socioeconomic status, and health: Complexities, ongoing challenges, and research opportunities. *Annals of the New York Academy of Sciences* 1186:69-101.

Yang, G., I. Cintina, A. Pariser, E. Oehrlein, J. Sullivan, and A. Kennedy. 2022. The national economic burden of rare disease in the United States in 2019. *Orphanet Journal of Rare Diseases* 17(1).

Zhou, G., and S.-C. Chow. 2023. Current issues in clinical trials utilizing master protocol design. *Clinical Trials and Bioavailability Research* 2:01-04

2

FDA Flexibilities, Authorities, and Mechanisms

> *FDA is adapting to this evolving world by embracing both the challenges and opportunities we face. We are leveraging flexibilities in our regulatory pathways to enable breakthroughs in medical science that can be translated into medical products that improve health outcomes. We are reshaping our regulatory processes and creating a nimble workforce that adapts to new technologies, medical products, biomedical science, food science, and public health.*[1]
>
> Robert Califf,
> Commissioner of Food and Drugs
> (Committee on Oversight and Accountability:
> U.S. House of Representatives, 2024)

In the United States, the Food and Drug Administration (FDA), has authority under the Federal Food, Drug, and Cosmetic Act (FD&C Act)[2] and Public Health Service Act[3] to regulate medical products and devices to ensure that they are safe and effective for their intended use. In addition to protecting the public health through regulation, the FDA mission also

---

[1] Robert Califf, testimony to Committee on Oversight and Accountability. Available at https://oversight.house.gov/wp-content/uploads/2024/04/FDA-House-Oversight-and-Accountability-Testimony.pdf (accessed June 26, 2024).

[2] P.L. 75–717. Federal Food, Drug, and Cosmetic Act (June 25, 1938).

[3] P.L. 78–410. Public Health Service Act (July 1, 1944).

states that it is "responsible for advancing the public health by helping to speed innovations that make medical products more effective, safer, and more affordable and by helping the public get the accurate, science-based information they need to use medical products and foods to maintain and improve their health" (FDA, 2023p).

Chapter 1 highlighted some of the many challenges faced by drug sponsors, researchers, and patients when it comes to generating evidence to support the approval of a drug to treat rare disease and conditions. The review and approval of such products by FDA likewise requires complex judgments, often based on limited information, about what it means for a drug product to be safe and effective.

FDA has long recognized the need to apply regulatory flexibility in the review and approval of marketing authorization applications. Analyses of noncancer orphan drugs have shown that over time FDA has continued to apply flexibility in the review of certain applications for orphan drug products (Sasinowski, 2011; Sasinowski et al., 2015; Valentine and Sasinowski, 2020). FDA's 2023 guidance for industry, *Rare Diseases: Considerations for the Development of Drugs and Biological Products*, reiterates the need for flexibility when it comes to applying statutory standards for drug development programs to rare disease, stating, "FDA has determined that it is appropriate to exercise the broadest flexibility in applying the statutory standards, while preserving appropriate standards of safety and effectiveness, for products that are being developed to treat severely debilitating or life-threatening rare diseases" (FDA, 2023l).

As specified in the statement of task, this report focuses on the flexibilities, authorities, and mechanisms available to regulators that are applicable to rare diseases or conditions. Where available, data are provided on the impact of these activities. For more general information on the FDA drug approval process please see FDA (2022b).

This chapter is organized into sections on the following topics: drug review and approval, designation for rare disease products, expedited regulatory programs, inclusion of pediatric populations, stakeholder engagement, rare disease programs, and transparency.

DRUG REVIEW AND APPROVAL

Before initiating a clinical trial of a drug or biological product in the United States, a sponsor generally must first submit an investigational new drug (IND) application to FDA. The proposed clinical trial is generally based on pre-clinical testing and includes plans for testing the drug in humans. FDA reviews the IND application to, among other things, ensure that the proposed clinical trials do not place trial participants at unreasonable risk of harm, and that the protocol and informed consent will be reviewed by an institutional review board (IRB) that meets FDA regulatory standards (FDA, 2014a). Although the IRB is responsible for reviewing the informed consent for all clinical trials under its jurisdiction, there are situations in which an FDA review of an informed consent document in addition to IRB review is particularly important to determine whether a clinical trial may safely proceed under 21 CFR part 312 (FDA, 2014a).

After carrying out clinical trials, FDA recommends, but does not require, that the drug sponsor meet with the agency before submitting a formal new drug application (NDA) or biologics license application (BLA); these applications include pre-clinical and clinical evidence for demonstrating the safety and effectiveness of the proposed drug or biological product. After FDA receives an NDA or BLA, the agency has 60 days to decide whether to file it for review. If FDA files the NDA or BLA, an FDA review team will evaluate the drug's safety and effectiveness. Drug products and some biological products are assigned to the Center for Drug Evaluation and Research (CDER), while other biological products (including gene therapies) and related products, including blood, vaccines, and allergenics, are assigned to the Center for Biologics Evaluation and Research (CBER). Within CDER, applications are assigned to the Office of New Drugs (OND), and then to a specific office and division within the OND based on the therapeutic area. Within CBER, applications are assigned to one of three program offices (the Office of Therapeutic Products [OTP], Office of Vaccines Research and Review [OVRR], or Office of Blood Research and Review [OBRR]) and then to a specific office and division within the OTP, OVRR, or OBRR, as appropriate, based on the treatment modality. Typically, the relevant office and division will have already been involved in the IND process. The FDA review team evaluates the NDA or BLA and decides whether to grant marketing approval (see Figure 2-1).

As part of the review process, FDA may seek external input through advisory committees, which include representatives from academia, industry, and patient groups. Other external input throughout the drug development lifecycle is typically collected through established governmental programs, public comment, or through special government employees. This input may be used to inform FDA's decision but the ultimate authority and decision making resides with FDA. While the regulatory process is the same for rare and common conditions, rare disease drug development is often dependent on a limited pool of experts, many of whom may be directly involved in drug development trials and considered to have a conflict of interest. This can make it challenging to populate advisory committees with people who have relevant expertise. Additionally, as described in Chapter 4, there are a number of considerations for data sourcing, trial design, and methodologies that are particularly relevant for rare disease marketing authorization applications.

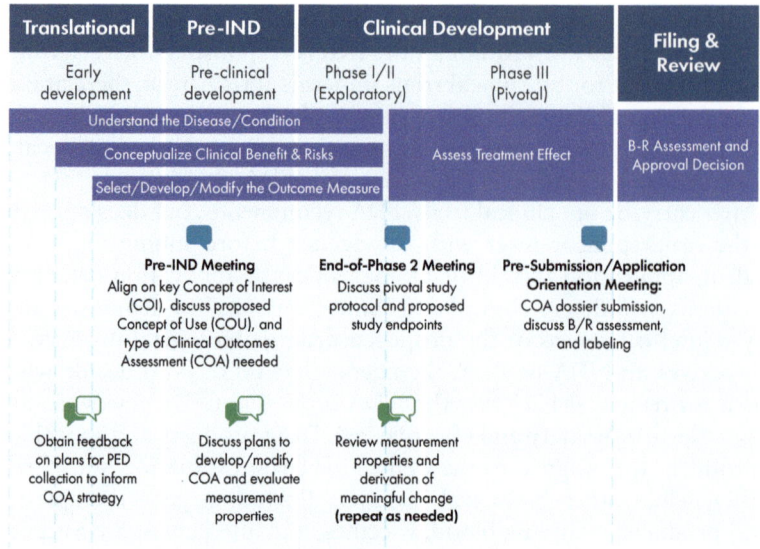

FIGURE 2-1 FDA drug review process.
NOTES: B-R = benefit/risk; COA = clinical outcomes assessment; COI = concept of interest; COU = concept of use; PED = patient experience data; Pre-IND = pre-investigational new drug application.
SOURCE: Adapted from Biotechnology Innovation Organization, 2022.

FDA strives to be transparent when sharing relevant documents following drug approval, such as letters, reviews, labels, and patient package inserts. At the same time, FDA is required by law to review and protect certain information from being released to the public, including confidential commercial information, trade secrets, and personal privacy information. FDA has stated that commercial information "is valuable data or information which is used in a business and is of such type that it is customarily held in strict confidence or regarded as privileged" (FDA, 2018c) There is an inherent tension between the legal limitations regarding the release of what could be considered confidential commercial information and FDA's obligation to share relevant information in the interest of public health. The Food and Drug Administration Amendments Act of 2007 requires that new molecular entities/new biological entities action packages be published on CDER's web page within 30 days after approval (see Table 2-1). However,

TABLE 2-1 Components of an Action Package for an NDA or BLA

Component	Examples
FDA-generated documents related to review of the marketing authorization application	Approval letter Summary minutes for meetings held with applicant Summary basis of regulatory action
Documents pertaining to the format and content of the application generated during the drug development phase (investigational new drug application)	Package insert
Certain documents submitted by the applicant	

NOTES: BLA = biologics license application; NDA = new drug application.
SOURCE: FDA, 2022a.

FDA is not required to publish complete response letters—a written response sent to sponsors to indicate that FDA's review of a marketing authorization application has been completed and the application is not ready for approval. Complete response letters usually describe "all of the specific deficiencies that the agency has identified in an application" (FDA, 2008).

Benefit–Risk Assessment

As articulated in the 2024 National Academies report, *Living with ALS*, there are trade-offs between enabling patient access to new medications and the degree of uncertainty when it comes to the assessment of benefit and risks for a given drug (NASEM, 2024). There are several factors involved in the assessment of the benefits and risks of a particular drug, including the clinical context, the availability of other treatments, and the seriousness of the condition (see Box 2-1). FDA guidance for industry, *Rare Diseases: Considerations for the Development of Drugs and Biological Products* (FDA, 2023l), notes that "a feasible and sufficient safety assessment is a matter of scientific and regulatory judgment based on the particular challenges posed by each drug and disease, including patients' tolerance and acceptance of risk in the setting of unmet medical need and the benefit offered by the drug." The benefit–risk assessment also involves an evaluation of the degree of uncertainty in the identified risks and benefits. For example, a small trial may not detect certain adverse events, or it may overestimate the effect of the drug. FDA guidance *Benefit–Risk Assessment for New Drug and Biological Products* (FDA, 2023c) states that a higher degree of uncertainty is common in rare disease drug development due to limitations on study size and that when drugs are being developed for serious diseases with few or no approved therapies, "greater uncertainty or greater risks

> **BOX 2-1**
> **Benefit–Risk Assessment**
>
> - "Benefit–risk assessment is an integral part of the U.S. Food and Drug Administration's (FDA's) regulatory review of marketing applications for new drugs and biologics. These assessments capture the Agency's evidence, uncertainties, and reasoning used to arrive at its final determination for specific regulatory decisions. Additionally, they serve as a tool for communicating this information to those who wish to better understand FDA's thinking" (FDA, 2022c).
> - All drugs can have adverse effects, so the demonstration of safety requires a showing that the benefits of the drug outweigh its risks (Fain, 2023; FDA, 2023c).
> - Benefit–risk assessment is integrated into FDA's regulatory review of marketing applications for new drugs (Fain, 2023).
> - Section 505(d) of the Federal Food, Drug, and Cosmetic Act requires FDA to "implement a structured risk-benefit assessment framework in the new drug approval process" and provides that this requirement does not alter the statutory criteria for evaluating an application for marketing approval of a drug (Fain, 2023).
> - FDA uses scientific assessment and regulatory judgment to determine whether the drug's benefits outweigh the risks, and whether additional measures are needed and able to address or mitigate this uncertainty (Fain, 2023; FDA, 2023c).
>
> SOURCES: Fain, 2023; FDA, 2022c, 2023c.

may be acceptable provided that the standard for substantial evidence of effectiveness has been met."

In the case of serious rare diseases, FDA may thus exercise regulatory flexibility by accepting clinical trials that have smaller sample sizes. Accepting smaller sample sizes for serious rare diseases places even greater importance on maximizing the trial's potential to provide interpretable scientific evidence about the drug's benefits and risks in order to be respectful of patients' willingness to participate in clinical trials. Patient contribution is optimized in clinical trials (and particularly in small sample size studies) by minimizing bias and maximizing precision with trial design features such as randomization, blinding, enrichment procedures, and adequate trial duration (FDA, 2023c).

Substantial Evidence of Effectiveness

Substantial evidence of effectiveness is defined in section 505(d) FD&C Act as:

> evidence consisting of adequate and well-controlled investigations, including clinical investigations, by experts qualified by scientific training and experience to evaluate the effectiveness of the drug involved, on the basis of which it could fairly and responsibly be concluded by such experts that the drug will have the effect it purports or is represented to have under the conditions of use prescribed, recommended, or suggested in the labeling or proposed labeling thereof.[4]

FDA has interpreted substantial evidence of effectiveness as generally requiring at least two adequate and well-controlled clinical investigations, each of which is convincing on its own (FDA, 2019a). Requiring two adequate and well-controlled clinical trials allows for independent substantiation of study results and protects against the possibility that a chance occurrence in one study would lead to an erroneous conclusion about the drug's effectiveness (FDA, 1998, 2019a; Freilich, 2024). However, there is regulatory flexibility available in some circumstances for the amount and type of evidence needed to meet the substantial evidence standard, as described further in the FD&C Act and FDA guidance documents and discussed below.

In 1997, Congress amended the FD&C Act to clarify that substantial evidence of effectiveness could also consist of a single adequate and well-controlled study and confirmatory evidence "if [FDA] determines, based on relevant science, that data from one adequate and well-controlled clinical investigation and confirmatory evidence (obtained prior to or after such investigation) are sufficient to establish effectiveness."[5]

This clarification reflected FDA's then-current thinking given the rapidly evolving science and practice of clinical research and drug development. In 1998, FDA released subsequent guidance[6] for industry, *Providing Clinical Evidence of Effectiveness for Human Drug and Biological Products* (FDA, 1998), to share the agency's thinking on the quantity and quality of data

---

[4] 21 U.S.C. § 355(d).
[5] 21 P.L. 105–115. Food and Drug Modernization Act (November 21, 1997).
[6] FDA develops guidance documents to share FDA's current thinking on a topic (FDA, 2023f). These documents are not legally binding for FDA or the public. To develop a guidance document, FDA first has the option to seek input from external stakeholders. FDA then prepares a draft version of the document which is posted publicly along with a notice in the *Federal Register*. The draft guidance is then open to public comment. FDA then reviews the comments and makes any necessary edits before posting the finalized guidance document (21 CFR §10.115).

that could be used for demonstrating effectiveness of drugs.[7] In this guidance, FDA provided several illustrations of the "types of evidence that could be considered confirmatory evidence, with a specific focus on adequate and well-controlled trials of the test agent in related populations or indications, as well as a number of illustrations of a single adequate and well-controlled trial supported by convincing evidence of the drug's mechanism of action in treating a disease or condition" (FDA, 2023f). For example, a pediatric indication might be approved based on a study on adults if the pathophysiology and drug effect are similar between the populations.

In December 2019, FDA issued draft guidance, *Demonstrating Substantial Evidence of Effectiveness for Human Drug and Biological Products*, which complemented and expanded on the 1998 guidance. The new draft guidance stated, "Although FDA's evidentiary standard for effectiveness has not changed since 1998, the evolution of drug development and science has led to changes in the types of drug development programs submitted to the Agency. Specifically, there are more programs studying serious diseases lacking effective treatment, more programs in rare diseases, and more programs for therapies targeted at disease subsets" (FDA, 2019a). Consequently, the 2019 guidance lists several illustrative examples of the types of evidence that could be considered as confirmatory of a single adequate and well-controlled study. Those examples included: (1) data from a single adequate and well-controlled study that demonstrated the drug's effectiveness in another closely related approved indication; (2) data providing strong mechanistic support; (3) natural history data from the disease, and (4) scientific knowledge about the effectiveness of other drugs in the same pharmacological class. A single study could be sufficient for demonstrating effectiveness if the study is a large multicenter, adequate, and well-controlled trial and "the trial has demonstrated a clinically meaningful and statistically very persuasive effect on mortality, severe or irreversible morbidity, or prevention of a disease with potentially serious outcome and confirmation of the result in a second trial would be impractical or unethical" (FDA, 2019a).[8]

In 2023, FDA issued a draft guidance, *Demonstrating Substantial Evidence of Effectiveness with One Adequate and Well-Controlled Clinical Investigation and Confirmatory Evidence,* which offers further clarification on when one study and confirmatory evidence may be sufficient for establishing effectiveness (FDA, 2023f). The guidance identifies types of confirmatory evidence that could be used to supplement one clinical investigation; FDA notes that the list is not exhaustive, and that each application is considered on a case-by-case basis. The types of confirmatory evidence

---

[7] This sentence was edited after release of the prepublication version of the report to reflect the nature of data used.

[8] This section was edited after release of the prepublication version of the report to clarify when a single trial approach could be sufficient for demonstrating effectiveness.

listed include clinical evidence from a related indication, mechanistic or pharmacodynamic evidence, evidence from a relevant animal model, evidence from other members of the same pharmacological class, natural history evidence, real-world data, and evidence from expanded access use of an investigational drug (see Chapter 4).

FDA conducts a thorough review of an application to determine whether the submitted data constitutes substantial evidence of effectiveness. FDA examines both final summaries and data from nonclinical and clinical studies, from which it determines the safety and effectiveness of the product through its own independent analysis. The review team replicates the applicant's analyses and, if necessary, conducts additional analyses to further inform the efficacy assessment (Bugin, n.d.).

Conclusion 2-1: While the statutory requirements for drug approval for rare diseases and conditions are the same as for non-rare diseases or conditions, FDA has long recognized the need to apply regulatory flexibility in the review and approval of marketing authorization applications.

DESIGNATION FOR RARE DISEASE PRODUCTS

As discussed in Chapter 1, FDA has the authority to grant orphan drug designation for products that are used to prevent, diagnose, or treat a rare disease or condition. Additionally, FDA can award "rare pediatric disease" designation for drug applications that meet certain criteria.[9] These designation programs, which are further described below, provide incentives for sponsors to develop drugs to treat rare diseases and conditions.

Orphan Drug Designation

The orphan drug designation is an FDA incentive that began in 1983 following the enactment of the Orphan Drug Act, with the goal of stimulating the development of drugs and biological products for rare diseases by lessening the financial burdens associated with orphan drug development. A drug may qualify for orphan-drug designation (ODD) if the targeted disease or condition affects fewer than 200,000 individuals in the United States at the time of the sponsor's request, or if it affects more than 200,000 individuals but there is no reasonable expectation that the cost of developing a drug for the condition would be recovered by sales of the drug.[10] To be eligible for ODD, a drug or biological product must be for a distinct rare disease or condition. FDA determines what the distinct disease or condition is by considering such factors as the pathogenesis of the condition, course

---

[9] P.L. 112–144. Food and Drug Administration Safety and Innovation Act (July 9, 2012).
[10] 21 CFR §316.20(b)(8); 21 U.S.C. § 360bb(a)(2).

of the condition, prognosis of the condition, and resistance to treatment.[11] These factors are assessed in the context of the specific drug seeking ODD.

A sponsor can receive multiple designations for the same drug if it can be shown to treat more than one distinct disease or condition. A sponsor can also receive ODD for its version of a drug that is otherwise the "same drug" as an already approved drug for the same disease or condition as long as the sponsor can present a plausible hypothesis that its drug may be clinically superior to the first drug.[12]

A sponsor may receive ODD for a drug designed to treat an "orphan subset"[13] of individuals with a disease that affects more than 200,000 people if it can be demonstrated that the subset affects less than 200,000 people in the United States and that the remaining individuals with the disease would not be appropriate candidates due to some property of the drug.[14] To be considered for ODD under this "orphan subset" provision, the demonstration that other patients would not be appropriate candidates must be based on pharmacologic or biopharmaceutical properties of the drug, or previous clinical experience with the drug.[15] For example, ODD could be granted if data demonstrate that the drug is only effective for patients with a certain biomarker, or that the toxicity of the drug makes it appropriate only for patients who do not respond to standard, less toxic treatments.[16] FDA has clarified that an orphan subset does not refer to a clinically distinguishable subset of persons with a particular condition; eligibility for ODD under an orphan subset must be based on a property of the drug itself, not a subset of patients.[17] A product targeted at just the pediatric population may be eligible for ODD in a number of ways (FDA, 2018a). First, if the disease is rare in the overall population, any product may be eligible. Second, if the disease is common in the general population, a product may be eligible for ODD if the affected pediatric population is less than 200,000 and is a valid orphan subset, meaning that the product would not be appropriate for use in the adult population owing to some property or properties of the drug; this would be considered an orphan subset designation. Third, a product may be eligible for ODD if the disease in the pediatric population is a different disease than in the adult population and the affected pediatric population is less than 200,000.

---

[11] 78 FR 35117(III)(A).
[12] 21 CFR §316.20(a).
[13] 78 FR 35117(III)(A) at 35119, explaining that: "orphan subset is a regulatory concept specific to the Orphan Drug regulations, and that it does not simply mean any medically recognizable or clinically distinguishable subset of persons with a particular disease or condition (as the term 'medically plausible' in this context may have been erroneously interpreted to imply)."
[14] 21 CFR §316.20(b)(6).
[15] 21 CFR §316.3(b)(13).
[16] 78 FR 35117(III)(A).
[17] 78 FR 35117(III)(A).

Process

Orphan drug designation is a separate process from drug approval or licensing. Sponsors seeking ODD submit a request to FDA that includes an explanation of the rare disease or condition the drug is intended to treat along with data (e.g., clinical, *in vivo*, and *in vitro*) to support the scientific rationale for using the drug in this population.[18] FDA reviews the request to assess whether the drug product meets the criteria for ODD and will send the sponsor a designation letter granting ODD, a deficiency letter that requests additional information, or a denial letter (FDA, 2023h). In 2017, according to FDA's Orphan Drug Modernization Plan, the agency aimed to complete all new ODD reviews within 90 days of receipt (FDA, 2017b).

Benefits

ODD qualifies sponsors for incentives which include tax credits of 25 percent of qualifying clinical trial expenses, a waiver of the user fee ($4 million for fiscal year 2024) (FDA, 2024o), and potentially 7-year market exclusivity—upon approval for an indication or use within the scope of the designation (Michaeli et al., 2023).[19,20] In addition, the Orphan Drug Act established the Orphan Product Grants Program to provide funding for developing products for rare diseases or conditions. The statutory authority for the Orphan Products Grants Program has been expanded to include support for "prospectively planned and designed observational studies and other analyses conducted to assist in the understanding of the natural history of a rare disease."[21]

Approvals of Drugs with Orphan Drug Designation

Prior to the Orphan Drug Act, few drugs were approved by FDA for rare diseases and conditions (Asbury, 1991). During the last 40 years, over 6,300 drugs have received ODD for over 1,000 rare diseases. Of the ODDs granted by FDA, 882 resulted in at least one drug approval for 392 diseases (Fermaglich and Miller, 2023). As of 2022, between 4 and 6 percent of rare diseases had an approved drug, while between 11 and 15 percent had received an ODD (Fermaglich and Miller, 2023).

In 2010, CDER approved six new molecular entities with ODD, representing 29 percent of approved new products. In 2022, CDER approved 20 new molecular entities for orphan conditions, constituting 54 percent of

---

[18] 21 CFR §316.20.
[19] This sentence was edited after release of the prepublication version of the report to more accurately reflect 21 USC § 360cc – Protection for drugs for rare diseases or conditions.
[20] 21 U.S.C §360cc(a).
[21] 21 U.S.C §360ee(b).

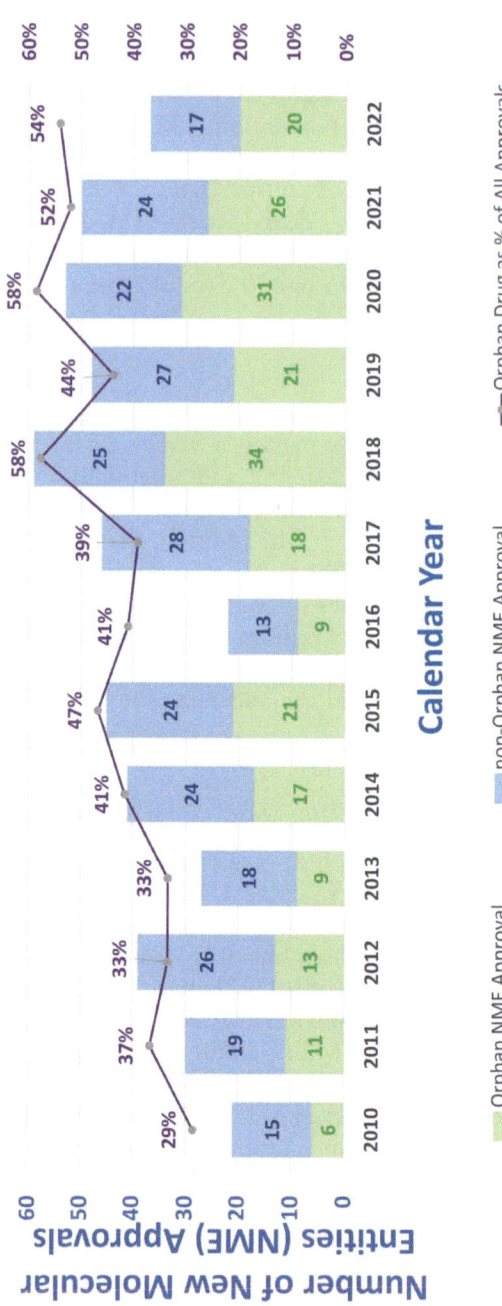

FIGURE 2-2 Proportion of CDER novel drug approvals that were orphan from 2010 to 2022.
NOTE: CDER = Center for Drug Evaluation and Research.
SOURCE: Presented to the Committee by Kerry Jo Lee, on November 6, 2023.

all center approvals (see Figure 2-2). CBER product approvals followed a similar trend, increasing from zero ODD approvals in 2010 to five in 2022, constituting 63 percent of all center approvals (see Figure 2-3). Overall, from 2010 to 2022, the number of orphan drug approvals increased in both number and percentage of the total approved new products for both CDER and CBER, with orphan drugs making up over half of approved new products for both centers in 2021 and 2022.

To understand the rates of FDA approvals for non-orphan and orphan drug products over time, the committee commissioned an analysis of marketing submissions, regulatory orphan designations, and marketing approvals of new drug products from 2013–2022 using new drug applications and biologics license applications (types 1 and 1,4). Due to a lack of available data on approval and non-approval rates, the committee requested information about new drug products received from 2013–2022. Data from 2015–2020 were obtained directly from the agency for CDER and CBER. Additional data on the therapeutic areas and use of expedited review pathways were obtained from agency public assessment reports (see Appendix D for full methodology). Overall, approval rates for orphan drug product applications received between 2015 and 2020 are higher than for non-orphan drug products at nearly all FDA offices, with approval rates ranging from 83 percent (Office of Cardiology, Hematology, Endocrinology, and Nephrology) to 100 percent (Office of Immunology and Inflammation) (see Figure 2-4). Despite the increasing number of ODD and associated drug approvals, much of the progress has been concentrated in a few therapeutic areas. Between 2013 and 2022, a large portion of orphan drug approvals were for anti-cancer and immunomodulator treatments, followed by alimentary and metabolism treatments and the blood and blood forming organs treatments (see Figure 2-5).[22]

Rare Pediatric Disease Priority Review Voucher Program

The rare pediatric disease priority review voucher (PRV) program, established in 2012 under section 908 of the Food and Drug Administration Safety and Innovation Act (FDASIA), was designed to incentivize the development of certain new drugs or biologics to prevent or treat rare diseases that affect pediatric populations.[23] Section 908 of FDASIA defines a rare pediatric disease as "a serious or life-threatening disease in which the serious or life-threatening manifestations primarily affect individuals aged from birth to 18 years, including age groups often called neonates, infants, children, and adolescents," and the disease is a rare disease or condition within the meaning of section 526 of the FD&C Act.[24] Under this program,

---

[22] This section was edited after release of the prepublication version of the report to more accurately describe the data requested and received.
[23] 21 U.S.C. § 360ff.
[24] 21 U.S.C. § 360ff(a)(3).

58

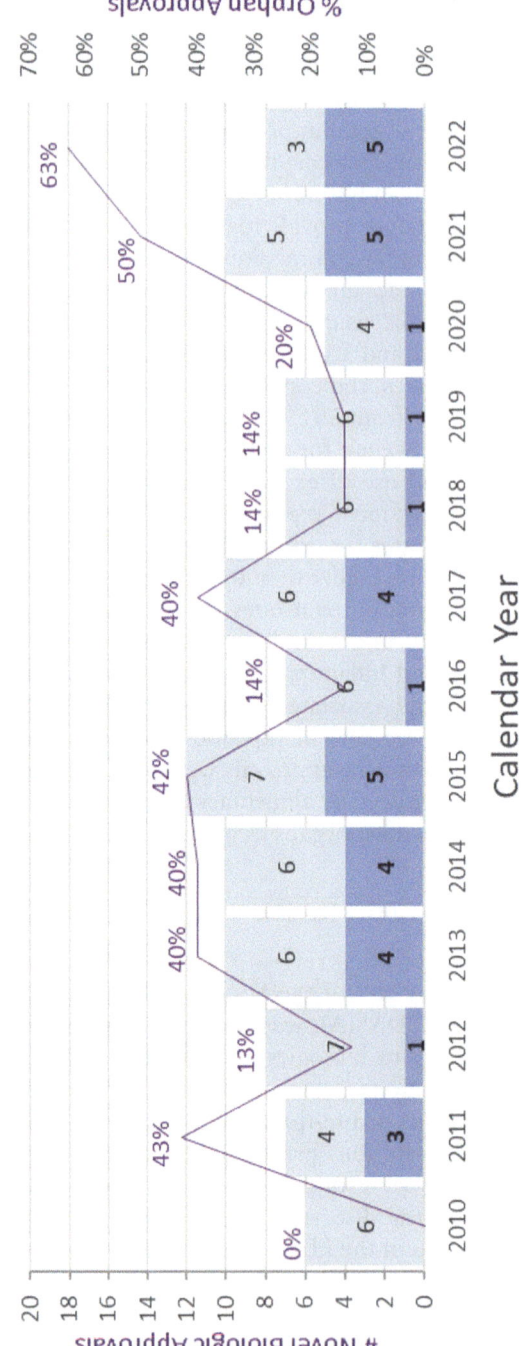

FIGURE 2-3 Proportion of CBER novel biologic approvals that were orphan from 2010 to 2022.
NOTES: These data exclude in vitro diagnostic products, reagents, and intermediate biological products approved for further manufacture, such as source plasma. CBER = Center for Biologics Evaluation and Research.
SOURCE: Presented to the Committee by Julienne Vaillancourt, on November 6, 2023.

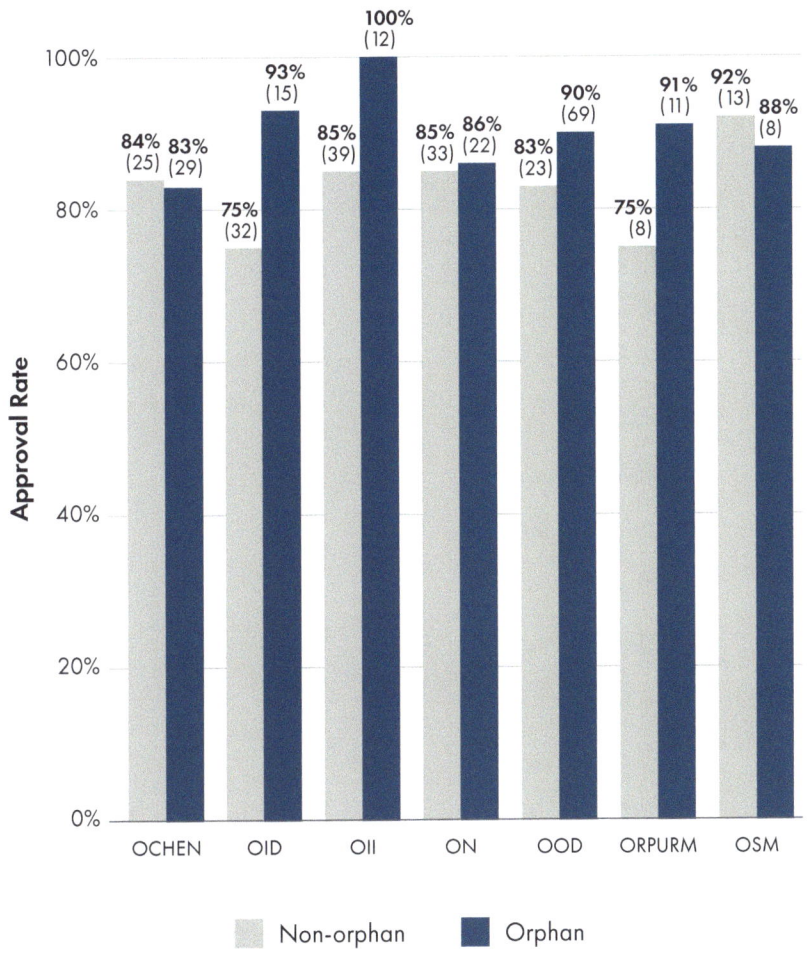

FIGURE 2-4 Novel approval rates for non-orphan and orphan new drug applications submitted to CDER from 2015 to 2020 by office.
NOTES: CDER = Center for Drug Evaluation and Research; OCHEN = Office of Cardiology, Hematology, Endocrinology and Nephrology; OID = Office of Infectious Diseases; OII = Office of Immunology and Inflammation; ON = Office of Neuroscience; OOD = Office of Oncologic Diseases; OROURM = Office of Rare Diseases, Pediatrics, Urologic and Reproductive Medicine; OSM = Office of Specialty Medicine.
SOURCE: CIRS Data Analysis, 2024; data directly provided by FDA.

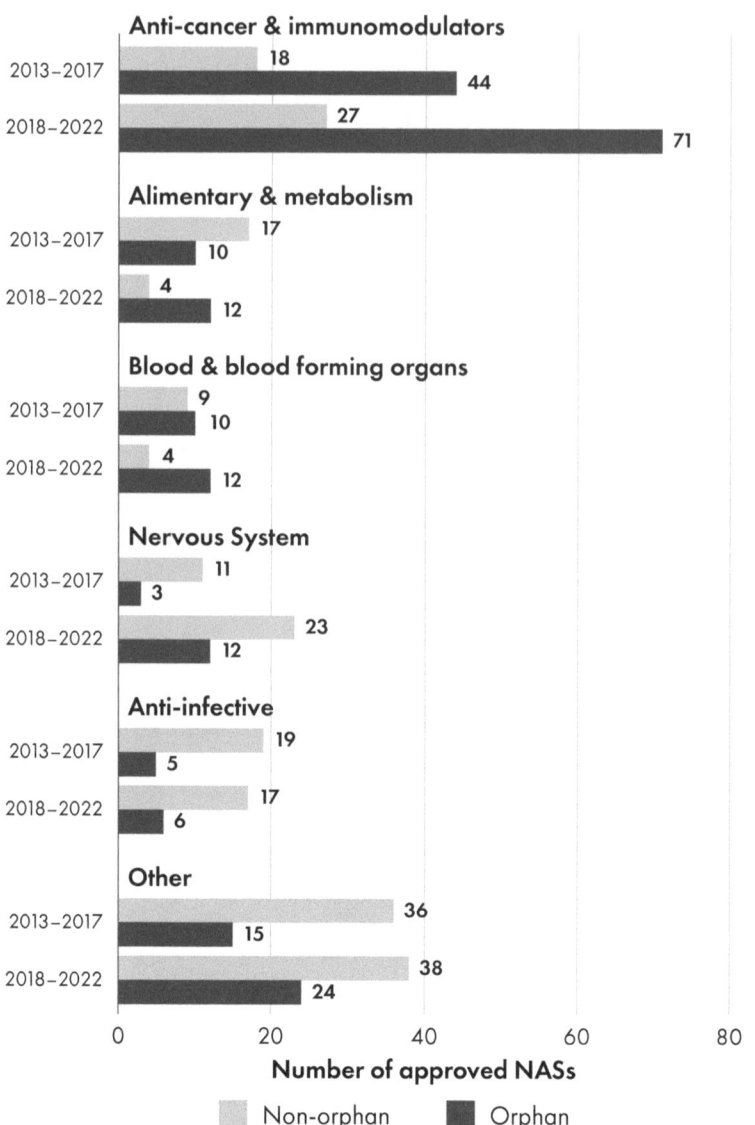

FIGURE 2-5 FDA approval of orphan and non-orphan drugs by therapeutic area from 2013 to 2022.
NOTES: FDA = U.S. Food and Drug Administration; NASs = new active substances; Other = other therapeutic areas not described in the top five therapeutic indications list.
SOURCE: CIRS Data Analysis, 2024.

sponsors who receive approval for a drug to treat a rare pediatric disease may qualify for a voucher for priority review of a subsequent product (FDA, 2019d). Priority review generally means a marketing authorization submission will be reviewed by FDA in 6 months rather than the standard 10-month period review time. The sponsor may transfer or sell the voucher to another sponsor. The program has been renewed by Congress in the past, typically for 4 years at a time. Under current legislation, the rare pediatric disease designation PRV program begins to sunset after September 30, 2024 (FDA, 2024q).

Process

FDA's draft guidance for industry *Rare Pediatric Disease Priority Review Vouchers* provides information on implementation of this program (FDA, 2019d). After a sponsor submits a request to FDA for rare pediatric disease designation the agency decides whether to grant the designation and whether to designate the marketing application as a "rare disease product application." If a sponsor submits the designation request at the same time as a request for ODD or fast-track review, the "review clock" is set at 60 days.[25] FDA will accept requests for rare pediatric disease designations at other times as long as requests are received prior to a filing of the NDA or BLA; these requests do not have a statutory review goal date. There are instances in which a drug may qualify for rare pediatric disease designation but not qualify for ODD and instances where a drug may qualify for ODD but not qualify for rare pediatric disease designation (FDA, 2019d). A rare pediatric disease PRV may be issued to a sponsor at the time of marketing approval if the application for the drug meets the criteria in section 529 of the FD&C Act (FDA, 2019d) and entitles the holder to priority review of an application regardless of whether the subsequent product is indicated for a rare disease.[26] Sponsors also have the option of requesting a PRV independently of submitting a designation request for a rare pediatric disease.

Benefits

Drug development is a costly and time-consuming process, including the time it takes for a drug marketing authorization submission to be reviewed by regulators. A PRV helps reduce the review time for a new drug application, which can help a sponsor bring a product to market sooner. PRVs can be used by the sponsor of the original product or sold to another

---

[25] 21 U.S.C. § 360ff(d)(3).
[26] 21 U.S.C. § 360ff(b).

party; purchase prices have ranged from $67.5 million to $350 million (GAO, 2020).

The first PRV for a rare pediatric disease was awarded in 2014 (Mease et al., 2024). A 2024 report by the National Organization for Rare Disorders (NORD) showed that since the rare pediatric disease PRV program was established in 2012, there have been more than 550 rare disease pediatric designations and over 50 rare disease pediatric PRVs awarded (NORD, 2024). During the first few years of the program, Hwang et al. (2019) found that after the voucher program was implemented, drugs likely to be eligible for rare pediatric disease designation had a greater likelihood of progressing from Phase 1 to Phase 2 trials than ineligible rare disease drug products. However, no association between the launch of the program and changes in the rate of new pediatric drugs starting or completing clinical testing was found (Hwang et al., 2019). According to a 2020 U.S. Government Accountability Office (GAO) study, drug sponsors indicated that PRVs were a factor in the decision-making process for drug development (GAO, 2020). A selection of researchers interviewed by GAO reported mixed views of the rare disease PRV program—some said that the program is a useful incentive, while others indicated that some sponsors received PRVs for products they would have likely developed anyway (GAO, 2020). Other stakeholders have also shared mixed views on the program, with some saying that PRVs have been important for small companies and others saying that PRVs are a source of additional revenue for companies that do not need the money to finance drug development (GAO, 2020). Since the last GAO report, the number of rare pediatric disease PRVs granted by FDA has more than doubled, suggesting an updated assessment of the program would be helpful (NORD, 2024).

Approvals of drugs with rare pediatric disease designation

Similar to ODD, rare pediatric disease designations are concentrated for a small number of diseases. Mease et al. (2024) found that of the 245 diseases that were granted rare pediatric disease designation between 2013 and 2022, 26 diseases accounted for 41 percent of all designations.

EXPEDITED REGULATORY PROGRAMS

FDA has four general expedited programs to facilitate and expedite the development and review of certain new drugs and biological products: (1) accelerated approval, (2) fast track, (3) breakthrough therapy, and (4) priority review (see Figure 2-6). Additionally, CBER has a designation available for biologics—regenerative medicine advanced therapy (RMAT)—and FDA's Oncology Center of Excellence has programs to expedite the review of medical products for oncologic indications. These programs are intended

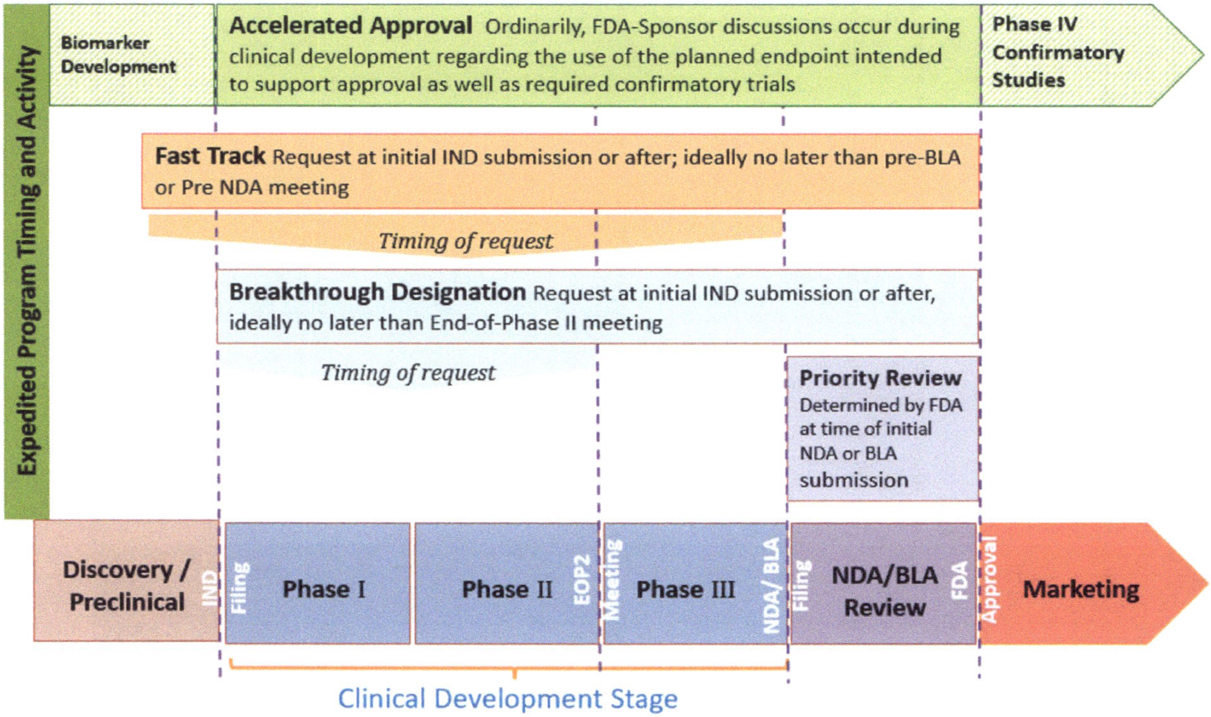

FIGURE 2-6 Entry points of expedited approval programs by clinical development stage.
NOTES: BLA = biologics license application; EOP2 = end of Phase 2; IND = investigational new drug; NDA = new drug application.
SOURCES: Presented to the Committee by Miranda Raggio, on November 6, 2023; created by Michael Lanthier; information derived from FDA, 2014b.

to facilitate and expedite the development and review of drugs that treat serious or life-threatening conditions (FDA, 2014b). FDA guidance for industry on expedited programs for serious conditions describes the eligibility criteria for expedited development and review and applies to both drugs and biologics under CDER and CBER (FDA, 2014b). Each program has its own criteria, timeline for request, and benefits, which are described in more depth below.

Expedited regulatory pathways may be used alone or in combination with ODD or with each other; the use of these programs, particularly in combination with ODD, has increased in recent years (see Figure 2-7). To be eligible for these expedited programs, a drug must be intended to treat a serious condition and generally must represent an improvement over existing therapies (e.g., must meet an "unmet need," show a "meaningful advantage" over existing therapies, or provide "a significant improvement in safety or

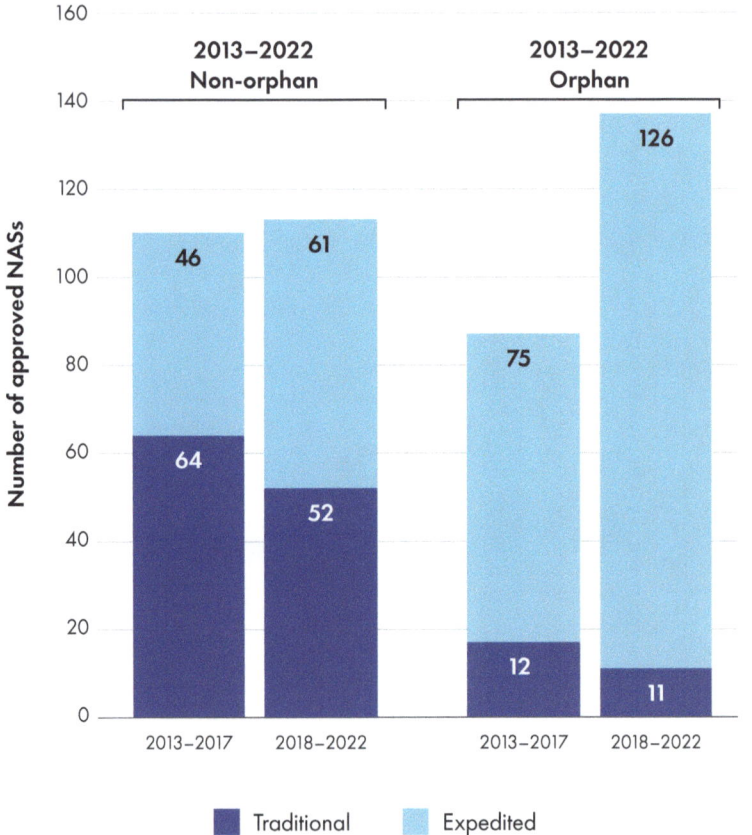

FIGURE 2-7 FDA approval rates for orphan and non-orphan drugs using expedited approval pathways from 2013 to 2022.
NOTES: FDA = U.S. Food and Drug Administration; NASs = new active substances.
SOURCE: CIRS Data Analysis, 2024.

effectiveness"). Due to the seriousness of and the lack of available therapies for many rare diseases, products developed to treat rare diseases may be eligible for one or more of the expedited programs offered by FDA (FDA, 2014b).

Accelerated Approval

The accelerated approval pathway was established by FDA in 1992 in response to the acquired immunodeficiency syndrome (AIDS) epidemic with the goal of bringing forward new therapies for patients who desperately needed treatment options. Today, the pathway is available for drugs that meet *all* of the following criteria (FDA, 2014b):

- The drug "treats a serious condition"; and
- The drug "generally provides a meaningful advantage over available therapies"; and
- The drug "demonstrates an effect on a surrogate endpoint that is reasonably likely to predict clinical benefit, or on a clinical endpoint that can be measured earlier than irreversible morbidity or mortality that is reasonably likely to predict an effect on irreversible morbidity or mortality or other clinical benefit (i.e., an intermediate clinical endpoint)."

The pathway allows the use of a surrogate endpoint (e.g., a biomarker) or an intermediate clinical endpoint for accelerated approval—an approach viewed by some critics as subjecting patients to unnecessary risks (Kesselheim and Darrow, 2015; Redberg, 2015). Confirmatory trials are also required to verify and describe the clinical benefit (FDA, 2014b).[27] In the early years of the accelerated approval program, the pathway was primarily used for drugs to treat human immunodeficiency virus (HIV) and cancer. Between 2013 and 2022, 86 percent of all drugs approved through this pathway were orphan designated drug products (see Figure 2-8). The vast majority of drugs approved through this pathway between 2010 and 2020 have been for oncology indications; 85 percent of accelerated approval drugs treated cancers (Temkin and Trinh, 2021). Although the accelerated approval pathway is not used as frequently for non-oncology rare diseases as it is for rare types of cancers, if applied appropriately, it can be a beneficial tool for bringing safe and effective drugs to patients who suffer from serious and life-threatening conditions and for whom there are no meaningful alternative treatment options (Temkin and Trinh, 2021).

---

[27] This sentence was edited after release of the prepublication version of the report to more accurately describe the accelerated approval process.

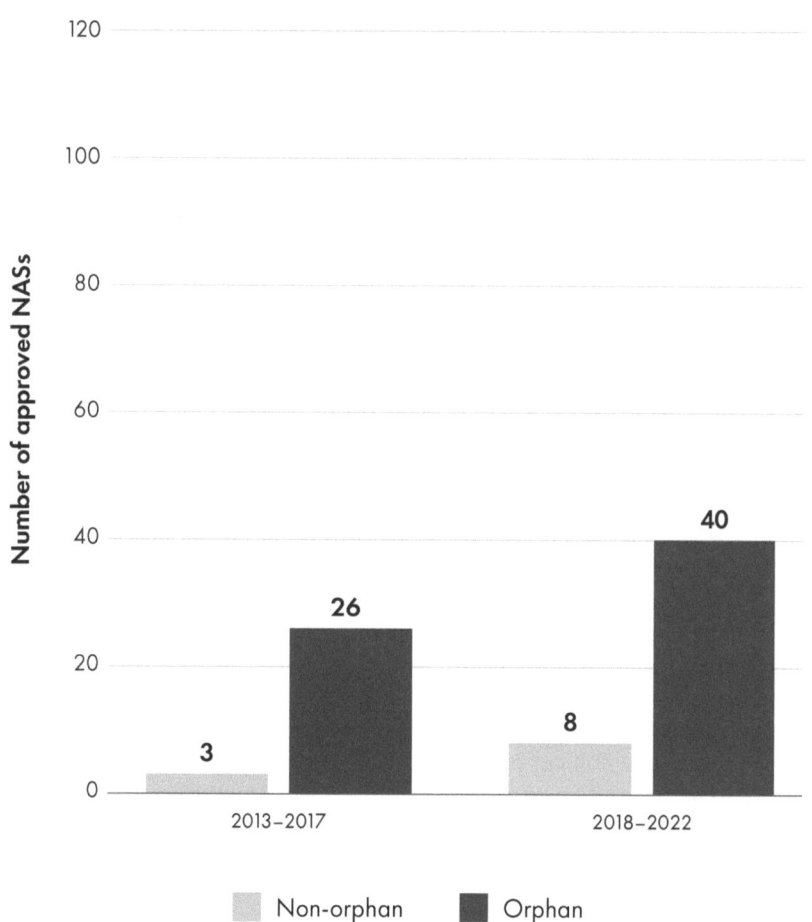

FIGURE 2-8 Number of orphan and non-orphan drug products that received accelerated approval designation by FDA between 2013 and 2022.
NOTES: FDA = U.S. Food and Drug Administration; NASs = new active substances.
SOURCE: CIRS Data Analysis, 2024.

As laid out in Chapter 1, the heterogeneity of rare diseases and conditions makes it difficult to identify and validate biomarkers for regulatory decision-making that are pertinent across the entire study population (Murray et al., 2023). To help fill this gap, efforts such as the Critical Path Institute's Biomarker Data Repository, seek to advance ongoing research to advance new biomarkers for rare diseases and conditions (Critical Path Institute, n.d.).[28] In 2022, Congress made several reforms to the accelerated approval program through the Food and Drug Omnibus Reform Act

---

[28] More information on the Critical Path Institute's Biomarker Data Repository can be found at https://c-path.org/program/biomarker-data-repository (accessed June 26, 2024).

of 2022 to help promote transparency and more accountable use of the pathway (see Box 2-2).

Fast Track

FDA offers fast track designation for drugs that meet *one* of the following criteria:

BOX 2-2
Reforms and Future Direction of Accelerated Approval

The accelerated approval pathway recently came under scrutiny following a 2022 Office of Inspector General report, which documented that over one-third of drugs granted accelerated approval have incomplete confirmatory trials (OIG, 2022). The Food and Drug Omnibus Reform Act of 2022 made several reforms to the accelerated approval program (Benjamin and Lythgoe, 2023). The first reform is focused on ensuring that confirmatory studies are conducted and submitted on time and providing new procedures for the U.S. Food and Drug Administration (FDA) to expedite withdrawal of approval if the sponsor fails to conduct the required studies. The second reform is aimed at improving transparency; sponsors will be required to submit progress reports on confirmatory studies every 180 days and these reports will be publicly available. Third, an Accelerated Approval Coordinating Council (AACC) will be formed to discuss issues related to the program and to implement necessary changes. Finally, if a sponsor is not required to conduct a post-approval study, FDA must publish a rationale for why a study is not appropriate or necessary.

In February 2024, Peter Marks, director of Center for Biologics Evaluation and Research, stated that accelerated approval is "going to be the norm for a lot of . . . initial approvals of gene therapies" (Brennan, 2024). The accelerated approval program is based on the use of a surrogate endpoint, and Marks has stated that biomarker qualification is not a requirement for the pathway; that is, biomarkers used as surrogate endpoints do not need to undergo the FDA biomarker qualification process (Brennan, 2024). Since establishment in early 2023, the AACC has held discussions on policies related to accelerated approval, including the dissemination of policy across FDA to ensure consistent and appropriate application of accelerated approval (Benjamin and Lythgoe, 2023).

- Intended to treat a serious or life-threatening disease or condition, and nonclinical or clinical evidence demonstrate the potential to address unmet medical need;[29] or
- Designated as a qualified infectious disease product[30] (section 505E of the FD&C Act).

Impact

Many products developed for rare diseases meet the criteria for fast track designation—targeted at a serious or life-threatening condition and having the potential to fill an unmet medical need—at a higher rate than products developed for non-rare diseases. Using the fast track program may benefit sponsors of rare disease products by facilitating earlier and more frequent communication so that unique study issues can be discussed, and problems can be identified and addressed early in the process. Since the launch of fast track designation, it has been used primarily by orphan products, which accounted for over 50 percent of all designated products between 1998 and 2014 (Miller and Lanthier, 2016) and 64 percent of all designated products between 2013 and 2022 (see Figure 2-9).

Breakthrough Therapy

Breakthrough therapy designation is available for drugs that meet *both* of the following criteria:

- Intended to treat a serious or life-threatening disease or condition; and
- Preliminary clinical evidence indicates that the drug may demonstrate substantial improvement on a clinically significant endpoint(s) over available therapies (FDA, 2014b).

FDA guidance for industry, *Expedited Programs for Serious Conditions* (FDA, 2014b), goes into detail about the criteria that must be met for breakthrough therapy designation. FDA explains that "preliminary clinical evidence" means evidence generally from Phase 1 or Phase 2 clinical trials that is sufficient to indicate that the drug substantially improves upon available therapies but in most cases is not sufficient to establish safety and effectiveness for purposes of approval (FDA, 2014b). In general, to demonstrate a "substantial improvement," preliminary clinical evidence should show a "clear advantage over available therapy." The determination of whether there is substantial improvement over available therapy is

---

[29] 21 U.S.C. § 356b(1).
[30] 21 U.S.C. § 355f(g).

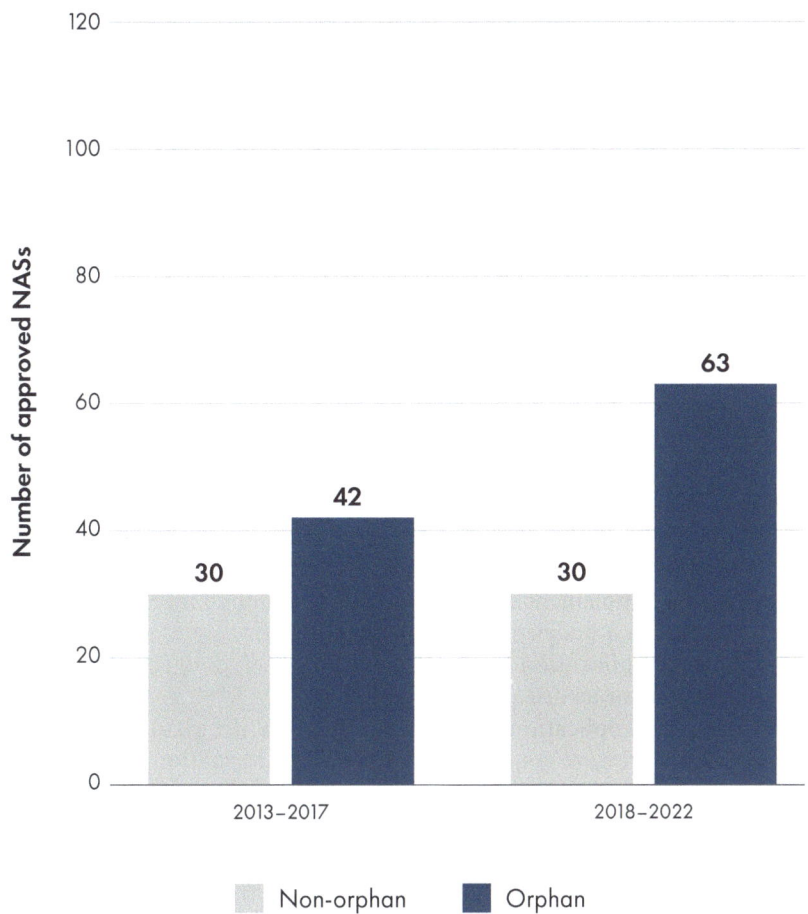

FIGURE 2-9 Number of orphan and non-orphan drug products that received fast track designation approved by FDA between 2013 and 2022.
NOTES: FDA = U.S. Food and Drug Administration; NASs = new active substances.
SOURCE: CIRS Data Analysis, 2024.

a matter of judgment and depends on the size of the treatment effect and the importance of the effect to the treatment of the condition (FDA, 2014b). The "clinically significant endpoint" could be a measure of irreversible morbidity or mortality, specific symptoms that represent serious consequences of the disease, or an effect on a biomarker that strongly suggests an impact on a serious aspect of the disease (FDA, 2014b).

Due to the serious nature of rare diseases and the lack of available or adequate therapies, products aimed at rare diseases have received breakthrough therapy designation at a higher rate than products aimed at common diseases (see Table 2-2 for data on non-oncology drugs and biologics). Between 2013 and 2022, orphan medical products accounted for 75 percent of all drug products that received the breakthrough therapy designation (see Figure 2-10). Moreover, between 2018 and 2022, over half (52 percent) of novel approved orphan drugs received the designation. Experience to date has shown that the breakthrough therapy designation can dramatically speed the development and approval for selected products, improving access to effective drugs for patients with difficult-to-treat conditions (Collins et al., 2023; Shea et al., 2016).

Priority Review

An application for a drug can receive a priority review designation if it meets *one* of the following criteria:

- It is an application (original or efficacy supplement) for a drug that treats a serious condition and, if approved, would provide a significant improvement in safety or effectiveness; or
- It is a supplement that proposes a labeling change pursuant to a report on a pediatric study under 505A; or
- It is an application for a drug that has been designated as a qualified infectious disease product; or
- It is an application or supplement for a drug submitted with a priority review voucher (see above for information about priority review vouchers).

TABLE 2-2 CDER Decisions to Grant or Deny Breakthrough Therapy Designation Requests for Non-Oncology Drugs and Biological Products from 2017 to 2019

Category; n (% of designation requests)	Designation Granted	Designation Denied
Orphan product, no therapy available for disease; n=63 (26%)	35 (56%)	28 (44%)
Non-orphan product, therapy available for disease; n=80 (33%)	18 (22.5%)	62 (77.5%)
Orphan product, therapy available for disease; n=27 (11%)	12 (44%)	15 (56%)
Non-orphan product, no therapy available for disease; n=70 (29%)	28 (40%)	42 (60%)
Total; N=240	93	147

NOTE: CDER = Center for Drug Evaluation and Research.
SOURCES: Presented to the Committee by Miranda Raggio, on November 6, 2023. Poddar et al., 2024. CC BY 4.0 http://creativecommons.org/licenses/by/4.0/.

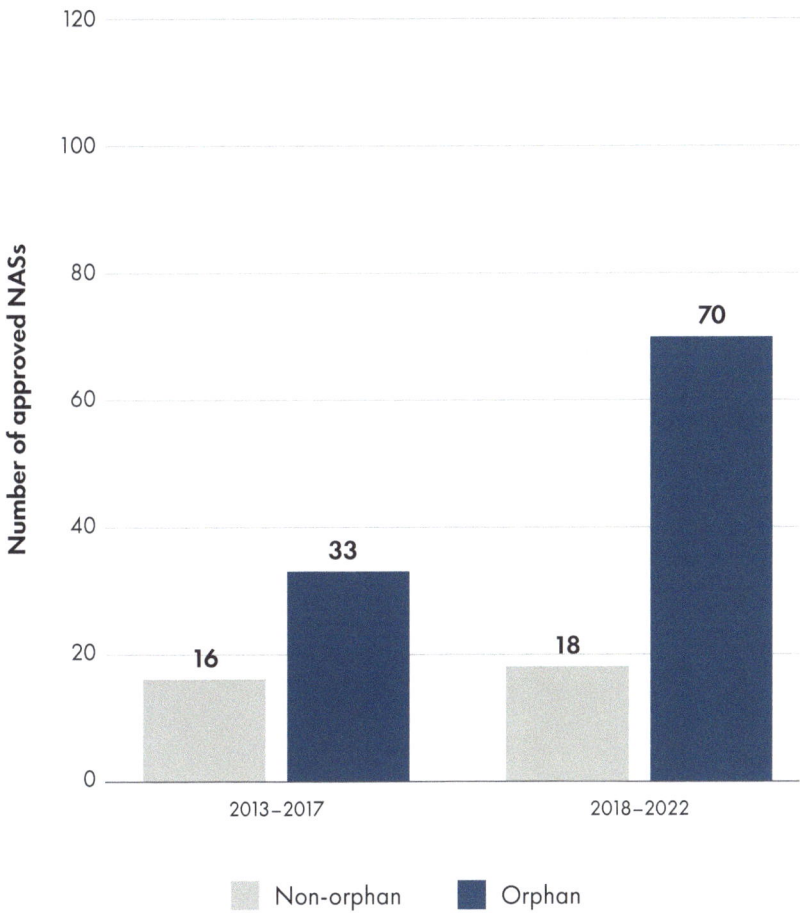

FIGURE 2-10 Number of orphan and non-orphan drug products that received breakthrough therapy designation approved by FDA between 2013 and 2022.
NOTES: FDA = U.S. Food and Drug Administration; NASs = new active substances.
SOURCE: CIRS Data Analysis, 2024.

"Significant improvement in safety or effectiveness" can be demonstrated in several ways, including with evidence of increased effectiveness of treatment, prevention, or diagnosis; substantial reduction of a treatment-limiting adverse drug reaction; improved patient compliance that is expected to lead to improvement in serious outcomes; or evidence of safety and effectiveness in a new subpopulation (FDA, 2014b).

Between 2008 and 2021, 62.4 percent of all drugs receiving priority review designation were orphan drugs (Monge et al., 2022). Between 2013 and 2022, 65 percent of the drug products approved through priority review received orphan designation (see Figure 2-11). Priority review can

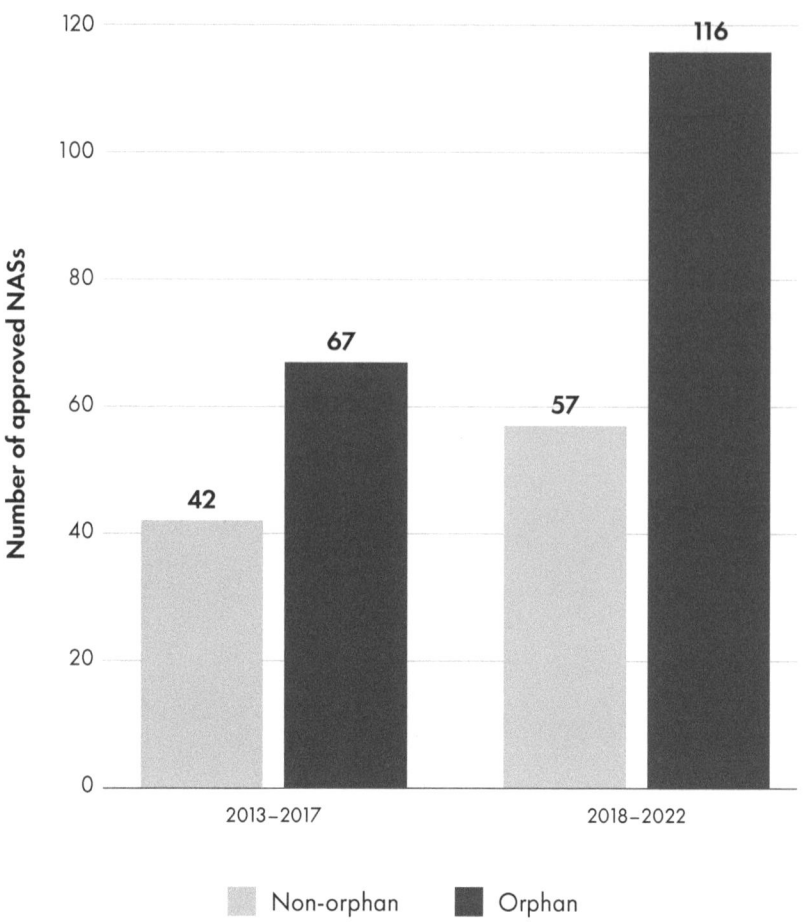

FIGURE 2-11 Number of orphan and non-orphan drug products that received priority review designation approved by FDA between 2013 and 2022.
NOTES: FDA = U.S. Food and Drug Administration; NASs = new active substances.
SOURCE: CIRS Data Analysis, 2024.

help treatments reach market more quickly, which can be critical in rare disease where there may not be another treatment option.

Regenerative Medicine Advanced Therapy

In addition to the programs discussed above, there is one expedited program available only for specific biologics. The 21st Century Cures Act included a provision to establish the RMAT designation to enable a new expedited option for products that meet the following criteria:

- "The drug is a regenerative medicine therapy, which is defined as a cell therapy, therapeutic tissue engineering product, human cell and tissue product, or any combination product using such therapies or products, except for those that are regulated solely under Section 361 of the Public Health Service Act and part 1271 of Title 21, Code of Federal Regulations;[31]
- "The drug is intended to treat, modify, reverse, or cure a serious or life-threatening disease or condition; and
- "Preliminary clinical evidence indicates that the drug has the potential to address unmet medical needs for such disease or condition." (FDA, 2023n)

RMAT designation is distinct from fast track and breakthrough therapy designation and has different requirements, but it includes the same benefits, such as early interactions with FDA to obtain advice on product development. In addition, there is potential for accelerated approval with post-approval requirements (FDA, 2019b). And during an open session of the committee, FDA staff reported that, as of December 31, 2022, of the 82 biologics that had received RMAT designation, 35 (43 percent) have been for orphan products (Raggio, 2023).

Oncology Center of Excellence Programs

FDA's Oncology Center of Excellence (OCE) was established in 2017 following its authorization by the 21st Century Cures Act of 2016. The OCE brings together experts from across the agency to conduct expedited review of medical products for oncologic indications (FDA, 2024l). Between 2013 and 2022, the majority of orphan designation applications approved by FDA were for anti-cancer and immunomodulator treatments (see Figure 2-5). During this time, FDA approved 2.5 times as many orphan applications for anti-cancer and immunomodulating treatments than for non-orphan treatments. Most of the orphan approvals during this time received an expedited review.

---

[31] Human cells, tissues, and cellular and tissue-based products that are regulated solely under Section 361 of the Public Health Service Act and 21 CFR, part 1271 (aka "361 HCT/Ps") do not undergo pre-market review. These products must meet the four criteria described in 21 CFR part 1271.10(a) (see https://www.ecfr.gov/current/title-21/chapter-I/subchapter-L/part-1271/subpart-A/section-1271.10) (accessed March 16, 2024).

Project Orbis

FDA's OCE launched an international collaborative review program called Project Orbis in 2019. Applicants submitting marketing applications for products with great potential to address unmet medical needs can be considered for eligibility. Project Orbis partners can opt in or out of participating in the review of each application. The process allows for collaborative exchange of information and regulatory perspectives during the review process, while each country retains independent decision making. As of October 31, 2023, there were 81 Project Orbis applications that have resulted in product approval, with approximately one-third of these being new molecular entities in the United States (Donoghue, 2024).[32] Project Orbis partners include representatives from Australia, Brazil, Canada, Israel, Singapore, Switzerland, and the United Kingdom. As of late 2023, the European Medicines Agency (EMA) and Pharmaceuticals and Medical Devices Agency (Japan's regulatory body) became observers of the program but are not full partners in Project Orbis.

Applications in Project Orbis can be identified by the FDA review team or a sponsor can request inclusion (FDA, 2022h). Applications identified by FDA are recommended based on a combination of "breakthrough designation, impressive results, and unmet need" (FDA, 2022h). When a sponsor requests inclusion, the application is considered based on various criteria, and "high impact, clinically significant applications, should generally qualify for priority review because of improvement in safety/efficacy" (FDA, 2022h). The project is open to NDAs, BLAs, and supplemental applications for oncology indications. Sponsors are encouraged to submit marketing applications to all Project Orbis partners but are not required to do so. While review is collaborative and agencies share analysis with partners, sponsors must work with each regulatory agency to comply with regulatory requirements and timelines.

As an example of how Project Orbis works, its first review in 2019 involved FDA, Health Canada, and the Australian Therapeutic Goods Administration. The three agencies collaboratively reviewed the application and identified all regulatory divergence; all three countries simultaneously approved the drug under their own accelerated approval programs. Each country used its own format for the drug label, although they exchanged labels to note any differences (FDA, 2022h). As a result of the collaborative process, the products—for a specific type of endometrial carcinoma—were approved. The approval came 3 months prior to the FDA goal date (FDA, 2019c). For rare disease patients and their families, gaining access to new treatments even a few months earlier can mean significantly improved health outcomes, reduced suffering, and a better quality of life.

---

[32] The sentence has been modified after release of the prepublication version of the report to provide temporal context.

The overarching intent of Project Orbis is to leverage a global patient population and evolve toward uniform global standards ("global regulatory convergence") for the evaluation of oncology-related orphan drugs and biologics. This is broadly applicable and appropriate for other rare diseases and aligns with the International Council for Harmonisation of Technical Requirements for Pharmaceuticals for Human Use (ICH). The framework of Project Orbis that informs the concurrent submission and collaborative review process will also help the community of potential Collaboration on Gene Therapies Global Pilot (CoGenT Global) stakeholders engage productively with the program by shaping their expectations (see Box 2-3).

BOX 2-3
Pilot Program: Collaboration on Gene Therapies Global Pilot

Over the past several decades, gene therapies have been developed for the treatment of rare diseases and conditions, including several products that received marketing authorization (Fox and Booth, 2024). Despite these successes, gene therapy for rare diseases has yet to meet the needs of most rare disease patients.

U.S. Food and Drug Administration/Center for Biologics Evaluation and Research (FDA/CBER) is conducting a pilot program, the Collaboration on Gene Therapies Global (CoGenT Global), where proactive sharing of review experiences between multiple regulators could allow for better leveraging of global patient populations with rare diseases and could attract more sponsor interest in developing a product for a particular disease. It is expected that such exchanges may also lead to increased convergence among international regulatory authorities and encourage sponsors to develop their rare disease products internationally, ultimately increasing the availability of important treatments to patients in medical need. The pilot will be initiated in 2024, starting with the European Medicines Agency, and could be expanded to other international regulatory partners in the future (Anatol, 2024; Eglovitch, 2024; Lu and Abbott, 2024). According to Peter Marks, director of CBER, "if [FDA and EMA] can harmonize our requirements and pull forces to review these products, we can make it much more attractive for people to go into this rare disease area" (Eglovitch, 2024).

Specific and detailed information on CoGenT is still pending and much will depend on the early results of the ability of this pilot program to drive private capital investments in the development of gene therapies and to streamline the conduct of associated regulatory reviews. However, this platform could be even more useful by expanding its scope to include collaborations on issues like harmonization of rare disease registries across jurisdictions and setting of uniform minimum standards of real-world data quality, among other drug development tools.

Real-Time Oncology Review

The real-time oncology review (RTOR) was implemented by OCE in 2018 to "facilitate earlier submission of top-line results." To be eligible for RTOR, a product must meet all of the following criteria (FDA, 2023m):

- Clinical evidence indicates that the drug demonstrates substantial improvement on a clinically relevant endpoint(s) over available therapies; and
- Clinical trial endpoints are easily interpreted; and
- No aspect of the submission is likely to require a longer review time.

Though focused on cancers, RTOR has benefited rare diseases. Of the 10 new molecular entity (NME) product applications accepted by the initial pilot, 8 received orphan designation (Gao et al., 2022). Additionally, 11 of the 13 approvals through RTOR between 2013 and 2022 were for orphan products (see Figure 2-12).

One lesson that is relevant to rare diseases is that the program's resource-intensive nature (e.g., submitting multiple application components at different time points as outlined in the RTOR operating procedures) means that it is key to have close coordination and alignment between the sponsors, which are often small biotech companies, and agency reviewers on expectations and submission timelines related to datasets, analysis, key claims in labels, and safety update reports among others. The RTOR program implementation has been associated with faster approval times (see Figure 2-13) although this may be confounded by the concurrent usage of other expedited programs such as breakthrough designation and priority review (Gao et al., 2022). The frequent interactions with FDA reviewers during the submission and review lifecycle due to the RTOR has meaningfully informed industry practice with respect to application preparation and FDA engagement (Kim, 2022). The abbreviated time from submission to approval means that this framework has considerable applicability to non-oncology rare diseases more broadly. Applying a similar framework may be beneficial for the advancement of rare disease drug development beyond rare cancers.

Orphan Drugs and Expedited Review

Orphan products use expedited programs more often than non-orphan products. Figure 2-14 shows the percentage of orphan drug approvals compared with non-orphan drug approvals for NMEs and new biologics in each of the four expedited development programs available to all drugs and

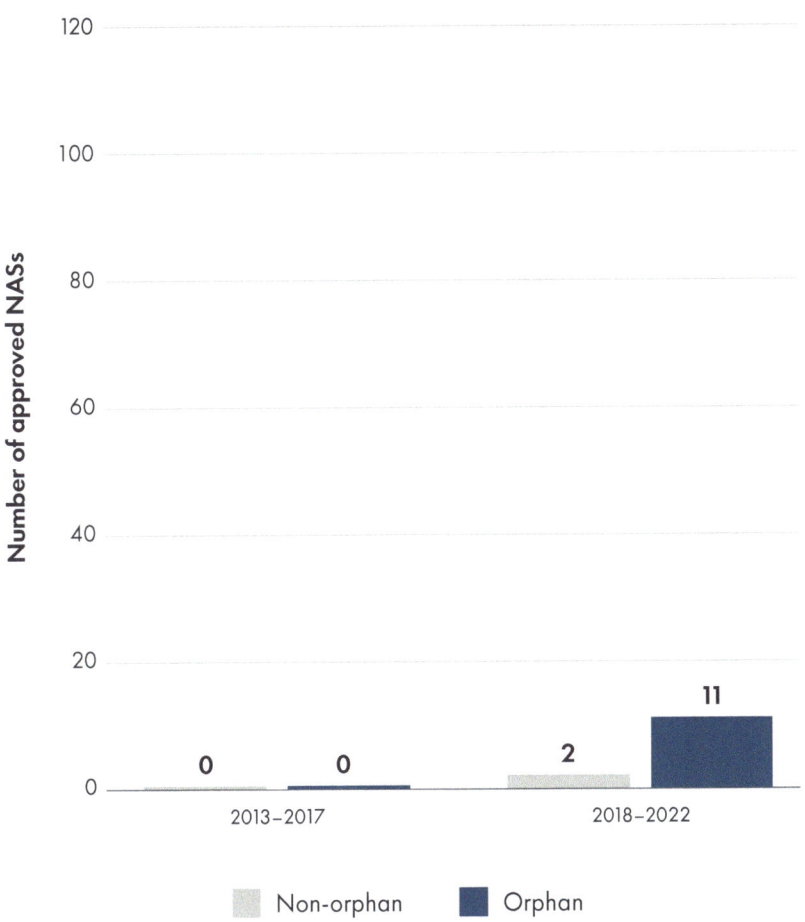

FIGURE 2-12 Number of orphan and non-orphan drug products using the real-time oncology review program approved by FDA between 2013 and 2022.
NOTES: FDA = U.S. Food and Drug Administration; NASs = new active substances.
SOURCE: CIRS Data Analysis, 2024.

biologics. The number of approvals of NMEs and new biologics through each program varies; for example, in 2022, there were 30 approvals for priority review, 19 breakthrough therapy approvals, 7 accelerated approvals, and 16 fast track approvals (see Figure 2-15). Drugs and biologics may be eligible for more than one expedited program (see Figure 2-14). Median approval times for orphan and non-orphan products are generally comparable within a given expedited development pathway (see Figure 2-14). Expedited approval programs do not change FDA's standards for approval. However, accelerated approval allows FDA to rely on a different evidence

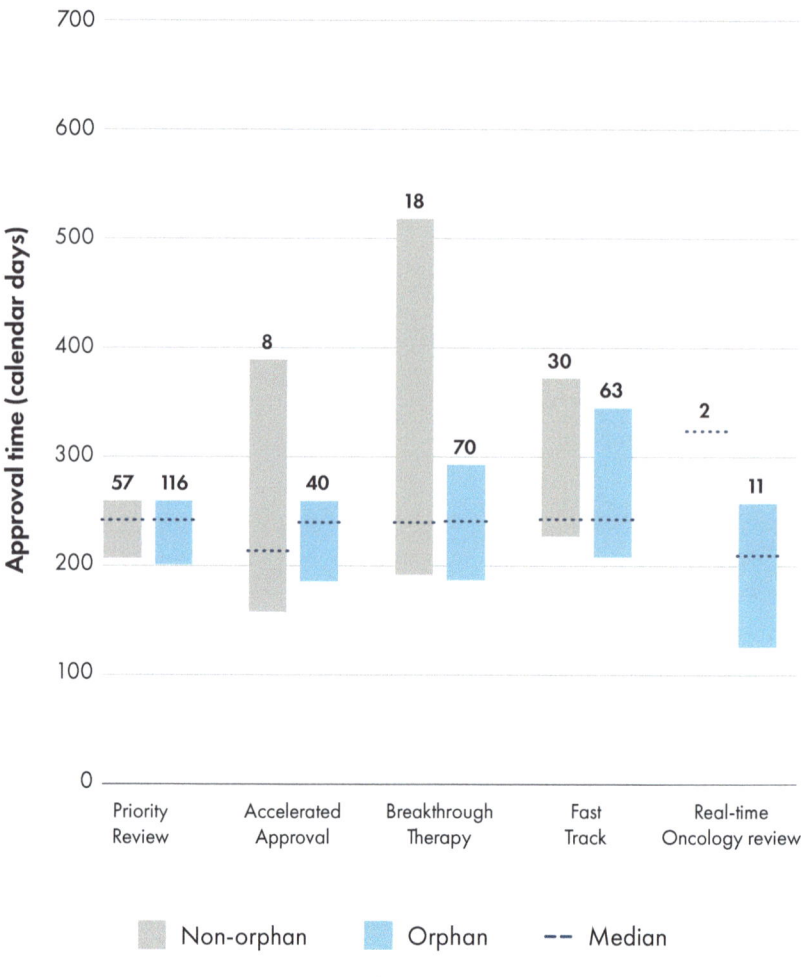

FIGURE 2-13 Approval time of orphan and non-orphan drug products approved by FDA from 2018 to 2022 by regulatory pathway.
NOTES: Box plot displays median approval time with 25–75% interquartile range. Range is not displayed when n < 3. FDA = U.S. Food and Drug Administration.
SOURCE: CIRS Data Analysis, 2024.

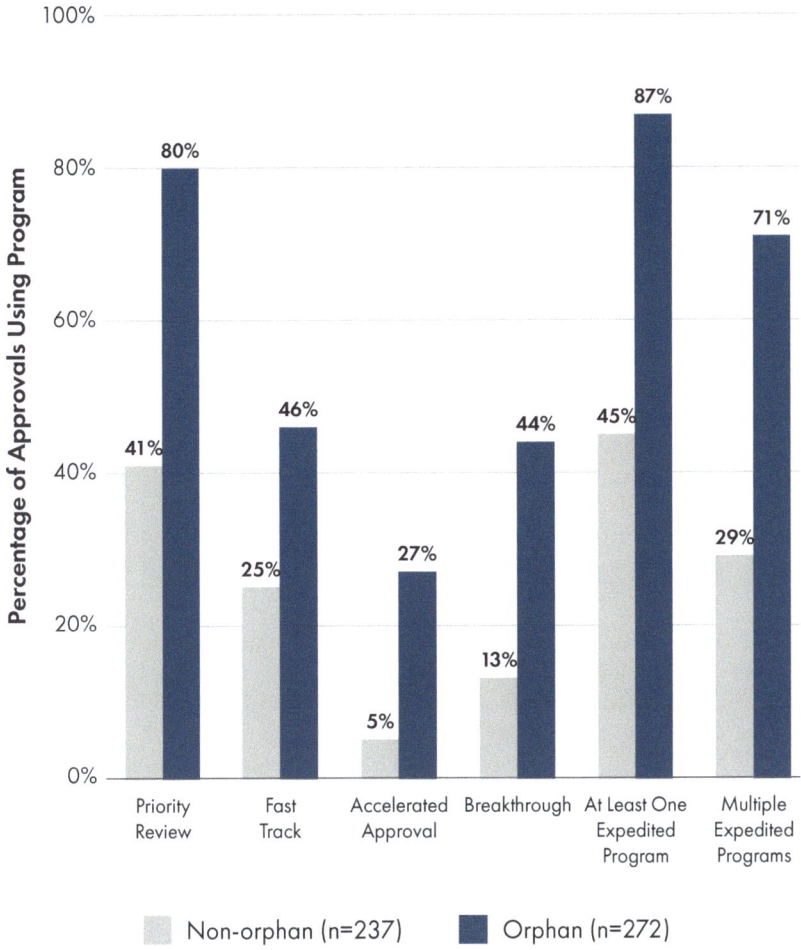

FIGURE 2-14 Use of expedited development programs in CDER and CBER from 2013 to 2022.
NOTES: CBER = Center for Biologics Evaluation and Research; CDER = Center for Drug Evaluation and Research.
SOURCES: Presented to the Committee by Miranda Raggio, on November 6, 2023; created by Michael Lanthier.

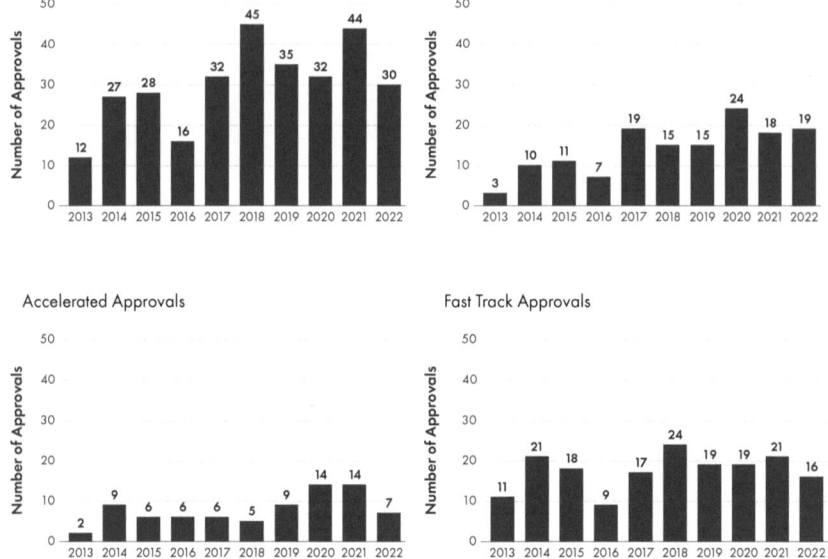

FIGURE 2-15 Expedited program approvals for new molecular entities and novel biologics in CDER and CBER from 2013 to 2022.
NOTES: CBER = Center for Biologics Evaluation and Research; CDER = Center for Drug Evaluation and Research.
SOURCES: Presented to the Committee by Miranda Raggio, on November 6, 2023; created by Michael Lanthier.

base. Surrogate endpoints or intermediate clinical endpoints can serve as the basis for accelerated approval with careful evaluation of the endpoints' effect on clinical benefit (FDA, 2014b).

INCLUSION OF PEDIATRIC POPULATIONS

The majority of rare diseases affect the pediatric population (Wright et al., 2018). Evidence has shown there can be substantial differences in the way that children respond to drug treatment compared to adults (IOM, 2008). Thus, the inclusion of pediatric populations in clinical trials should be a core component for rare disease drug development. Epps et al. (2022) list the following challenges for rare pediatric disease drug development: "(1) garnering interest from sponsors, (2) small numbers of children affected by a particular disease, (3) difficulties with study design, (4) lack of definitive outcome measures and assessment tools, (5) the need for additional safeguards for children as a vulnerable population, and (6) logistical hurdles to completing trials, especially with the need for longer term follow-up to establish safety and efficacy." These challenges are common across all therapeutic areas, but are amplified for rare diseases and conditions.

Over the past several decades, a combination of legislation, regulatory action (see Table 2-3 for list of guidances on pediatric drug development), and the accumulation of scientific evidence has enabled what some have considered a to be a "revolutionary change" in pediatric drug development—a shift from considering pediatric populations as "therapeutic orphans" to a current state in which the number of drug products approved for use in children continues to increase (FDA, 2024m; Fung et al., 2021).

Two laws—the Pediatric Research Equity Act (PREA) of 2003 (FDA, 2024n), the Best Pharmaceuticals for Children Act (BPCA) of 2002 (NICHD, n.d.)—work together to address the need for pediatric drug development. Pediatric provisions in FDASIA further strengthened these laws (FDA, 2018b). BPCA provides incentives (additional marketing exclusivity) to encourage sponsors to carry out studies in pediatric populations, and PREA authorizes FDA to require pediatric studies for certain drugs and biological products (FDA, 2018b, n.d.-a; PhRMA, 2020; Sachs et al., 2012) (see Box 2-4).

Following enactment of BPCA and PREA, FDA has reported "significant progress in the number, timeliness, and successful completion of studies in pediatric populations" (FDA, n.d.-a). The number of pediatric labeling changes—updates to a drug product's labeling to add information on safety, effectiveness, or dosing for children—has continued to increase

TABLE 2-3 FDA Guidance on Pediatric Drug Development

Guidance	Source
Pediatric Drug Development: Regulatory Considerations — Complying With the Pediatric Research Equity Act and Qualifying for Pediatric Exclusivity Under the Best Pharmaceuticals for Children Act	FDA (2023j)
Pediatric Drug Development Under the Pediatric Research Equity Act and the Best Pharmaceuticals for Children Act: Scientific Considerations	FDA (2023i)
ICH Pediatric Extrapolation: E11A	ICH (2022)
Ethical Considerations for Clinical Investigations of Medical Products Involving Children	FDA (2022d)
General Clinical Pharmacology Considerations for Pediatric Studies of Drugs, Including Biological Products	FDA (2022g)
General Clinical Pharmacology Considerations for Neonatal Studies for Drugs and Biological Products	FDA (2022f)
Considerations for Long-Term Clinical Neurodevelopmental Safety Studies in Neonatal Product Development	FDA (2023e)

NOTE: FDA = U.S. Food and Drug Administration.

over time. Between 2010 and 2018, approximately one-third of the orphan drug indications approved by FDA were approved for use in children or targeted a pediatric disease (Kimmel et al., 2020). A more recent analysis showed that the percentage of orphan indications for rare pediatric diseases has continued to increase over time (Fung et al., 2021).

In 2020, PhRMA cited the following numbers:

- "Since 1998, there have been over 750 labeling changes reflecting pediatric information.
- "Since the reauthorization of BPCA and PREA in 2007, more than 680 pediatric studies have been completed under BPCA and PREA.
- "Over 250 drugs have been granted pediatric exclusivity under BPCA.
- "There are currently more than 2100 industry sponsored pediatric clinical trials underway, involving more than 1.2 million pediatric patients across a variety of therapeutic areas, including diseases

---

BOX 2-4
Best Pharmaceuticals for Children Act (BPCA)
and Pediatric Research Equity Act (PREA)

BPCA

"BPCA exists to improve the safety and efficacy of drug use and dosage for children.

"The overarching goals of BPCA are to:

- "Encourage the pharmaceutical industry to perform pediatric studies to improve labeling for patented drug products used in children, by granting an additional 6 months of patent exclusivity
- "Authorize NIH, through Section 409I, to prioritize needs in various therapeutic areas and sponsor clinical trials of off-patent drug products that need further study in children, as well as training and other research that addresses knowledge gaps in pediatric therapeutics" (NICHD, n.d.).

PREA:

"PREA gives FDA the authority to require pediatric studies in certain drugs and biological products. Studies must use appropriate formulations for each age group. The goal of the studies is to obtain pediatric labeling for the product" (FDA, 2024n).

where there is significant unmet need, such as infectious diseases, neurologic conditions, genetic disorders, and several forms of cancer" (PhRMA, 2020).

Notably, orphan designated drug products are generally exempted from PREA requirements. PREA states, "Unless the Secretary requires otherwise by regulation, this section does not apply to any drug for an indication for which orphan designation has been granted under section 526" (FDA, 2005). While the intent of this provision may have been to incentivize the development of drugs to treat rare diseases and conditions, patient groups, such as the Treatment Action Group and Elizabeth Glaser Pediatric AIDS Foundation, have argued that the exemption has led to the opposite result—delays or complete lack of research on the safety and efficacy of rare disease drug products for pediatric populations (Treatment Action Group and Elizabeth Glaser Pediatric AIDS Foundation, 2019).

PREA requires sponsors to submit an initial pediatric study plan (iPSP) "before the date on which the sponsor submits the required assessments or investigation and no later than either 60 days after the date of the end-of-Phase 2 meeting or such other time as agreed upon between FDA and the sponsor" (FDA, 2020b). The iPSP must include the following:
- "an outline of the pediatric study or studies that the sponsor plans to conduct (including, to the extent practicable, study objectives and design, age groups, relevant endpoints, and statistical approach);
- "any request for a deferral or waiver. . .if applicable, along with any supporting information; and
- "other information specified in the regulations promulgated under paragraph (7)"[a]

A sponsor should not submit a marketing application or supplement until FDA confirms agreement on the iPSP, and the total review period for iPSPs should not exceed 210 days. PREA provides an exemption from iPSP requirements for applications for drugs that have orphan designation. In 2017, PREA was amended by the FDA Reauthorization Act of 2017, by including RACE for Children Act to lift the orphan exemption for rare pediatric cancers, requiring sponsors to submit iPSPs for these indications. This amendment has required that sponsors submit a planned approach for studying drugs in pediatric populations if they intend to apply for approval of adult cancer drugs (GAO, 2023).

---

[a] 21 U.S.C. § 355c(e)(2)(B).

The 2017 Research to Accelerate Cures and Equity (RACE) for Children Act[33] amended PREA to remove the exemption for orphan designated drugs, but only for certain cancer drugs. A 2024 FDA briefing document to the Pediatric Oncology Subcommittee of the Oncologic Drugs Advisory Committee stated that:

"Based upon the updated FDA analysis of initial pediatric study plans for molecularly targeted drugs and the results of the GAO audit, it appears that the RACE Act has contributed to an increase in the number of planned studies to test certain molecularly targeted drugs in pediatric patients with cancer. However, given the amount of time needed to design and conduct clinical trials evaluating new drugs for the treatment of pediatric cancers, it is too early to determine the extent to which implementation of the Food and Drug Reauthorization Act of 2017 (FDARA) provisions of PREA will advance the development of new treatments for pediatric cancers" (FDA, 2024g)

Closing the Gap

Despite legislative, regulatory, and scientific advances, meta-analysis has shown that off-label prescriptions for children accounted for up to 38 percent of all pediatric prescriptions between 2007 to 2017 (Allen et al., 2018). To this day, off-label drug use remains an issue for pediatric populations, particularly those living with rare diseases and conditions for which there is no available treatment on the market (Committee on Drugs et al., 2014). More is needed to meet the needs of children living with rare diseases and conditions.

In addition to measures taken by Congress to incentivize the inclusion of pediatric populations in rare disease drug development, FDA and NIH, in partnership with nongovernmental organizations—including patient and disease advocacy groups, academic clinical investigators, and biopharmaceutical companies—have an opportunity to better collaborate on approaches to include pediatric populations as early as possible in rare disease clinical trials.

During an open session held by the committee on February 7, 2024, senior representatives from CDER, CBER, and OCE all stated the agency's view concerning the inclusion of pediatric participants early in clinical trials is "evolving." This sentiment has been echoed by FDA in other venues. On FDA Rare Disease Day, February 27, 2023, Martha Donoghue, the associate director for pediatric oncology and rare cancers in OCE, stated that "over the past decade, this tendency to think about protecting pediatric patients from clinical trials has shifted to thinking that we can best protect

---

[33] H.R.1231—RACE for Children Act—115th Congress (2017–2018).

pediatric patients with cancer through more timely and thoughtful conduct of pediatric clinical trials. In essence, to give them a chance to benefit through participation in clinical trials as soon as it is scientifically justified and feasible, with the ultimate goal of providing increased access to new, safe, and effective treatment that are approved for pediatric patients with cancer" (FDA, 2023g).

Dr. Nicole Verdun, director, Office of Therapeutic Products, CBER, FDA, stated publicly on March 8, 2024, "…traditionally, the thought has been that you should try things in adults before children…what I hear from patient communities is that we have diseases, especially in the rare disease space, that affect children from birth, and we want to prevent those conditions from happening. We do not want to wait to have to enroll a young child in a trial…we have to pivot a little in mindset and be comfortable with starting sometimes in areas where there is some uncertainty… it really depends on the program, but we are looking for ways to enroll pediatric patients earlier in the development process" (The Alliance for a Stronger FDA, 2024).

Such sentiments have been reiterated in other public meetings, including a 2024 Roundtable on Effective Inclusion of Children Early in Clinical Trials hosted by Leavitt Partners and the Friedreich's Ataxia Research Alliance, during which senior FDA leadership at the office, division, and center level discussed the need to pivot toward earlier inclusion of pediatric populations in clinical trials. The committee recognizes the need to focus on protecting children living with rare diseases and conditions through clinical trials, so they have access to safe and effective therapies.

> **RECOMMENDATION 2-1:** Congressional action is needed to encourage and incentivize more studies that provide information about the use of rare disease drug products in pediatric populations. To that end, Congress should remove the Pediatric Research Equity Act orphan exemption and require an assessment of additional incentives needed to spur the development of drugs to treat rare diseases or conditions.[34]
>
> Additionally, the U.S. Food and Drug Administration (FDA) and the National Institutes of Health in partnership with nongovernmental organizations, including patient groups, clinical investigators, and biopharmaceutical companies, should work to provide clarity regarding the evolving regulatory policies and practices for the inclusion of pediatric populations as early as possible in rare disease clinical trials. Actions should include, but are not limited to the following:

---

[34] This sentence was edited after release of the prepublication version of the report to clarify the intent of the recommendation.

- FDA should convene a series of meetings with relevant stakeholders and participate in relevant meetings convened by others to clarify what data are required to support the early inclusion of pediatric populations in clinical trials for rare diseases as well as other key considerations.
- Publish or revise guidance for industry on pediatric study plans for rare disease drug development programs.

STAKEHOLDER ENGAGEMENT

As laid out in Chapter 1, rare disease drug development faces multiple challenges: lack of understanding of the underlying disease, a lack of defined endpoints, and limited patient populations.

FDA has recognized the need for its employees to supplement their knowledge, particularly for "new and emerging fields of science, pioneering technologies, and the increasing complexity of medical devices and pharmaceuticals" (FDA, 2024k). Drugs intended to treat rare diseases fall under each of these umbrellas.

FDA has a number of mechanisms in place to leverage the experience and expertise of external stakeholders, including public workshops on novel and evolving areas of development (e.g., disease-specific or method-based approaches), advisory committee meetings, and public comment on proposed regulations or guidances. Additionally, FDA can appoint special government employees, recruit qualified experts to serve on advisory committees, and collaborate with other organizations (FDA, 2016). The agency has used all of these mechanisms to support the review and approval of drugs to treat rare disease and conditions, though some of these approaches can be slow and onerous to implement.

FDASIA, signed into law in 2012, includes sections aimed at expanding the role of external stakeholders in FDA regulatory processes. Section 1137 directs the Secretary of Health and Human Services (HHS) to "develop and implement strategies to solicit the views of patients during the medical product development process and consider the perspectives of patients during regulatory discussions."[35] This provision assists FDA in developing strategies for integrating the input of patients in regulatory decision-making.

Section 1138 of FDASIA "requires the Secretary of Health and Human Services (HHS), acting through the Commissioner of Food and Drugs, review and modify as necessary, FDA's communication plan to inform and educate health care practitioners and patients on the benefits and risks of medical products, with particular focus on underrepresented subpopulations, including racial subgroups" (FDA, 2013a). While these provisions are

---

[35] 21 U.S.C. 360bbb–8c.

complementary, they serve different purposes in aiding the agency better integrate the critical input of patients and ensuring adequate communication of information about drug development.

Patient Engagement

FDA has made important strides to engage people with lived experience throughout the regulatory review process. Guidance documents, patient focused drug development (PFDD) meeting summaries, direct interaction with patients, and other resources have helped to bridge the gaps among regulators, sponsors, and people with lived experience.

An FDA guidance for industry, *Rare Diseases: Considerations for the Development of Drugs and Biological Products*, encourages sponsors to discuss trial design with patients and caregivers early in the planning stages, and to consider modifying designs to address patient and family concerns (FDA, 2023l). For example, the guidance notes that endpoint selection can be informed by understanding what aspects of the disease are meaningful to patients and caregivers. In addition, the guidance emphasizes the importance of centering patients in the process. Patient engagement is a critical aspect of the regulatory review process as it provides decision makers with information on lived experience, meaningful outcome measures, therapeutic context, and benefits and risks.

Patients and caregivers are experts in their own experience of living with or caring for someone with a disease or condition and their perspectives and insights should be valued alongside those of regulators, sponsors, and researchers when it comes to informing the development of drugs to meet their needs. A 2015 *JAMA* article by Hunter, O'Callaghan, and Califf (Hunter et al., 2015) stated that "the FDA is working to give patients a greater voice in medical product development and evaluation" (p. 2500). FDA has several avenues for patient and caregiver input to inform regulatory decision-making. These include the PFDD initiative, the FDA Patient Listening Session program, the FDA Patient Representative Program, and the FDA–Clinical Trials Transformation Initiative (CTTI) Patient Engagement Collaborative (PEC). Information shared via these avenues can provide key insights on disease course and variability, disease outcomes, patient preferences, desired benefits, and acceptable risks and has increasingly become a component of regulatory science at FDA (Kuehn, 2018).

Patient-Focused Drug Development

FDA's PFDD initiative, which was established under the fifth authorization of the Prescription Drug User Fee Act (PDUFA), is a "systematic approach to help ensure that patients' experiences, perspectives, needs, and priorities are meaningfully incorporated into drug development and evaluation" (FDA, 2024d) (see Box 2-5). PFDD initially included a series of FDA-hosted disease-specific meetings, which were held between 2012 and 2017, in which FDA and other key stakeholders, including medical product developers, health care providers, and federal partners, heard directly from patients, their families, caregivers, and patient advocates about the symptoms that matter most to them, the impact the disease has on patients' daily lives, and patients' experiences with currently available treatments. Following each meeting, FDA published a summary of the input shared by meeting participants (FDA, 2024f).

PFDD has since expanded to include externally-led PFDD meetings (FDA, 2022e), the development of guidance documents, and other initiatives to facilitate the incorporation of patient input into medical product decision making. Patient listening sessions, similar to PFDD meetings, serve

---

BOX 2-5
What is Patient-Focused Drug Development?

"Patient-focused drug development (PFDD) is a systematic approach to help ensure that patients' experiences, perspectives, needs, and priorities are captured and meaningfully incorporated into drug development and evaluation. As experts in what it is like to live with their condition, patients are uniquely positioned to inform the understanding of the therapeutic context for drug development and evaluation.

The primary goal of patient-focused drug development is to better incorporate the patient's voice in drug development and evaluation, including but not limited to:

- Facilitating and advancing use of systematic approaches to collecting and utilizing robust and meaningful patient and caregiver input to more consistently inform drug development and regulatory decision-making.
- Encouraging identification and use of approaches and best practices to facilitate patient enrollment and minimizing the burden of patient participation in clinical trials.
- Enhancing understanding and appropriate use of methods to capture information on patient preferences and the potential acceptability of tradeoffs between treatment benefit and risk outcomes.
- Identifying the information that is most important to patients related to treatment benefits, risks, and burden, and how to best communicate the information to support their decision making."

SOURCE: FDA, 2024d.

to inform FDA on the concerns of the patient community. However, patient listening sessions are nonpublic, only FDA, patients, caregivers, advocates, and community representatives can participate in the sessions, and they are non-interactive in that the agency participants are listening but not conversing with other participants (FDA, 2024h). There have been over 35 rare disease-specific patient listening sessions since they began in October 2018 (FDA, 2024e) (see Appendix F for a full list of rare disease-specific PFDD meetings and patient listening sessions).

During a series of qualitative interviews with industry representatives, interviewees suggested that PFDD meetings are an adequate mechanism for FDA to gather patient input on disease-specific drug development (see Appendix E for full methodology and results). At the same time, during committee meeting open sessions, a few speakers suggested that the one-way nature of PFDD meetings and patient listening sessions makes it hard for participants to understand the value of their contributions during these convenings. The committee did not find adequate evidence to assess the impact of PFDD meetings and patient listening sessions one way or the other.

PFDD meetings and patient listening sessions provide a pathway for patient input to be considered during the review process, but patient groups often face barriers to effectively leverage these opportunities. Challenges cited in a study by Kuehn (2018) include "resources capacity, . . . policy knowledge, and regulatory culture [at FDA]" (p. 663). There is a perception that well-funded patient groups are more capable than smaller groups of generating data that meet FDA regulatory standards. Smaller advocacy groups may have limited resources to host PFDD meetings and lack full knowledge of regulatory processes and data requirements for decision making.

A broader issue raised by Kuehn (2018) was a perception on the part of interviewees that FDA did not give adequate weight to patient experience data (PED) and should put in place more practical conflict of interest policies for patient groups, which often depend on industry engagement and funding support.[36]

Conclusion 2-2: FDA is using available mechanisms to gather patient input. However, there are opportunities to better ensure that patient input informs the development of treatments for rare diseases as well as the design and conduct of clinical trials for rare diseases. More clarity is needed on the part of patient groups and people with lived experience on how the agency is using patient input to inform regulatory decision-making and what types of patient input are most relevant.

---

[36] This section was edited after release of the prepublication version of the report to more accurately reflect the article cited.

FDA Patient Listening Sessions

FDA patient listening sessions are small, informal meetings between FDA staff and patient communities that allow staff in various centers and review divisions the opportunity to hear patient and caregiver perspectives on a range of topics (e.g., disease/treatment, burden, impact on daily activities/quality of life, meaningful outcomes in managing their disease, perspectives on clinical trial participation) related to their experiences with a disease/condition or health care consideration for specific populations (FDA, 2024h).

FDA–CTTI Patient Engagement Collaborative

The PEC was established in 2018 as a joint project of FDA and CTTI, a public-private partnership of Duke University and FDA (CTTI, 2023). The PEC serves as a setting for patients, FDA, and CTTI to discuss patient engagement during medical product regulation. The idea for the PEC came out of public comments related to how FDA could develop strategies to solicit the views of patients (as well as a joint structure between FDA and EMA known as the Pediatric Cluster; see Chapter 5); many commenters suggested that a group outside FDA would be best suited to providing ideas about how to do so. Members of the PEC are representatives of the patient community. Meetings are held up to six times per year and may cover topics such as exploring creative ideas to enhance patient engagement, identifying needs for tools and resources for patient communities, and engaging in two-way education about medical product regulation. In 2022 the PEC held a joint meeting with EMA Patients and Consumers Working Party (see Chapter 3) to discuss common issues in patient engagement.[37]

Patient Representative Program

The Patient Representative Program allows for patients, caregivers, and advocates representing selected disorders chosen by FDA to serve on FDA advisory committees via appointment as a special government employee and provide advice to FDA on the regulation of medical products (FDA, 2024b).

---

[37] For more information, see https://www.ema.europa.eu/en/events/meeting-ctti-fda-patient-engagement-collaborative-pec-and-ema-patients-and-consumers-working-party-pcwp-0 (accessed March 19, 2024).

Patient Experience Data

Patient experience data[38] provide information about the experiences, perspectives, needs, and priorities of people living with a disease or condition. These data can be used to inform clinical trial design, endpoint selection, and regulatory review, including benefit–risk assessments (FDA, n.d.-b).

An analysis of NMEs approved by FDA in 2018 found that of the 59 NMEs approved, 48 contained a patient experience data table within the review documentation and 34 reported using patient experience data in the drug review process. Within this group of NMEs, 28 had received an orphan designation. However, only 17 of the 28 (60.7 percent) orphan designated NMEs used PED in the review. In comparison, 17 of the other 20 (85 percent) non-orphan reviews used PED. Sponsor-submitted patient-reported outcomes (PROs) were the most significant source of patient experience data and were used in over half of approved drug reviews. Non-PRO patient experience data used in reviews were qualitative studies, PFDD meeting summary reports, observational survey studies, natural history studies, and patient preference studies (Kieffer et al., 2019).

The 21st Century Cures Act directs FDA to report on the use of patient experience data in regulatory decision-making. A 2021 report by Eastern Research Group (ERG) showed that while patient experience data play an important role in FDA decisions about when to use PROs or other types of clinical outcome assessments, they "generally provide supporting information in situations where the condition is not well characterized, as with some rare diseases" (Eastern Research Group Inc., 2021). The report included interviews with external stakeholders, including patients and their caregivers, clinicians, and representatives of patient and disease advocacy organizations, which indicated a lack of understanding about how FDA uses patient experience data. Similar statements were made by Kara Berasi, the chief executive officer of the Haystack Project, at a committee meeting open session. The ERG report offered recommendations for FDA and other stakeholders to provide more clarity and consistency on whether and how FDA uses patient experience data in regulatory decision-making (see Box 2-6).

---

[38] Title III, Section 3001(c) of the 21st Century Cures Act defines patient experience data as data that "(1) are collected by any persons (including patients, family members and caregivers of patients, patient advocacy organizations, disease research foundations, researchers, and drug manufacturers); and (2) are intended to provide information about patients' experiences with a disease or condition, including—(A) the impact of such disease or condition, or a related therapy, on patients' lives; and (B) patient preferences with respect to treatment of such disease or condition."

BOX 2-6
Select Eastern Research Group Report Findings and Recommendations

Finding 3: Whether and how the U.S. Food and Drug Administration (FDA) uses patient experience data in application approval decisions varies widely. In part, this is because (1) applications vary in the need for clinical and patient experience data, (2) applicants vary in whether and how they develop and use patient experience data, (3) the availability of fit-for-purpose Patient-Focused Drug Development (PFDD) tools varies by therapeutic context, and (4) the quality, completeness, and relevance of submitted patient experience data vary. In addition, FDA staff openness to use of patient experience data varies across (and sometimes within) Center for Biologics Evaluation and Research (CBER) and Center for Drug Evaluation and Research (CDER) review divisions.

Recommendation for Applicants: When pursuing a drug/biologic development program, consult FDA guidance, other PFDD resources, and FDA staff early and often to discuss the potential value of patient experience data, types of data to develop, fit-for-purpose tools to use, approaches to collecting complete data, and a data analysis plan.

Recommendation for FDA: Continue or expand collaborative programs to foster development of PFDD tools and Clinical Outcome Assessments (COAs). Internally and externally, provide models of applicant development and presentation of patient experience data in marketing applications and FDA use of these data in various therapeutic contexts. Within and across review divisions, encourage sharing of additional examples of use of patient experience data in regulatory decision-making.

Finding 4: Applicants, patients, caregivers, and other stakeholders cannot easily determine how FDA uses patient experience data in regulatory decision-making.

Recommendation for FDA: In the Patient Experience Data Table, add a column for "Use in Review" with a straightforward list of options (e.g., Background/Context, Risk-Benefit Analysis, Factor in Decision, and Not Used). In the Patient Experience Data Table, add a column for Not Used: Reason with a straightforward list of options (e.g., Tool not Fit-For-Purpose, Data Incomplete, and Data not for Primary or Key Endpoint). As noted above, provide models of applicant development and presentation of patient experience data in marketing applications and FDA use of these data in various therapeutic contexts.

SOURCE: Eastern Research Group Inc., 2021.

Opportunity to Enhance Patient Input

Taken together, FDA has demonstrated a commitment to engaging people with lived experience. While there are numerous programs, collaborations, and partnerships in place that value the experience and perspectives of people living with rare diseases and conditions and their caregivers, more is needed to fully implement Section 1137 of FDASIA. This is particularly the case for patient groups that are small and under resourced. Strategies are needed to better solicit input from people no matter their race, ethnicity, ability, socio-economic level, or geography with particular consideration for enabling the participation of those who come from marginalized communities.

FDA advisory committees offer independent expert advice and recommendations on scientific, technical, and policy matters related to FDA-regulated products. In addition to including a patient representative who provides lived experience with a particular disease, condition, or medical product, all advisory committee meetings include an open public hearing session during which patients and their caregivers have an opportunity to share relevant information about a given drug and disease or condition.[39] In principle, open public hearing sessions should inform the advisory committee on the particular drug product under consideration. In practice, information shared may not be relevant or balanced.

Given limited time, speakers are typically allotted 5–10 minutes each to share their perspective with the advisory committee. Selection of the speakers is typically done on a lottery basis, which means that anyone may have the opportunity to share a point of view whether or not they have relevant experience with a given disease or the drug product being discussed (FDA, 2013b). For example, at the advisory committee meeting for Elevidys for Duchenne muscular dystrophy (DMD), of the 18 public commenters, 8 were not patients or their caregivers (FDA, 2023a). For rare disease patients and their families who have worked hard to reach this point and who depend on the expertise and evidence-based consideration of advisory committees, it can be defeating to share equal time with people who do not have relevant experience or expertise.

In keeping with patient focused drug development, FDA has an opportunity to shape open public hearings so that they provide better input from patients on clinically meaningful benefit and risk tolerance. This is particularly the case for drug development for rare diseases and conditions—patients are often the experts on the disease because, so little is known. Providing a more structured format for selecting speakers who have lived experience with a rare disease or condition or have experience

---

[39] 21 CFR §14.25(a).

with a given treatment and managing the session to ensure that speakers are contributing valuable information that is relevant to the marketing authorization application may enable a more focused and streamlined approach for seeking public input. Furthermore, better engagement and inclusion of people with lived experience throughout the regulatory lifecycle could help to ensure that the regulatory process is meeting the needs of patients with rare diseases.

A 2013 guidance for the public, FDA advisory committee members, and FDA staff specifies information that speaker requests should include name and affiliation, contact information, and a general description of the nature of the presentation (FDA, 2013b). It does not indicate that speakers should have firsthand experience with a given disease or condition or with the product under consideration. For rare disease patients and caregivers with lived experience, FDA should provide materials on the types of insights and perspectives that would be most beneficial for the advisory committee. This may include reference to relevant PFDD listening sessions or data relevant to the disease indication. For example, speakers could be asked to demonstrate how the primary or secondary outcomes relate to their ability to perform activities of daily living or other challenges or limitations they perceive of these measures.

Advisory committees should be well informed by the community of people most affected by the disease, and they need to listen to the patient voice when making evaluations about a drug to treat a rare disease or condition. In addition to speaking at an open hearing sessions, there are opportunities for patients and caregivers to submit written or electronic comments through the *Federal Register*. Taken together, these mechanisms are insufficient compared to the opportunity that FDA and the applicant have to speak with the advisory committee, each of which are guaranteed time on the agenda for formal presentation, including a question-and-answer period. Patients and their caregivers should have this dedicated allotted time as well, so their insights and perspectives can be weighted similarly to those of other key stakeholders at the table.

> *Conclusion 2-3: The strategic engagement of people who have rare diseases and their caregivers with lived experience throughout the drug review and approval process can help regulatory agencies facilitate the development of drug products that meet the needs of patients living with rare diseases and conditions.*

RECOMMENDATION 2-2: The U.S. Food and Drug Administration (FDA) should strengthen mechanisms to integrate input from people living with a rare disease or condition, their caregivers, and patient representatives, especially patient groups that are small and under-resourced, throughout the full continuum of the drug development process. To that end, FDA should take the steps necessary to fully implement Section 1137 of the Food and Drug Administration Safety and Innovation Act (Public Law 112-144), which directs the Secretary of Health and Human Services to develop and implement strategies to solicit the views of rare disease patients during the full range of regulatory review discussions. This should include but not be limited to:

- Implementing strategies to meaningfully engage people living with a rare disease or condition, their caregivers, and patient representatives throughout the review process, from initial review discussions to final regulatory decision.
- Ensuring equitable representation of people living with a rare disease or condition, their caregivers, and patient representatives throughout the review process by actively recruiting and supporting participation from underrepresented and under-resourced patient groups, providing necessary support and accommodations to enable their full participation.
- Developing a structured approach to directly engage people with lived experience (those living with or caring for someone living with a rare disease or condition), including in all open public hearing sessions of advisory committee meetings by establishing a mechanism to prioritize and provide speaking opportunities for people with lived experience, particularly patients and caregivers, to inform advisory committees on how primary or secondary outcome measures relate to functional status and quality of life.
- Developing in-person and hybrid education and training programs to assist rare disease patient groups in creating and maintaining tools (e.g., patient registry, natural history data, translational tools) that can contribute to research and development.

Sponsor Engagement

Sponsors developing new drugs must navigate a range of complex challenges when designing and conducting a study for regulatory submission. Clinical trials for regulatory submission require a combination of clinical, safety, biostatistical, and regulatory expertise, as well an understanding of the patient populations a drug is intended to treat to maximize the likelihood that study results meet regulatory requirements to gain market approval (FDA, 2017a). These challenges are heightened when it comes to rare diseases and conditions. Additionally, many companies developing rare disease drugs are small and medium-sized enterprises, which may have fewer resources and less in-house expertise than large pharmaceutical companies. For these reasons it is critically important for sponsors developing rare disease drug products to engage with the agency early and often.

Sponsors may request a meeting with FDA at any time during drug development; FDA may communicate with a sponsor at any time during the process about the need for more data or information. Regulatory project managers (RPMs) located within the clinical review divisions serve an important role as the main point of contact between FDA and sponsors, while nonclinical review division RPMs focus on specific issues (e.g., proprietary names, manufacturing, and controls) (FDA, 2017a).

Sponsors are encouraged to contact FDA through the appropriate RPM, and they are strongly discouraged from directly contacting reviewers assigned to their IND. The 2017 guidance for industry and review staff, *Best Practices for Communication Between IND Sponsors and FDA During Drug Development*, states, "CDER and CBER strive to provide timely and accurate advice and feedback to sponsors that represent the review teams' current thinking on the issue, and this is best accomplished by adhering to the communication procedures described above and throughout this guidance" (FDA, 2017a). When appropriate, sponsors may solicit advice on issues including regulatory, clinical and statistical, safety, pharmacology and pharmacokinetics, toxicology, and product quality. In addition to communications between the sponsor and the RPM, sponsors may also request a formal meeting; these can be particularly useful at critical junctures or "milestone meetings" (FDA, 2017a).

> *Conclusion 2-4: FDA engagement with rare disease drug development sponsors is of particular importance because compared with common diseases, rare diseases are less well understood, more often do not have regulatory precedent, and more commonly lack validated endpoints and outcome measures and involve small patient populations which limit the size and number of clinical trials that can be conducted.*

As discussed above, there are opportunities to better ensure that sponsors and other stakeholders, particularly small companies, have access to the knowledge, expertise, and tools to advance new drugs for the treatment of rare diseases and conditions.

> **RECOMMENDATION 2-3:** The U.S. Food and Drug Administration and the National Institutes of Health in collaboration with the European Medicines Agency, nongovernmental organizations, patient groups, and biopharmaceutical sponsors, should implement a sponsor, investigator, and patient group navigation service to support the development of drugs to treat rare diseases and conditions (1) by advising on the range of available regulatory pathways and flexibilities and (2) by providing clarity on how to comply with regulatory policies, apply

guidances, and meet requirements in rare disease drug development. Actions should include:
- Facilitation including, but not limited to, consultation, referral to other organizations, services to identify and overcome regulatory barriers, needs assessment, and regular follow-up; and
- The development of educational materials and tools.

SELECT RARE DISEASE PROGRAMS

In addition to its programs focused on the approval process for rare disease products, FDA has several other programs relevant to rare diseases. These programs, several of which are in pilot form, are described below.

The Rare Disease Innovation Hub

In 2024, FDA announced a plan to establish a Rare Disease Innovation Hub (the Hub) to establish a new model for FDA to leverage cross-agency expertise and enhance shared learnings to spur drug development for rare diseases and conditions (FDA, 2024i). The Hub, which will be co-led by the director of CDER and the director of CBER, will provide services across all rare diseases with a special focus on treatments of smaller populations where natural history and disease progression is not fully understood (FDA, 2024i). This will include three primary functions:

- "Serve as a single point of connection and engagement with the rare disease community, including patient and caregiver groups, trade organizations, and scientific/academic organizations, for matters that intersect CDER and CBER. The Hub will help the larger rare disease community navigate important intersections across FDA that affect patients with rare diseases, such as medical devices, including diagnostic tests, and combination products.
- "Enhance intercenter collaboration to address common scientific, clinical and policy issues related to rare disease product development, including relevant cross-disciplinary approaches related to product review, and promote consistency across offices and Centers.
- "Advance regulatory science with dedicated workstreams for consideration of novel endpoints, biomarker development and assays, innovative trial design, real world evidence, and statistical methods" (FDA, 2024i).

In addition to enabling more collaboration across ongoing FDA rare disease programs, the Hub will seek to expand collaborative opportunities with patient groups, sponsors, researchers, and other interested parties (FDA, 2024i). Patients will have an opportunity to shape the Hub's priorities through and open public meeting that will take place in the fall of 2024.

Accelerating Rare Disease Cures Program

CDER launched the Accelerating Rare disease Cures (ARC) Program in 2022; its mission is "to drive scientific and regulatory innovation and engagement to accelerate the availability of treatments for patients with rare diseases" (FDA, 2024c). The program is governed by senior leaders from the Office of New Drugs, the Office of the Center Director, and the Office of Translational Science and managed by CDER's Rare Diseases Team; the Rare Diseases Team, established after the fifth reauthorization of PDUFA, is committed in the sixth and seventh reauthorizations of PDUFA to connect rare disease initiatives and programs across CDER. In addition to these groups that lead the ARC program, many other offices, divisions, and programs within FDA contribute and are connected to the work.

In the first year since its inception, ARC focused on stakeholder outreach and education, including FDA patient listening sessions, quarterly newsletters, and new initiatives aimed at gathering stakeholder input and making the rare disease drug approval process more transparent (FDA, 2023b). ARC launched its Learning and Education to Advance and Empower Rare Disease Drug Developers (LEADER 3D) initiative in 2023. Through LEADER 3D, FDA seeks input from stakeholders who design and conduct rare disease drug development programs in order to identify gaps in knowledge about the regulatory process. Input is curated and documented in a public report by FDA (FDA, 2024j) and will be used to create or expand educational resources for stakeholders. Also in 2023, ARC added two new filters to CDER's Drugs and Biologics Dashboard hosted on FDA-TRACK (FDA, 2024a). This dashboard serves as a management program to report on performance measures and key projects at FDA. The new filters, "Original Rare Disease Application Approval" and "Novel Rare Disease Drugs Approval," allow users to view information about the development and approval of products for rare diseases (FDA, 2023b).

In addition to these stakeholder-focused efforts, the ARC program has also supported scientific and regulatory initiatives, including the development of platforms to facilitate natural history studies, exploring methodologies to construct novel endpoints, the expansion of the use of drug/disease modeling; establishing efficient approaches to dose-selection for drugs for small population diseases, exploring innovative methodologies to trial design and interpretation for very small populations, and expanding efforts to support in translational medicine approaches for individual rare disease programs (FDA, 2023b).

Rare Disease Endpoint Advancement Pilot Program

The Rare Disease Endpoint Advancement (RDEA) Pilot Program is a joint CDER and CBER program that is intended to advance rare disease drug development by providing a mechanism for sponsors to collaborate with FDA throughout the efficacy endpoint development process. Sponsors submit a proposal for development of a novel efficacy endpoint for consideration to the RDEA pilot program; proposed endpoints are eligible for selection into the program if:

- The associated drug or biological product development program is active and addresses a rare disease (or a common disease where the endpoint or methodology could be applicable to a rare disease);
- The associated drug or biological product has an active IND or pre-IND for this treatment (with the exception of the endpoint being studied through natural history studies); and
- The proposed endpoint is a novel efficacy endpoint intended to establish substantial evidence of effectiveness for rare disease treatment. A novel endpoint is one that has never been used to support drug development or one that has been modified from its prior use (FDA, 2024p).

Announced in October 2022, the RDEA pilot will accept proposals through fiscal year 2027. When a proposal is admitted into the RDEA pilot program, FDA conducts an initial meeting and up to three follow-up meetings with the sponsor. At these meetings, sponsors can engage in focused discussion with interdisciplinary FDA experts and talk through the development of novel efficacy endpoints intended to establish evidence of effectiveness (FDA, 2023k). The RDEA meetings are in addition to other interactions with FDA that are conducted through the IND submission process.

The RDEA pilot program is intended to serve an educational purpose and encourage transparency and collaboration among the rare disease community (Lee et al., 2023). To this end, FDA conducts public workshops to discuss topics related to endpoint development for rare disease and can share information about the novel endpoints developed through the RDEA pilot program in various public-facing materials, such as in guidance documents and on the RDEA pilot program webpage. Sponsors who submit proposals to the RDEA pilot program for novel endpoints must agree to disclose certain elements of their endpoint development program prior to a product's approval.

Support for clinical Trials Advancing Rare disease Therapeutics

Support for clinical Trials Advancing Rare disease Therapeutics (START) is a joint CBER and CDER pilot program that was launched in late 2023. It augments currently available formal meetings by addressing issues through more rapid, ad hoc communication mechanisms (FDA, 2023o; Lee et al., 2023). To be eligible, a drug development program must be under an active IND that is in electronic common technical document (eCTD) format, unless the IND is of a type granted a waiver from eCTD format and must have a chemistry manufacturing and controls development strategy that aligns with clinical development plans. For CBER-regulated products, the product must be a cell or gene therapy under IND being developed toward a BLA and must be intended to address an unmet medical need as a treatment for a rare disease or serious condition that is likely to lead to significant disability or death within the first decade of life. For CDER-regulated products, the product must be intended to treat rare neurodegenerative conditions, including those of rare genetic metabolic etiology (FDA, 2023o).

Sponsors who are selected to participate in START will receive enhanced communications with FDA review staff, including an initial meeting to review features of the pilot, discuss a pathway to support a marketing application, and to identify specific issues about which the sponsor would like further communication (FDA, 2023o). Additional communications may be conducted via email or teleconference, which will be scheduled or held as needed as agreed upon by the sponsor and FDA. The program is designed to be milestone-driven; that is, it is intended to help a product reach a significant regulatory milestone, such as initiation of a pivotal clinical study stage or the pre-BLA or pre-NDA meeting stage (FDA, 2023o). The additional communication provided to sponsors is intended to address issues that would otherwise delay or prevent a promising product from progressing along the pathway toward approval (FDA, 2023o).

Complex Innovative Trial Design Meeting Program

Due to the complex biology underpinning rare diseases and conditions, low disease prevalence, and patient heterogeneity, it is often challenging to design traditional randomized controlled trials for studying drugs that treat rare diseases or conditions. As such, clinical trials for rare diseases and conditions are often smaller than for other more prevalent conditions and may require the use of novel design elements to meet evidentiary standards. To assist sponsors, FDA's Complex Innovative Trial Design Meeting program (also referred to as the Complex Innovative Trial Paired Meeting Program) offers sponsors up to two meetings with FDA to discuss their proposed complex innovative design elements during late-stage clinical development.

In guidance, FDA explains that there is no fixed definition of a complex innovative design because what is considered innovative may change over time, and that the determination of whether a specific novel design is appropriate for regulatory use is made on a case-by-case basis (FDA, 2020a). The guidance provides examples of innovative design approaches (e.g., adaptive designs, Bayesian inference), and gives sponsors suggestions on common elements that should be included in a proposal for this program (FDA, 2020a). Like RDEA, the Complex Innovative Trial Design (CID) meeting program has educational components and requires sponsors to sign a disclosure agreement so that certain information can be shared publicly. FDA held several meetings on CIDs on diseases during which FDA and sponsors discussed trial design elements such as:

- Use of information from historical studies to increase the study power;
- Use of an active-controlled non-inferiority design;
- Model-based extrapolation from adults to the pediatric population; and
- Use of Bayesian methods and response adaptive randomization (FDA, 2023d).

In the first year of its existence, the CID meeting program selected five meeting requests, all of which were related to the use of Bayesian methods. Two of the requests were from sponsors developing products for rare diseases: Duchenne muscular dystrophy and pediatric multiple sclerosis (Price and Scott, 2021). Other CID meetings that supported rare disease drug product development focused on pediatric multiple sclerosis, lupus, epilepsy with myoclonic-atonic seizures (FDA, 2023d).

Bespoke Gene Therapy Consortium

FDA serves an advisory role in the Accelerating Medicines Partnership® Program Bespoke Gene Therapy Consortium, which is a public–private partnership aimed at facilitating the development of adeno-associated virus (AAV) gene therapies for individuals or small populations with very rare diseases.[40] The consortium is involved in two concurrent and interrelated projects aimed at making AAV technology more broadly applicable and advancing scientific and regulatory approaches to AAV gene therapies:

1. Further the understanding of AAV technology for gene therapy by supporting research in areas including enhancing vector generation

---

[40] This sentence was edited after release of the prepublication version of the report to more clearly describe FDA's role.

and transgene expression for AAV gene therapies. Though AAV has been successfully used to treat genetic diseases, there is a need to better understand the underlying biology and how to best leverage this tool.
2. Develop a standard operational playbook for developing these "bespoke" gene therapies for very rare diseases. The playbook will contain approaches to streamlining product development and navigating the regulatory pathway and standardized submission package templates to create a repeatable process for the development and regulatory approval of AAV gene therapies.

The first version of the playbook was released in February 2024 and focused on potential for streamlining pre-clinical and product testing, navigating the regulatory pathway, and standardized regulatory submissions (Bespoke Gene Therapy Consortium, 2024). The playbook serves as a guide for developers, with notes about best practices, decision trees to guide the submission process, and templates for submission requirements.

Opportunities for Expanding FDA Rare Disease Programs

Although the programs described above are welcome developments, most remain limited in scope and scale compared with the vastness of need in rare disease drug development. Some programs have existed for enough time to assess their effectiveness and strengths and weaknesses. Several programs are still early on in their implementation, making it difficult to assess their impact on orphan product development. For instance, the RDEA pilot as conceived will address only an exceedingly small fraction of the endpoint challenges that exist in rare disease development. Furthermore, while the START pilot program holds great promise, participant selection was only just publicly announced earlier this year, and, as such, the committee was unable to assess the program's effectiveness or impact on orphan approvals.

Each of these special programs is intended to strengthen the overall orphan drug development and review, but their recency and proliferation present analytical challenges for program assessment. The lack of a track record makes it challenging for sponsors to choose the best path forward, increasing the complexity of designing an orphan drug development program.

Recommendation 2-4: The U.S. Food and Drug Administration (FDA) should assess the impact of new and ongoing programs and approaches that support drug development for rare diseases and conditions to improve the regulatory decision-making process; publicly share the results of these assessments in a timely manner; take steps to ensure that

lessons learned across different programs are disseminated throughout FDA centers and divisions, including a summary of regulatory flexibilities and novel innovative approaches that were considered acceptable; scale up and expand successful programs across therapeutic areas; and modify or sunset programs that are not improving the regulatory decision-making process. Programs and regulatory approaches should include, but not be limited to:
- Rare Disease Endpoint Advancement Pilot Program
- Support for clinical Trials Advancing Rare disease Therapeutics pilot program
- Complex Innovative Trial Design meeting program
- FDA-NIH Bespoke Gene Therapy Consortium
- Programs and pilots led by the Oncology Center of Excellence (e.g., real-time oncology review, Project Orbis);
- Flexibility and leadership in the review and oversight of genetically-targeted advanced therapeutics (e.g., genetic therapies), especially for very low-prevalence patient populations;
- Adoption and support of master protocols, particularly basket trials, to support mutationally defined product approvals;
- Guidance development on cutting-edge topics to support drug research and development, such as the use of accelerated approval in tissue-agnostic drug development (i.e., drugs that target specific molecular alterations) and master protocols, among others.

TRANSPARENCY

In addition to public meetings, guidance documents, and other materials on regulatory policy, FDA makes certain information about approved drugs available on its public website Drugs@FDA.[41] The database has records for drugs approved as early as 1939, but it does not contain FDA-approved products that are regulated by CBER. However, external parties can access records of approvals for CBER-regulated products via the Licensed Biological Products with Supporting Documents database. The availability of review documents can vary by drug. While review documents are helpful for third parties to understand FDA decision making, they are redacted to protect confidential information. There are several elements of medical product submissions and regulatory decisions that are not publicly released, including:

---

[41] Users can search by drug name or by month of approval, and can access information on drug name, active ingredients, patient labeling, marketing status, regulatory history, priority review and orphan designation status, and therapeutic equivalents. Available at https://www.accessdata.fda.gov/scripts/cder/daf/index.cfm (accessed March 19, 2024).

- Filing of an application;
- Patient-level datasets, clinical study reports, or other post-marketing reports associated with an application;
- Justification for orphan designation;
- Rationale for complete response;
- Safety or efficacy reasons for a clinical hold;
- Key milestones in product approval; and
- Underlying decisions for non-approval (Sharfstein et al., 2017).

While the elements above are not released, when the agency holds an advisory committee meeting, minutes of the meeting and commentary on the sponsors application are made public (Sharfstein et al., 2017).

SUMMARY OF CONCLUSIONS AND RECOMMENDATIONS

Conclusion 2-1: While the statutory requirements for drug approval for rare diseases and conditions are the same as for non-rare diseases or conditions, FDA has long recognized the need to apply regulatory flexibility in the review and approval of marketing authorization applications.

Conclusion 2-2: FDA is using available mechanisms to gather patient input. However, there are opportunities to better ensure that patient input informs the development of treatments for rare diseases as well as the design and conduct of clinical trials for rare diseases. More clarity is needed on the part of patient groups and people with lived experience on how the agency is using patient input to inform regulatory decision-making and what types of patient input are most relevant.

Conclusion 2-3: The strategic engagement of people who have rare diseases and their caregivers with lived experience throughout the drug review and approval process can help regulatory agencies facilitate the development of drug products that meet the needs of patients living with rare diseases and conditions.

Conclusion 2-4: FDA engagement with rare disease drug development sponsors is of particular importance because compared with common diseases, rare diseases are less well understood, more often do not have regulatory precedent, and more commonly lack validated endpoints and outcome measures and involve small patient populations which limit the size and number of clinical trials that can be conducted.

RECOMMENDATION 2-1: Congressional action is needed to encourage and incentivize more studies that provide information about the use of rare disease drug products in pediatric populations. To that end, Congress should remove the Pediatric Research Equity Act orphan exemption and require an assessment of additional incentives needed to spur the development of drugs to treat rare diseases or conditions.[42]

Additionally, the U.S. Food and Drug Administration (FDA) and the National Institutes of Health in partnership with nongovernmental organizations, including patient groups, clinical investigators, and biopharmaceutical companies, should work to provide clarity regarding the evolving regulatory policies and practices for the inclusion of pediatric populations as early as possible in rare disease clinical trials. Actions should include, but are not limited to the following:
- FDA should convene a series of meetings with relevant stakeholders and participate in relevant meetings convened by others to clarify what data are required to support the early inclusion of pediatric populations in clinical trials for rare diseases as well as other key considerations.
- Publish or revise guidance for industry on pediatric study plans for rare disease drug development programs.

RECOMMENDATION 2-2: The U.S. Food and Drug Administration (FDA) should strengthen mechanisms to integrate input from people living with a rare disease or condition, their caregivers, and patient representatives, especially patient groups that are small and under-resourced, throughout the full continuum of the drug development process. To that end, FDA should take the steps necessary to fully implement Section 1137 of the Food and Drug Administration Safety and Innovation Act (Public Law 112-144), which directs the Secretary of Health and Human Services to develop and implement strategies to solicit the views of rare disease patients during the full range of regulatory review discussions. This should include but not be limited to:
- Implementing strategies to meaningfully people living with a rare disease or condition, their caregivers, and patient representatives throughout the review process, from initial review discussions to final regulatory decision.
- Ensuring equitable representation of people living with a rare disease or condition, their caregivers, and patient representatives throughout the review process by actively recruiting and supporting participation from underrepresented and under-resourced

---

[42] This sentence was edited after release of the prepublication version of the report to clarify the intent of the recommendation.

patient groups, providing necessary support and accommodations to enable their full participation.
- Developing a structured approach to directly engage people with lived experience (those living with or caring for someone living with a rare disease or condition), including in all open public hearing sessions of advisory committee meetings by establishing a mechanism to prioritize and provide speaking opportunities for people with lived experience, particularly patients and caregivers, to inform advisory committees on how primary or secondary outcome measures relate to functional status and quality of life.
- Developing in-person and hybrid education and training programs to assist rare disease patient groups in creating and maintaining tools (e.g., patient registry, natural history data, translational tools) that can contribute to research and development.

RECOMMENDATION 2-3: The U.S. Food and Drug Administration and the National Institutes of Health in collaboration with the European Medicines Agency, nongovernmental organizations, patient groups, and biopharmaceutical sponsors, should implement a sponsor, investigator, and patient group navigation service to support the development of drugs to treat rare diseases and conditions (1) by advising on the range of available regulatory pathways and flexibilities and (2) by providing clarity on how to comply with regulatory policies, apply guidances, and meet requirements in rare disease drug development. Actions should include:
- Facilitation including, but not limited to, consultation, referral to other organizations, services to identify and overcome regulatory barriers, needs assessment, and regular follow-up; and
- The development of educational materials and tools.

RECOMMENDATION 2-4: The U.S. Food and Drug Administration (FDA) should assess the impact of new and ongoing programs and approaches that support drug development for rare diseases and conditions to improve the regulatory decision-making process; publicly share the results of these assessments in a timely manner; take steps to ensure that lessons learned across different programs are disseminated throughout FDA centers and divisions, including a summary of regulatory flexibilities and novel innovative approaches that were considered acceptable; scale up and expand successful programs across therapeutic areas; and modify or sunset programs that are not improving the regulatory decision-making process. Programs and regulatory approaches should include, but not be limited to:

- Rare Disease Endpoint Advancement Pilot Program
- Support for clinical Trials Advancing Rare disease Therapeutics pilot program
- Complex Innovative Trial Design meeting program
- FDA-NIH Bespoke Gene Therapy Consortium
- Programs and pilots led by the Oncology Center of Excellence (e.g., real-time oncology review, Project Orbis);
- Flexibility and leadership in the review and oversight of genetically-targeted advanced therapeutics (e.g., genetic therapies), especially for very low-prevalence patient populations;
- Adoption and support of master protocols, particularly basket trials, to support mutationally defined product approvals;
- Guidance development on cutting-edge topics to support drug research and development, such as the use of accelerated approval in tissue-agnostic drug development (i.e., drugs that target specific molecular alterations) and master protocols, among others.

REFERENCES

Allen, H. C., M. C. Garbe, J. Lees, N. Aziz, H. Chaaban, J. L. Miller, P. Johnson, and S. DeLeon. 2018. Off-label medication use in children, more common than we think: A systematic review of the literature. *Journal of the Oklahoma State Medical Association* 111(8):776-783.

Anatol, R. 2024. Regulatory flexibilities for cell and gene therapies for rare diseases: Processes to Evaluate the Safety and Efficacy of Drugs for Rare Diseases or Conditions in the United States and the European Union (Meeting 3 - Virtual).

Asbury, C. H. 1991. The Orphan Drug Act: The first 7 years. *JAMA* 265(7):893-897.

Benjamin, D. J., and M. P. Lythgoe. 2023. Modernising the US FDA's accelerated approval pathway. *Lancet Oncology* 24(3):203-205.

Bespoke Gene Therapy Consortium. 2024. *Regulatory playbook version 1.0.* https://fnih.org/wp-content/uploads/2024/04/BGTC-Regulatory-Playbook-Version-1.0.pdf (accessed August 1, 2024).

Biotechnology Innovation Organization. 2022. *FDA—sponsor engagement framework: Clinical outcomes assessments.* https://www.bio.org/sites/default/files/2023-06/BIO_FDA_Sponsor_Engagement_Framework_for_COA_Development.pdf (accessed August 15, 2024).

Brennan, Z. 2024. Accelerated approval will be 'the norm' for gene therapies, FDA's Peter Marks says. *Endpoints News.* https://endpts.com/accelerated-approval-will-be-the-norm-for-gene-therapies-fdas-peter-marks-says/ (accessed February 27, 2024).

Bugin, K. n.d. *What does FDA do during review? How do we use the patient voice during review?* U.S. Food and Drug Administration. https://www.fda.gov/media/176607/download (accessed August 1, 2024).

CIRS (Centre for Innovation in Regulatory Science). 2024. Data analysis and summary to help inform the National Academies committee on Processes to Evaluate the Safety and Efficacy of Drugs for Rare Diseases or Conditions in the United States and the European Union. Data analysis commissioned by the Committee on Processes to Evaluate the Safety and Efficacy of Drugs for Rare Diseases or Conditions in the United States and the European Union. National Academies of Sciences, Engineering, and Medicine, Washington, DC.

Collins, G., M. Stewart, B. McKelvey, H. Stires, and J. Allen. 2023. Breakthrough therapy designation criteria identify drugs that improve clinical outcomes for patients: A case for more streamlined coverage of promising therapies. *Clinical Cancer Research* 29(13):2371-2374.

Committee on Drugs, K. A. Neville, D. A. C. Frattarelli, J. L. Galinkin, T. P. Green, T. D. Johnson, MMM, I. M. Paul, and J. N. Van Den Anker. 2014. Off-label use of drugs in children. *Pediatrics* 133(3):563-567.

Committee on Oversight and Accountability: U.S. House of Representatives. 2024. *Testimony of Dr. Robert Califf.* https://oversight.house.gov/wp-content/uploads/2024/04/FDA-House-Oversight-and-Accountability-Testimony.pdf (accessed August 1, 2024).

Critical Path Institute. n.d. *Biomarker data repository.* https://c-path.org/program/biomarker-data-repository/ (accessed August 15, 2024).

CTTI (Clinical Trials Transformation Initiative). 2023. *Patient Engagement Collaborative.* https://ctti-clinicaltrials.org/wp-content/uploads/2023/05/PEC-Framework_Compliant-Apr-10-2023_FINAL.pdf (accessed March 10, 2024).

Donoghue, M. 2024. Rare Cancer Drug Development. *Processes to Evaluate the Safety and Efficacy of Drugs for Rare Diseases or Conditions in the United States and the European Union* (Meeting 3 - Virtual).

Eastern Research Group Inc. 2021. *Assessment of the use of patient experience data in regulatory decision-making.* https://www.fda.gov/media/150405/download?attachment (accessed August 1, 2024).

Eglovitch, J. 2024. *FDA eyes collaborative review pilot for gene therapies.* https://www.raps.org/news-and-articles/news-articles/2024/1/fda-eyes-collaborative-review-pilot-for-gene-thera (accessed January 12, 2024).

Epps, C., R. Bax, A. Croker, D. Green, A. Gropman, A. V. Klein, H. Landry, A. Pariser, M. Rosenman, M. Sakiyama, J. Sato, K. Sen, M. Stone, F. Takeuchi, and J. M. Davis. 2022. Global regulatory and public health initiatives to advance pediatric drug development for rare diseases. *Therapeutic Innovation & Regulatory Science* 56(6):964-975.

Fain, K. 2023. FDA approval standards for new drugs and biological products: Processes to Evaluate the Safety and Efficacy of Drugs for Rare Diseases or Conditions in the United States and the European Union (Meeting 1 - Virtual).

FDA (U.S. Food and Drug Administration). 1998. *Providing clinical evidence of effectiveness for human drug and biological product: Guidance for industry.* https://www.fda.gov/media/71655/download (accessed August 1, 2024).

FDA. 2005. *How to comply with the Pediatric Research Equity Act.* https://www.fda.gov/media/72274/download (accessed August 1, 2024).

FDA. 2008. Applications for approval to market a new drug; complete response letter; amendments to unapproved applications. *Federal Register* 73(133). https://www.govinfo.gov/content/pkg/FR-2008-07-10/pdf/E8-15608.pdf (accessed August 1, 2024).

FDA. 2013a. *FDA report: Ensuring access to adequate information on medical products for all - with a special focus on underrepresented subpopulations, including racial subgroups.* https://www.fda.gov/media/86023/download (accessed August 1, 2024).

FDA. 2013b. *The open public hearing at FDA advisory committee meetings: Guidance for the public, FDA advisory committee members, and FDA staff.* https://www.fda.gov/media/79874/download (accessed August 1, 2024).

FDA. 2014a. *CDER MAPP 6030.2 Rev. 1: INDs: Review of Informed Consent Documents.* https://www.fda.gov/media/72752/download (accessed August 1, 2024).

FDA. 2014b. *Expedited programs for serious conditions—drugs and biologics: Guidance for industry.* https://www.fda.gov/media/86377/download (accessed August 1, 2024).

FDA. 2016. *Advisory committees: Critical to the FDA's product review process.* https://www.fda.gov/drugs/information-consumers-and-patients-drugs/advisory-committees-critical-fdas-product-review-process (accessed July 11, 2024).

FDA. 2017a. *Best practices for communication between IND sponsors and FDA during drug development guidance for industry and review staff: Good review practice.* https://www.fda.gov/media/94850/download (accessed August 1, 2024).

FDA. 2017b. *Orphan Drug Modernization Plan.* https://www.fda.gov/industry/designating-orphan-product-drugs-and-biological-products/orphan-drug-modernization-plan (accessed March 19, 2024).

FDA. 2018a. *Clarification of orphan designation of drugs and biologics for pediatric subpopulations of common diseases: Guidance for industry.* https://www.fda.gov/media/109496/download (accessed March 19, 2024).

FDA. 2018b. *Fact sheet: Pediatric provisions in the Food and Drug Administration Safety and Innovation Act (FDASIA).* https://www.fda.gov/regulatory-information/food-and-drug-administration-safety-and-innovation-act-fdasia/fact-sheet-pediatric-provisions-food-and-drug-administration-safety-and-innovation-act-fdasia (accessed August 1, 2024).

FDA. 2018c. *Information sharing.* https://www.fda.gov/federal-state-local-tribal-and-territorial-officials/communications-outreach/information-sharing (accessed August 15, 2024).

FDA. 2019a. *Demonstrating substantial evidence of effectiveness for human drug and biological products: Guidance for industry.* https://www.fda.gov/media/133660/download (accessed August 1, 2024).

FDA. 2019b. *Expedited programs for regenerative medicine therapies for serious conditions: Guidance for industry.* https://www.fda.gov/media/120267/download (accessed August 1, 2024).

FDA. 2019c. *FDA takes first action under new international collaboration with Australia and Canada designed to provide a framework for concurrent review of cancer therapies, approving treatment for patients with endometrial carcinoma: News release.* https://www.fda.gov/news-events/press-announcements/fda-takes-first-action-under-new-international-collaboration-australia-and-canada-designed-provide (accessed August 1, 2024).

FDA. 2019d. *Rare pediatric disease priority review vouchers guidance for industry.* https://www.fda.gov/media/90014/download (accessed August 1, 2024).

FDA. 2020a. *Interacting with the FDA on complex innovative trial designs for drugs and biological products: Guidance for industry.* https://www.fda.gov/media/130897/download (accessed August 1, 2024).

FDA. 2020b. *Pediatric study plans: Content of and process for submitting initial pediatric study plans and amended initial pediatric study plans: Guidance for industry.* https://www.fda.gov/media/86340/download (accessed August 1, 2024).

FDA. 2022a. *Action package for posting* SOPP 8401.7. https://www.fda.gov/media/82426/download (accessed August 1, 2024).

FDA. 2022b. *Development & approval process | drugs.* https://www.fda.gov/drugs/development-approval-process-drugs (accessed June 12, 2024).

FDA. 2022c. *Enhancing benefit-risk assessment in regulatory decision-making.* https://www.fda.gov/industry/prescription-drug-user-fee-amendments/enhancing-benefit-risk-assessment-regulatory-decision-making (accessed August 15, 2024).

FDA. 2022d. *Ethical considerations for clinical investigations of medical products involving children.* https://www.fda.gov/media/161740/download (accessed August 1, 2024).

FDA. 2022e. *Externally-led patient-focused drug development meetings.* https://www.fda.gov/industry/prescription-drug-user-fee-amendments/externally-led-patient-focused-drug-development-meetings (accessed August 7, 2024).

FDA. 2022f. *General clinical pharmacology considerations for neonatal studies for drugs and biological products: Guidance for industry.* https://www.fda.gov/media/129532/download (accessed August 1, 2024).

FDA. 2022g. *General clinical pharmacology considerations for pediatric studies of drugs, including biological products.* https://www.fda.gov/media/90358/download (accessed August 1, 2024).

FDA. 2022h. *Project Orbis frequently asked questions.* https://www.fda.gov/about-fda/oncology-center-excellence/project-orbis-frequently-asked-questions (accessed August 1, 2024).

FDA. 2023a. *74th Cellular, Tissue, and Gene Therapies Advisory Committee (CTGTAC).* https://www.fda.gov/media/169105/download (accessed August 1, 2024).

FDA. 2023b. *Accelerating Rare disease Cures (ARC) Program: Year one anniversary update.* https://www.fda.gov/media/169429/download (accessed August 1, 2024).

FDA. 2023c. *Benefit-risk assessment for new drug and biological products: Guidance for industry.* https://www.fda.gov/media/152544/download (accessed August 1, 2024).

FDA. 2023d. *Complex Innovative Trial Design meeting program.* https://www.fda.gov/drugs/development-resources/complex-innovative-trial-design-meeting-program (accessed March 19, 2024).

FDA. 2023e. *Considerations for long-term clinical neurodevelopmental safety studies in neonatal product development.* https://www.fda.gov/media/165239/download (accessed August 1, 2024).

FDA. 2023f. *Demonstrating substantial evidence of effectiveness with one adequate and well-controlled clinical investigation and confirmatory evidence: Guidance for industry.* https://www.fda.gov/media/172166/download (accessed August 1, 2024).

FDA. 2023g. *FDA Rare Disease Day 2023: "Intersections with rare diseases—a patient focused event."* https://www.youtube.com/watch?v=ylk7eYTgUMM (accessed August 1, 2024).

FDA. 2023h. *Frequently asked questions (FAQ) about designating an orphan product.* https://www.fda.gov/industry/designating-orphan-product-drugs-and-biological-products/frequently-asked-questions-faq-about-designating-orphan-product (accessed March 19, 2024).

FDA. 2023i. *Pediatric drug development under the Pediatric Research Equity Act and the Best Pharmaceuticals for Children Act: Scientific considerations.* https://www.fda.gov/media/168202/download (accessed August 1, 2024).

FDA. 2023j. *Pediatric drug development: Regulatory considerations—Complying with the Pediatric Research Equity Act and qualifying for pediatric exclusivity under the Best Pharmaceuticals for Children Act.* https://www.fda.gov/media/168201/download (accessed August 1, 2024).

FDA. 2023k. *Rare Disease Endpoint Advancement pilot program frequently asked questions.* https://www.fda.gov/drugs/development-resources/rare-disease-endpoint-advancement-pilot-program-frequently-asked-questions (accessed August 15, 2024).

FDA. 2023l. *Rare diseases: Considerations for the development of drugs and biological products: Guidance for industry.* https://www.fda.gov/media/119757/download (accessed August 1, 2024).

FDA. 2023m. *Real-time oncology review (RTOR): Guidance for industry.* https://www.fda.gov/media/173641/download (accessed August 1, 2024).

FDA. 2023n. *Regenerative medicine advanced therapy designation.* https://www.fda.gov/vaccines-blood-biologics/cellular-gene-therapy-products/regenerative-medicine-advanced-therapy-designation (accessed July 19, 2024).

FDA. 2023o. *Support for clinical Trials Advancing Rare disease Therapeutics pilot program; program announcement.* https://www.federalregister.gov/documents/2023/10/02/2023-21235/support-for-clinical-trials-advancing-rare-disease-therapeutics-pilot-program-program-announcement (accessed August 1, 2024).

FDA. 2023p. *What we do.* https://www.fda.gov/about-fda/what-we-do (accessed July 19, 2024).

FDA. 2024a. *About FDA-TRACK.* https://www.fda.gov/about-fda/fda-track-agency-wide-program-performance/about-fda-track (accessed August 15, 2024).

FDA. 2024b. *About the FDA patient representative program.* https://www.fda.gov/patients/learn-about-fda-patient-engagement/about-fda-patient-representative-program (accessed March 10, 2024).

FDA. 2024c. *Accelerating Rare disease Cures (ARC) program.* https://www.fda.gov/about-fda/center-drug-evaluation-and-research-cder/accelerating-rare-disease-cures-arc-program (accessed February 20, 2024).

FDA. 2024d. *CDER patient-focused drug development.* https://www.fda.gov/drugs/development-approval-process-drugs/cder-patient-focused-drug-development (accessed March 05, 2024).

FDA. 2024e. *Condition-specific meeting reports and other information related to patients' experience.* https://www.fda.gov/industry/prescription-drug-user-fee-amendments/condition-specific-meeting-reports-and-other-information-related-patients-experience (accessed August 15, 2024).

FDA. 2024f. *FDA-led Patient-Focused Drug Development (PFDD) public meetings.* https://www.fda.gov/industry/prescription-drug-user-fee-amendments/fda-led-patient-focused-drug-development-pfdd-public-meetings (accessed August 7, 2024).

FDA. 2024g. *FDA briefing document: Pediatric oncology subcommittee of the Oncologic Drugs Advisory Committee (ODAC).* https://www.fda.gov/media/178681/download (accessed August 1, 2024).

FDA. 2024h. *FDA patient listening sessions.* https://www.fda.gov/patients/learn-about-fda-patient-engagement/fda-patient-listening-sessions (accessed August 7, 2024).

FDA. 2024i. *FDA Rare Disease Innovation Hub to enhance and advance outcomes for patients.* https://www.fda.gov/news-events/fda-voices/fda-rare-disease-innovation-hub-enhance-and-advance-outcomes-patients (accessed August 15, 2024).

FDA. 2024j. *LEADER 3D: Learning and Education to Advance and Empower Rare Disease Drug Developers: Public report of external stakeholder analysis.* https://www.fda.gov/media/176557/download?attachment= (accessed August 15, 2024).

FDA. 2024k. *Network of experts program: Connecting the FDA with external expertise.* https://www.fda.gov/about-fda/center-devices-and-radiological-health/network-experts-program-connecting-fda-external-expertise (accessed August 15, 2024).

FDA. 2024l. *Oncology Center of Excellence.* https://www.fda.gov/about-fda/fda-organization/oncology-center-excellence (accessed May 29, 2024).

FDA. 2024m. *Pediatric labeling changes.* https://www.fda.gov/science-research/pediatrics/pediatric-labeling-changes (accessed August 8, 2024).

FDA. 2024n. *Pediatric Research Equity Act.* https://www.fda.gov/drugs/development-resources/pediatric-research-equity-act-prea (accessed August 1, 2024).

FDA. 2024o. *Prescription Drug User Fee Amendments.* https://www.fda.gov/industry/fda-user-fee-programs/prescription-drug-user-fee-amendments (accessed June 25, 2024).

FDA. 2024p. *Rare Disease Endpoint Advancement pilot program.* https://www.fda.gov/drugs/development-resources/rare-disease-endpoint-advancement-pilot-program (accessed August 6, 2024).

FDA. 2024q. *Rare pediatric disease designation and priority review voucher programs.* https://www.fda.gov/industry/medical-products-rare-diseases-and-conditions/rare-pediatric-disease-designation-and-priority-review-voucher-programs (accessed August 15, 2024).

FDA. n.d.-a. *Best Pharmaceuticals for Children Act and Pediatric Research Equity Act - Status Report to Congress: July 1, 2015—June 30, 2020.* https://www.fda.gov/media/157840/download (accessed August 1, 2024).

FDA. n.d.-b. *Collecting patient experience data: How you can best help FDA?* https://www.fda.gov/media/112163/download (accessed August 1, 2024).

Fermaglich, L. J., and K. L. Miller. 2023. A comprehensive study of the rare diseases and conditions targeted by orphan drug designations and approvals over the forty years of the Orphan Drug Act. *Orphanet Journal of Rare Diseases* 18(1):163.

Fox, T. A., and C. Booth. 2024. Improving access to gene therapy for rare diseases. *Disease Models & Mechanisms* 17(6).

Freilich, E. R. 2024. Rare disease drug development: Processes to Evaluate the Safety and Efficacy of Drugs for Rare Diseases or Conditions in the United States and the European Union (Meeting 3 - Virtual).

Fung, A., X. Yue, P. R. Wigle, and J. J. Guo. 2021. Off-label medication use in rare pediatric diseases in the United States. *Intractable & Rare Diseases Research* 10(4):238-245.

GAO (U.S. Government Accountabilty Office). 2020. *FDA's priority review voucher programs.* https://www.gao.gov/assets/gao-20-251.pdf (accessed August 1, 2024).

GAO. 2023. *Pediatric cancer studies: Early results of the Research to Accelerate Cures and Equity for Children Act.* https://www.gao.gov/products/gao-23-105947 (accessed August 1, 2024).

Gao, Y. G., S. Roberts, and A. Guy. 2022. Maximizing regulatory review efficiency: The evolution of the FDA OCE RTOR pilot. *Therapeutic Innovation & Regulatory Science* Oct 9: 56(2):212-219.

Hunter, N. L., K. M. O'Callaghan, and R. M. Califf. 2015. Engaging patients across the spectrum of medical product development: View from the US Food and Drug Administration. *JAMA* 314(23):2499-2500.

Hwang, T. J., F. T. Bourgeois, J. M. Franklin, and A. S. Kesselheim. 2019. Impact of the priority review voucher program on drug development for rare pediatric diseases. *Health Affairs* 38(2):313-319.

ICH (International Council for Harmonsation of Technical Requirements for Pharmaceuticals for Human Use). 2022. *Pediatric extrapolation - E11A.* https://www.fda.gov/media/161190/download (accessed August 1, 2024).

IOM (Institute of Medicine). 2008. *Addressing the barriers to pediatric drug development: Workshop summary.* Edited by C. Vanchieri, A. S. Butler and A. Knutsen. Washington, DC: The National Academies Press.

Kesselheim, A. S., and J. J. Darrow. 2015. FDA designations for therapeutics and their impact on drug development and regulatory review outcomes. *Clinical Pharmacology & Therapeutics* 97(1):29-36.

Kieffer, C. M., A. R. Miller, B. Chacko, and A. S. Robertson. 2019. FDA reported use of patient experience data in 2018 drug approvals. *Therapeutic Innovation & Regulatory Science*:2168479019871519.

Kim, T. 2022. *Oncology Center for Excellence (OCE) regulatory programs.* https://www.fda.gov/media/165674/download (accessed August 1, 2024).

Kimmel, L., R. M. Conti, A. Volerman, and K. P. Chua. 2020. Pediatric orphan drug indications: 2010-2018. *Pediatrics* 145(4).

Kuehn, C. M. 2018. Patient experience data in US Food and Drug Administration (FDA) regulatory decision making: A policy process perspective. *Therapeutic Innovation & Regulatory Science* 52(5):661-668.

Lee, K. J., R. Bent, and J. Vaillancourt. 2023. Selected FDA programs on rare disease: Processes to Evaluate the Safety and Efficacy of Drugs for Rare Diseases or Conditions in the United States and the European Union (Meeting 1 - Virtual).

Lu, C.-F., and C. K. Abbott. 2024. *FDA takes first step toward international regulation of gene therapies to treat rare diseases.* https://natlawreview.com/article/fda-takes-first-step-toward-international-regulation-gene-therapies-treat-rare#google_vignette (accessed July 19, 2024).

Mease, C., K. L. Miller, L. J. Fermaglich, J. Best, G. Liu, and E. Torjusen. 2024. Analysis of the first ten years of FDA's rare pediatric disease priority review voucher program: Designations, diseases, and drug development. *Orphanet Journal of Rare Diseases* 19(1):86.

Michaeli, T., H. Jürges, and D. T. Michaeli. 2023. FDA approval, clinical trial evidence, efficacy, epidemiology, and price for non-orphan and ultra-rare, rare, and common orphan cancer drug indications: Cross sectional analysis. *BMJ* 381:e073242.

Miller, K. L., and M. Lanthier. 2016. Trends in orphan new molecular entities, 1983-2014: Half were first in class, and rare cancers were the most frequent target. *Health Affairs (Millwood)* 35(3):464-470.

Monge, A. N., D. W. Sigelman, R. J. Temple, and H. S. Chahal. 2022. Use of US Food and Drug Administration expedited drug development and review programs by orphan and nonorphan novel drugs approved from 2008 to 2021. *JAMA Network Open* 5(11):e2239336.

Murray, L. T., T. A. Howell, L. S. Matza, S. Eremenco, H. R. Adams, D. Trundell, S. J. Coons, and Rare Disease Subcommittee of the Patient-Reported Outcome Consortium. 2023. Approaches to the assessment of clinical benefit of treatments for conditions that have heterogeneous symptoms and impacts: Potential applications in rare disease. *Value Health* 26(4):547-553.

NASEM (National Academies of Sciences, Engineering and Medicine). 2024. *Living with ALS*. Edited by A. I. Leshner, R. A. English and J. Alper. Washington, DC: The National Academies Press.

NICHD (Eunice Kennedy Shriver National Institute of Child Health and Human Development). n.d. *About BPCA*. https://www.nichd.nih.gov/research/supported/bpca/about#:~:text=The%20latest%20renewal%20of%20the,6%20months%20of%20patent%20 exclusivity (accessed August 1, 2024).

NORD (National Organization for Rare Disorders). 2024. *Impact of the rare pediatric disease priority review voucher program on drug development 2012 - 2024*. https://rarediseases.org/wp-content/uploads/2024/07/NORD-Pediatric-PRV-Report.pdf (accessed August 1, 2024).

OIG (U.S. Office of Inspector General). 2022. *Delays in confirmatory trials for drug applications granted FDA's accelerated approval raise concerns*. https://oig.hhs.gov/oei/reports/OEI-01-21-00401.pdf (accessed August 1, 2024).

PhRMA (Pharmaceutical Research and Manufacturers of America). 2020. *PREA and BPCA: Spurring pediatric drug development*. https://phrma.org/-/media/Project/PhRMA/PhRMA-Org/PhRMA-Org/PDF/P-R/PREA-and-BPCA-Doc-2022_2.pdf (accessed August 6, 2024).

Poddar, A., M. Raggio, and J. Concato. 2024. Decisions on non-oncology breakthrough therapy designation requests in 2017-2019. *Therapeutic Innovation & Regulatory Science* 58(1):214-221.

Price, D., and J. Scott. 2021. The U.S. Food and Drug Administration's complex innovative trial design pilot meeting program: Progress to date. *Clinical Trials* 18(6):706-710.

Raggio, M. 2023. FDA expedited programs: Processes to Evaluate the Safety and Efficacy of Drugs for Rare Diseases or Conditions in the United States and the European Union (Meeting 1 - Virtual).

Redberg, R. F. 2015. Faster drug approvals are not always better and can be worse. *JAMA Internal Medicine* 175(8):1398.

Sachs, A. N., D. Avant, C. S. Lee, W. Rodriguez, and M. D. Murphy. 2012. Pediatric information in drug product labeling. *JAMA* 307(18):1914-1915.

Sasinowski, F. J. 2011. *Quantum of effectiveness evidence in FDA's approval of orphan drugs*. https://cdn.rarediseases.org/wordpresscontent/wp-content/uploads/2014/12/NORD-study-of-FDA-approval-of-orphan-drugs.pdf (accessed August 1, 2024).

Sasinowski, F. J., E. B. Panico, and J. E. Valentine. 2015. Quantum of effectiveness evidence in FDA's approval of orphan drugs: Update, July 2010 to June 2014. *Therapeutic Innovation & Regulatory Science* 49(5):680-697.

Sharfstein, J. M., J. D. Miller, A. L. Davis, J. S. Ross, M. E. McCarthy, B. Smith, A. Chaudhry, G. C. Alexander, and A. S. Kesselheim. 2017. Blueprint for transparency at the US Food and Drug Administration: Recommendations to advance the development of safe and effective medical products. *The Journal of Law, Medicine & Ethics* 45(2_suppl):7-23.

Shea, M., L. Ostermann, R. Hohman, S. Roberts, M. Kozak, R. Dull, J. Allen, and E. Sigal. 2016. Impact of breakthrough therapy designation on cancer drug development. *Nature Reviews Drug Discovery* 15(3):152.

Temkin, E., and J. Trinh. 2021. *FDA's accelerated approval pathway: A rare disease perspective—history and opportunities for reform.* https://rarediseases.org/wp-content/uploads/2022/10/NRD-2182-Policy-Report_Accelerated-Approval_FNL.pdf (accessed August 1, 2024).

The Alliance for a Stronger FDA. 2024. *Alliance webinar series: Webinar transcript with Nicole Verdun, head of the new CBER Office of Therapeutic Products.* https://acrobat.adobe.com/id/urn:aaid:sc:va6c2:8a91f106-2820-47a4-b90b-eef42686d6ff?viewer%21megaVerb=group-discover (accessed August 1, 2024).

Treatment Action Group and Elizabeth Glaser Pediatric AIDS (acquired immunodeficiency syndrome) Foundation. 2019. *Ensuring treatment for children with orphan diseases: Ending exemptions from the Pediatric Research Equity Act (PREA).* https://www.treatmentactiongroup.org/wp-content/uploads/2019/08/prea_brief_2019_final.pdf (accessed August 1, 2024).

Valentine, J. E., and F. J. Sasinowski. 2020. Orphan drugs and rare diseases. In *Principles and Practice of Clinical Trials*, edited by S. Piantadosi and C. L. Meinert. Cham: Springer International Publishing. Pp. 1-19.

Wright, C. F., D. R. FitzPatrick, and H. V. Firth. 2018. Paediatric genomics: Diagnosing rare disease in children. *Nature Reviews Genetics* 19(5).

3

EMA Flexibilities, Authorities, and Mechanisms

> *[The European Medicines Agency]... facilitates research into new medicines and encourages development, thereby translating progress in medical science into medicines with real health benefits for patients. In particular, it promotes the development of medicines for children and drugs to tackle rare diseases.*
>
> European Medicines Agency (n.d.-o)

The European Medicines Agency (EMA) is a decentralized agency of the European Union (EU) that is responsible for evaluating the safety and efficacy of human and veterinary drugs in Europe. As stated on its public website, the agency also serves to protect and promote human health (EMA, n.d.-o). Unlike the U.S. Food and Drug Administration (FDA), EMA does not have the authority to approve medications. Instead, the agency issues guidance and makes authorization recommendations on medical products that the European Commission ultimately approves for marketing in the European Union (EMA, n.d.-o). Day-to-day operations at EMA are carried out by staff who rely on a network of experts from across Europe and collaboration with national competent authorities of EU member states to pool resources and coordinate work to regulate medicines for use in humans (EMA, n.d.-ad) (collectively called the EU medicines regulatory network, which is a World Health Organization–listed authority like FDA).

EMA has regulatory policies in place to support and incentivize drug development for rare diseases and conditions, including an orphan designation program, mechanisms for expedited review, and opportunities for sponsors and people with lived rare disease experience to engage with the agency. These programs may be used separately or in combination; each has its own eligibility criteria and benefits. This chapter examines the regulatory processes, authorities, and mechanisms used by the agency to approve drug products that are relevant to rare diseases. Where available, data are provided on the potential impact of these activities. The chapter is divided into sections on the drug review and approval, standards of evidence, orphan medicine designation, expedited regulatory programs, stakeholder engagement, rare disease programs, and transparency.

DRUG REVIEW AND APPROVAL

In the EU, EMA is responsible for assessing the benefits and risks of medicines. The 27 member states of the EU each have their own regulatory authority for licensing drugs, but EMA provides a centralized procedure that allows a sponsor to apply to one authority, undergo one scientific evaluation, and receive one marketing authorization (EMA, n.d.-s). Once the Committee for Medicinal Products for Human Use (CHMP), which is convened by EMA and made up of experts selected from the 27 member states, issues a positive opinion on a marketing authorization application, the European Commission (EC) makes a final legally binding decision on whether a medicine can be marketed in the EU. This authorization is legally binding and valid in all 27 member states, as well as the other states of the European Economic Area (Iceland, Norway, and Liechtenstein) (EMA, n.d.-e, n.d.-s).

This centralized procedure through EMA is mandatory for certain categories of products, including orphan medicines, advanced therapies (e.g., tissue-engineered medicines, cell- and gene-therapy), medicines derived from biotechnology processes, and medicines with new active substances to treat human immunodeficiency virus (HIV), cancer, diabetes, neurodegenerative diseases, auto-immune and other immune dysfunctions, and viral diseases (EMA, n.d.-e).[1]

The CHMP is responsible for assessing drug marketing authorization applications and making recommendations regarding those applications to the European Commission (EMA, n.d.-k). The CHMP works with other EMA committees, including the "Committee for Advanced Therapies, which leads the assessment of advanced therapy medicines (gene therapy, tissue engineering and cell-based medicines); the Pharmacovigilance and Risk Assessment Committee for aspects related to the medicine's safety and

---

[1] For more information on the scope of EMA centralised procedure, see https://www.ema.europa.eu/en/about-us/what-we-do/authorisation-medicines (accessed June 13, 2024).

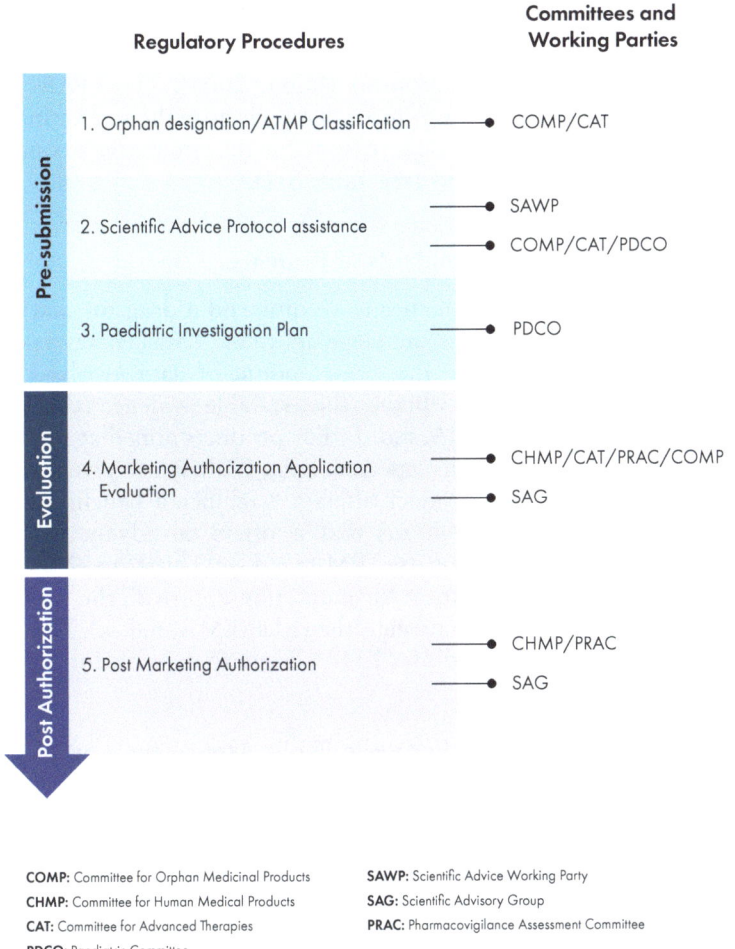

FIGURE 3-1 EMA committees in human medicines regulatory process.
SOURCE: Adapted from European Medicines Agency: Presentation—Centralised procedure at the European Medicines Agency, https://www.ema.europa.eu/system/files/documents/presentation/wc500201043_en.pdf (accessed March 15, 2024).

risk management; the Paediatric Committee (PDCO) for aspects related to the medicine's use in children; and the Committee for Orphan Medicinal Products (COMP) for orphan-designated medicines" (EMA, n.d.-r). During an assessment of a marketing authorization application, the CHMP is supported by a team of assessors from membership state agencies with relevant expertise (e.g., pharmaceutical, clinical, statistical), and the EMA secretariat provides technical, scientific, and administrative support (EMA, n.d.-r). See Figure 3-1 for an illustrative overview of the EMA process and the committees involved in each stage.

The EMA secretariate is required to publish a European public assessment report (EPAR) for all medicines that have been granted or refused marketing authorization[2] (European Union, 2004). The EPAR includes information about the drug product, including how the marketing authorization submission was assessed, reasons for the committee's conclusions, and a public-friendly overview (see Table 3-1).

Standards of Evidence

EMA's decision about whether to recommend a drug for marketing is based on whether its benefits outweigh its risks. This benefit–risk assessment can be complex due to the large amount of data involved and the inherent uncertainty around whether the available evidence is sufficient to assess benefits and risks (EMA, n.d.-f). For products aimed at rare disease, there are two types of "benefit" assessed. First, COMP may give the product orphan designation if the product offers a "significant benefit" compared with other treatments; this means that it offers an advantage in terms of efficacy, safety, or mode of use (EMA, n.d.-u; Thirstrup, 2023). Next, CHMP evaluates the application for marketing approval; the product can be approved if the benefits outweigh the risks (EMA, n.d.-k). The benefit–risk assessment framework allows EMA review to account for factors like

TABLE 3-1 Components of European Public Assessment Reports

Section	Type of information
Overview	Public-friendly overview in question-and-answer format.
Authorisation details	Key details about the product and the marketing authorisation holder.
Product information	Package leaflet and summary of product characteristics; labelling; list of all authorised presentations; pharmacotherapeutic group; therapeutic indications.
Assessment history	Public assessment report for the initial authorisation; public assessment report(s) for any variation concerning major changes to the marketing authorisation; orphan maintenance assessment report or withdrawal assessment report (as of 17 January 2018); tabulated overview of procedural steps taken before and after authorisation.

SOURCE: European Medicines Agency: European public assessment reports: background and context, https://www.ema.europa.eu/en/medicines/what-we-publish-medicines-and-when/european-public-assessment-reports-background-and-context (accessed March 15, 2024).

---

[2] Regulation (EC) No. 726/2004. Available at https://eur-lex.europa.eu/LexUriServ/LexUriServ.do?uri=OJ:L:2004:136:0001:0033:en:PDF (accessed July 5, 2024).

small patient populations and limited data within the context of the specific rare disease.

EMA has not issued guidance on drug development for rare diseases and conditions. However, EMA has issued several disease-specific guidelines, many of which concern rare diseases, and held a workshop in 2015 on the demonstration of significant benefit of orphan medicines (EMA, 2016). In addition, there are EMA guidelines and reflection papers on a number of topics that are relevant to the collection of data on rare disease drug development. The details of these guidelines are discussed further in Chapter 4. Table 3-2 includes some guidelines:

Inclusion of Pediatric Populations

In EMA, the paediatric investigation plan (PIP) serves to ensure that all needed data to support a marketing authorization for children are collected. PIPs are required to be submitted when the Phase 2 dose is selected at the end of Phase 1 (Ungstrup and Vanags, 2023). All medicines seeking marketing authorization have to include a PIP unless the treatment is exempt due to referral or waiver (EMA, n.d.-h). Typically, waivers are provided to treatments that are likely to be ineffective or unsafe in children, intended for adult-only conditions, or unlikely to provide significant benefit over current treatment available to children (EMA, n.d.-h). The PIP is reviewed and agreed upon by the drug sponsor and EMA's PDCO (EMA, n.d.-v). In early 2023, EMA launched a stepwise PIP pilot program which is designed to allow greater flexibility for sponsors that are developing innovative treatments. The stepwise PIP will allow sponsors to continue with development with a partial PIP in place rather than waiting for more data to support a full PIP (Al-Faruque, 2023). In qualitative interviews, sponsors indicated that the PIP can be restrictive to drug development and expect the stepwise program to ease some of the issues (see Appendix E for full methodology and results).

TABLE 3-2 EMA Guidelines on Collection of Data

Guideline	Source
Reflection Paper on Use of Real-World Data in Non-Interventional Studies to Generate Real-World Evidence	EMA (2024)
Guideline on Registry-Based Studies	EMA (2021)
Reflection Paper on Establishing Efficacy Based on Single-Arm Trials Submitted as Pivotal Evidence in a Marketing Authorisation	EMA (2023a)
Points To Consider On Application With 1. Meta-Analyses; 2. One Pivotal Study	EMA (2001)
Guideline on Clinical Trials in Small Populations	EMA (2006)

NOTE: EMA = European Medicines Agency.

ORPHAN MEDICINE DESIGNATION

In 1999, the European Parliament adopted Regulation (EC) 141/2000, which established the COMP, laid out the process for the designation of orphan medicines, and identified the incentives available to designated products. An "orphan medicine" is defined as one that is intended to treat a life-threatening or chronically debilitating condition for which there is no satisfactory method of diagnosis or treatment available, and which affects not more than 5 in 10,000 people in the European Union community. Alternatively, if it is intended to treat a condition that affects more than 5 in 10,000 people, it can still be eligible for orphan designation if the market is unlikely to generate sufficient return on the investment without incentives (European Commission, n.d.).

To receive orphan designation, a drug usually must be targeted at a disease or condition for which there is no treatment available; if a treatment is available, a drug may still be eligible if it provides "significant benefit" to those affected by the condition. Significant benefit is defined as either a "clinically relevant advantage" or "a major contribution to patient care." A clinically relevant advantage means that compared with previously approved treatments, the product offers either improved efficacy or improved safety and there is a reasonable probability that the patient will actually experience this benefit[3] (Thirstrup, 2023). A product that represents a "major contribution to patient care" is one with improved availability or ease of use. For example, a product that does not require refrigeration would be an improvement over one that does require refrigeration, or a product that can be taken by pill would be an improvement over one that requires an injection. As noted in a presentation to the committee, the determination of "major contribution to patient care" can be more difficult than the determination of a "clinically relevant advantage" because it depends in part on what patients consider to be important (Thirstrup, 2023). A "significant benefit" cannot be claimed based on an "alternative mode of action *per se*, an increase in supply or availability due to a shortage of existing products, or higher pharmaceutical quality" (Thirstrup, 2023).

The condition at which an orphan drug is targeted must be clearly distinct from other conditions; differences in severity or stages do not make a condition distinct from others. "Condition" is defined under EC Guideline (ENTR/6283/00) as "any deviation(s) from the normal structure or function of the body, as manifested by a characteristic set of signs and symptoms (typically a recognized distinct disease or a syndrome)" (European Commission, 2014b). If the targeted condition is a subtype of a more common condition, there must be justification for restricting the medicine

---

[3] Regulation (EC) No. 847/2000.

to the subgroup of patients. The patients must have "distinct and unique evaluable characteristics," and such characteristics must be essential for the action of the medicine such that the medicine would not be effective in the larger group of patients with the common condition (European Commission, 2014a). According to Steffan Thirstrup, chief medical officer of EMA, in open session with the committee, differences in biomarkers are currently not accepted as evidence of a distinct condition (Thirstrup, 2023). The determination of whether a condition is considered distinct enough to qualify for orphan designation may change over time as the understanding of disease progresses and new therapies are developed (Thirstrup, 2023).

Process

Orphan medicine designation is a separate process from marketing authorization, with the orphan designation coming before marketing authorization. Sponsors submit a request for orphan medicine designation to the COMP, which examines applications for orphan designation from EMA (EMA, n.d.-d). During the 90-day evaluation process, the COMP reviews the application to assess whether the drug product meets the criteria for orphan medicine designation. The COMP examines whether the condition is life-threatening or chronically debilitating, determines the prevalence of the condition, assesses the medical plausibility that the product will treat the condition, and compares the proposed treatment with existing treatments, if any (EMA, n.d.-u). Typically, products are designated as orphan early in the drug development process, although designation may happen as late as the marketing authorization application (see Figure 3-2). The COMP will adopt a positive opinion or provide a list of questions and invite the sponsor to provide an oral explanation at the next COMP meeting (EMA, n.d.-d). There is an appeals process if the COMP opinion is negative. Following a COMP positive opinion, EMA sends the opinion to the European Commission, which is responsible for issuing a decision within 30 days of receipt (EMA, n.d.-d).

Once a product is designated as orphan, it undergoes the same quality, safety, and efficacy assessment as any other medical product. The CHMP is responsible for assessing the product for authorization, while the COMP is responsible for determining whether an orphan product can maintain its orphan designation (EMA, n.d.-k, n.d.-r). A product could lose its orphan designation if, for example, another product received marketing authorization first and the second product cannot demonstrate a significant benefit over the already-authorized product (EMA, n.d.-c; Thirstrup, 2023).

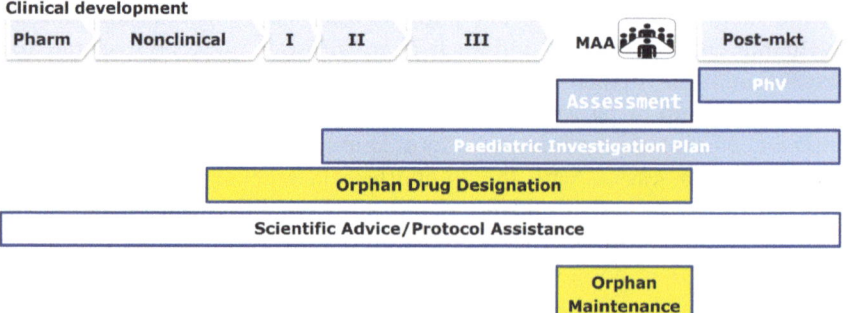

FIGURE 3-2 Orphan product designation and maintenance along drug life cycle.
NOTES: I = Phase 1 clinical trials; II = Phase 2 clinical trials; III = Phase 3 clinical trials; MAA = marketing authorization application; Pharm = pharmacology studies; PhV = pharmacovigilance; Post-mkt = post-marketing authorization.
SOURCE: Presented to the Committee by Steffan Thirstrup, on December 4, 2023.

Benefits

Products that receive orphan designation can access a number of incentives (EMA, n.d.-t). First, sponsors can request protocol assistance from EMA at a reduced fee; this allows sponsors to get answers to questions about what types of studies are necessary to demonstrate the quality, benefits, risks, and significant benefit of the drug. Second, a product with orphan designation is mandated to use the centralized marketing approval process conducted by EMA. Third, products maintaining orphan designation at the time of approval receive 10 years of market exclusivity; this is extended to 12 years for products with an approved pediatric investigation plan. Fourth, sponsors applying for orphan designation pay reduced fees for regulatory activities, including marketing authorization application fees, fees for inspections before authorization, and fees for applications for post-approval changes. In addition, sponsors may be eligible for incentives available through individual EU member states. For companies classified as small and medium-sized enterprises (SMEs) that are developing a product with orphan designation, there may also be administrative and procedural assistance from EMA's SME office and fee reduction (EMA, n.d.-t).

Approvals of Drugs with Orphan Designation

In the 20 years that EMA has issued orphan designation, over 2,730 products have received orphan designation, and over 230 of these have been

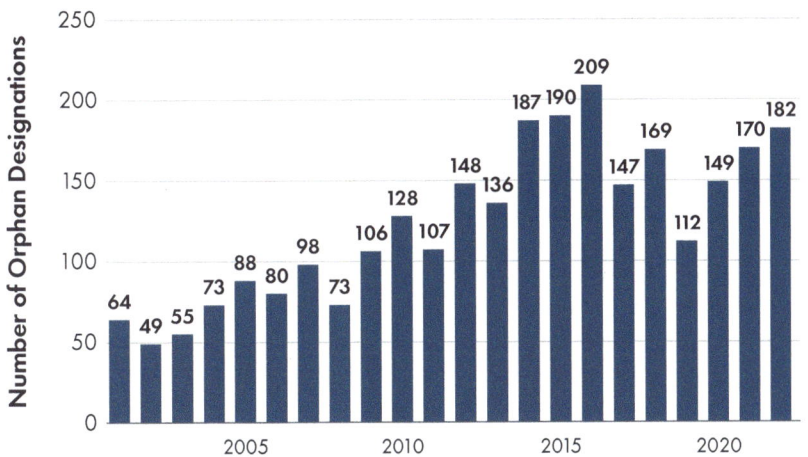

Number of orphan medicines recommended for authorization (2001–2022)

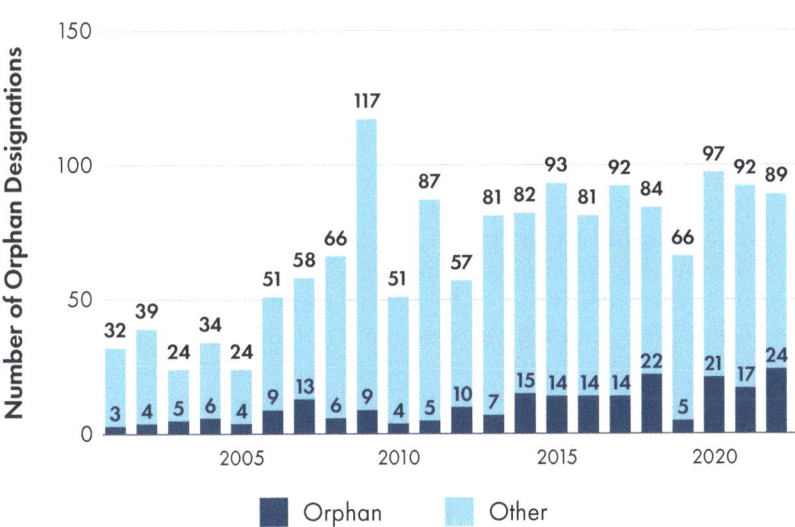

FIGURE 3-3 Designation and authorization of orphan medicines in the EU from 2001 to 2022.
NOTE: EU = European Union.
SOURCES: Presented to the Committee by Steffan Thirstrup, *EMA*, on December 4, 2023; adapted from European Medicines Agency: Orphan medicines in the EU, https://www.ema.europa.eu/en/documents/leaflet/infographic-orphan-medicines-eu_en.pdf (accessed March 15, 2024).

recommended for marketing authorization (see Figure 3-3). As of 2023, 142 orphan designations are still active (Thirstrup, 2023). Of the active orphan designations, 98 received full authorization, 26 are under conditional authorization pending confirmatory data, and 18 were approved under "exceptional circumstances" in which the applicant is unlikely to be able to generate more data (Thirstrup, 2023). The largest number of orphan product designations are for congenital, familial, and genetic disorders, with significant numbers of products for blood and lymphatic systems disorders as well as neoplasms (Thirstrup, 2023). Orphan designations are published on the EMA website, along with minutes and agendas of the scientific committee meetings. Reports are published for both the initial assessment of orphan designation, and the assessment of orphan maintenance (Thirstrup, 2023).

As described in Chapter 2, the committee examined the approval rates for orphan and non-orphan medicine applications between 2015 and 2020 (see Appendix D for full methodology). Overall, there was little difference in EMA approval rates for orphan and non-orphan medicine applications (see Figure 3-4) and no discernable differences in approval rates across therapeutic areas (see Figure 3-5).

EXPEDITED REGULATORY PROGRAMS

There are four expedited authorization pathways for drugs available through EMA. Each program has its own eligibility criteria, process, and benefits. While these pathways are available for any medicine that meets the criteria, they may be particularly relevant for products with orphan designation because orphan products are more likely to meet the criteria of the programs (e.g., meeting an unmet need, intended to treat a life-threatening disease, extremely rare indication). Expedited pathway programs and orphan medicine designation may be used separately or in combination; medicines targeted at rare, serious diseases—particularly those that have no existing treatment—may be eligible for multiple programs.

Priority Medicines

The Priority Medicines (PRIME) program is targeted at medicines with an unmet need—that is, where no treatment option exists or where a new therapy can offer a major benefit over existing therapies. Applicants must provide data that demonstrate a meaningful improvement of clinical outcomes (e.g., affecting morbidity or mortality of a disease) (EMA, n.d.-y).

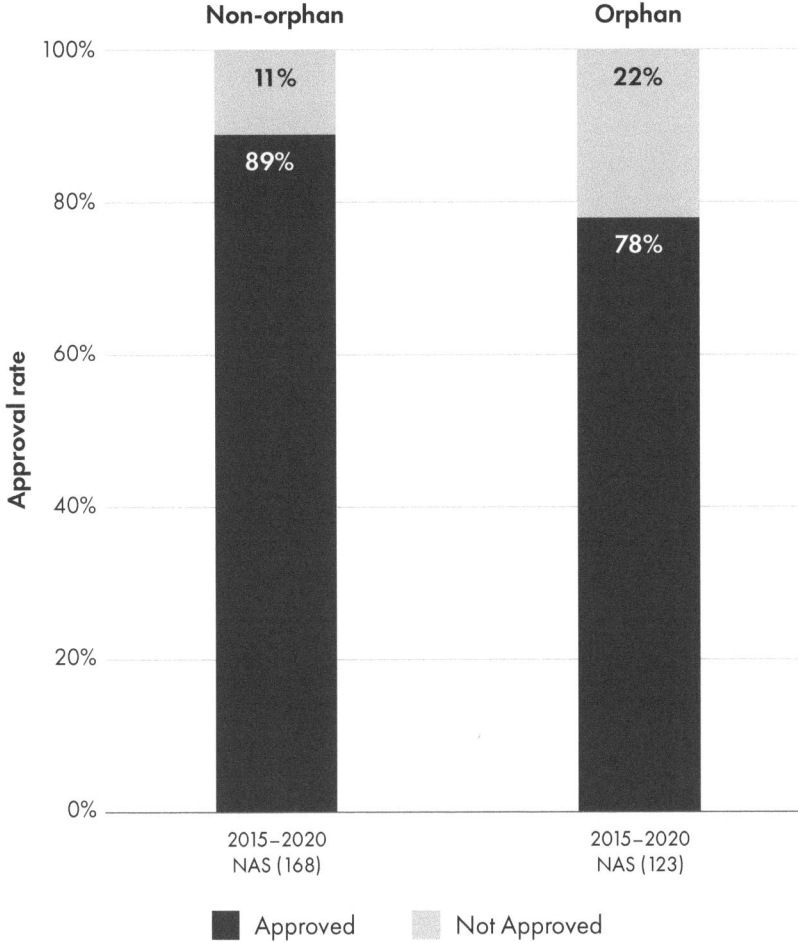

FIGURE 3-4 EMA approval rates for orphan and non-orphan drugs using expedited approval pathways from 2015 to 2020.
NOTES: EMA = European Medicines Agency; NAS = new active substance.
SOURCE: CIRS Data Analysis, 2024.

Process

Sponsors must apply for PRIME during the early stages of clinical research. It is designed to help sponsors who have preliminary clinical evidence that demonstrates promising potential of the medicine to significantly address an unmet need. Applicants from small businesses and academia, who may have less experience in the regulatory world, can apply for early entry PRIME if they have compelling nonclinical data in a relevant model

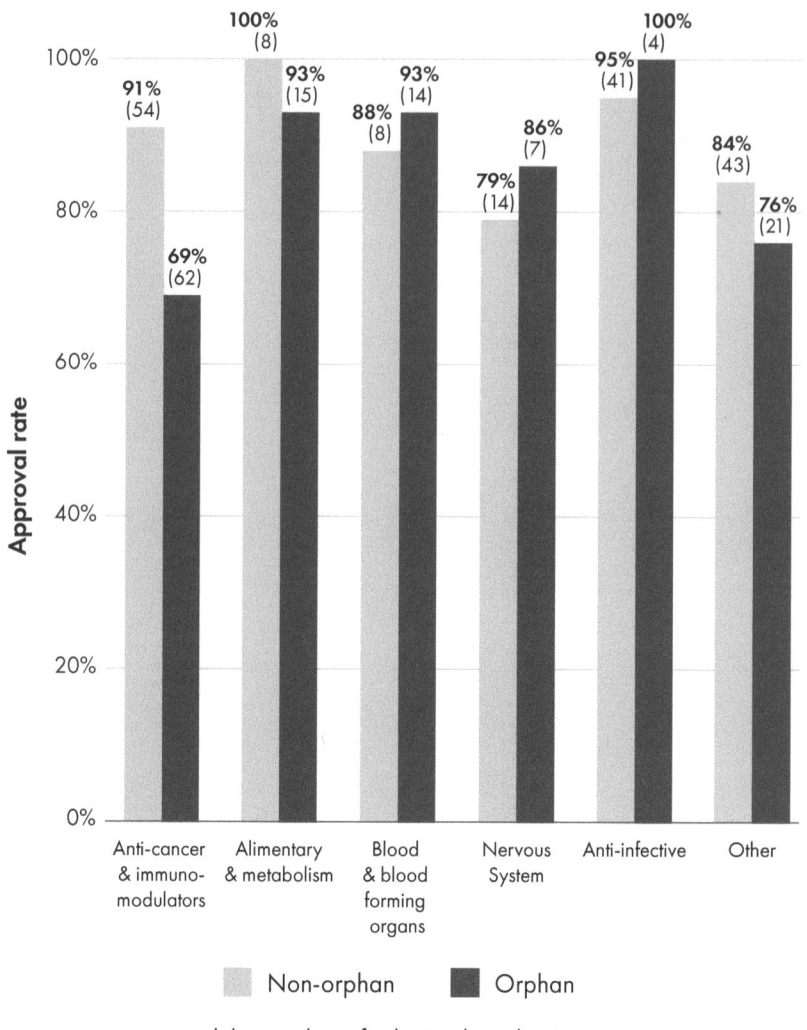

FIGURE 3-5 Approval rates for non-orphan and orphan NAS applications submitted to EMA from 2015 to 2020 per therapeutic area.
NOTES: EMA = European Medicines Agency; NAS = new active substance; Other = other therapeutic areas not described in the top 5 therapeutic indications list.
SOURCE: CIRS Data Analysis, 2024.

that shows proof of principle or if first-in-human studies demonstrate the desired effects and safety (EMA, n.d.-y).

Benefits

Applicants selected for the PRIME program receive a number of benefits throughout the regulatory process, including:

- Early appointment of a committee rapporteur
- Meeting with rapporteur and group of experts from EMA
- Appointment of PRIME scientific coordinator
- Iterative scientific advice on development and key issues
- Expedited follow-up scientific advice
- Submission readiness meeting
- Confirmation of potential for accelerated assessment (EMA, n.d.-y)

Applicants who are granted early entry PRIME status receive additional benefits, including an EMA product team, an introductory meeting about regulatory requirements, and total fee exemption for scientific advice for applicants from the European Economic Area (EMA, n.d.-y).

Impact

An EMA analysis of the PRIME program found that since its inception in 2016, PRIME has resulted in reduced overall time to marketing authorization, with PRIME products more likely to be granted accelerated assessment (EMA, 2022c). The analysis found that the benefits of PRIME were most pronounced for more complex products or applications that depend on smaller datasets, such as orphan diseases. EMA analysis found that 56 percent of PRIME products granted eligibility were orphan products (EMA, 2022c).

Accelerated Assessment

Medical products that are expected to be of "major public health interest," particularly with respect to therapeutic innovation, may be approved for accelerated assessment, which reduces the timeframe for assessment and approval. There is no specific definition of "major public health interest;" each application is reviewed on a case-by-case basis. In general, a product eligible for accelerated assessment is one that involves new methods of therapy or improves on existing methods in order to address unmet needs (EMA, n.d.-a).

Process

Applicants must apply for accelerated assessment at least 2 or 3 months before submitting the application for marketing authorization. EMA recommends that applicants request a pre-submission meeting several months before requesting accelerated assessment in order to discuss their proposal and plan. Applicants who have already received PRIME status may receive confirmation during the clinical development phase that their product is eligible for accelerated assessment (EMA, n.d.-a).

Benefits

Assessment of a marketing authorization application typically takes 210 days (excluding "clock stops" for requests of additional information). Under accelerated assessment, this timeframe is reduced to 150 days (EMA, n.d.-a).

Impact

A study of orphan medicinal product (OMP) approvals in the EU between 2010 and 2022 found that about 24 percent of OMPs were eligible for accelerated assessment, and that use of accelerated assessment for OMPs increased significantly around 2015 (see Figure 3-6). The study found that the use of accelerated assessment is more frequent in OMPs than in non-orphan medicinal products (Bouwman et al., 2024).

Conditional Marketing Authorization

The conditional marketing authorization program is available for products for which the available clinical data are less comprehensive than usual but for which the benefits of providing the public access to the medicine immediately outweigh the risks inherent in approving a product with fewer clinical data. Medicines that are eligible for conditional marketing authorization are those that are intended to treat, prevent, or diagnose seriously debilitating or life-threatening diseases (including orphan medicines), or those that are needed for a public health emergency (e.g., a pandemic) (EMA, n.d.-l). Specifically, products must meet all of the following criteria:

- "the benefit-risk balance of the medicine is positive;
- "it is likely that the applicant will be able to provide comprehensive data post-authorization;
- "the medicine fulfills an unmet medical need;

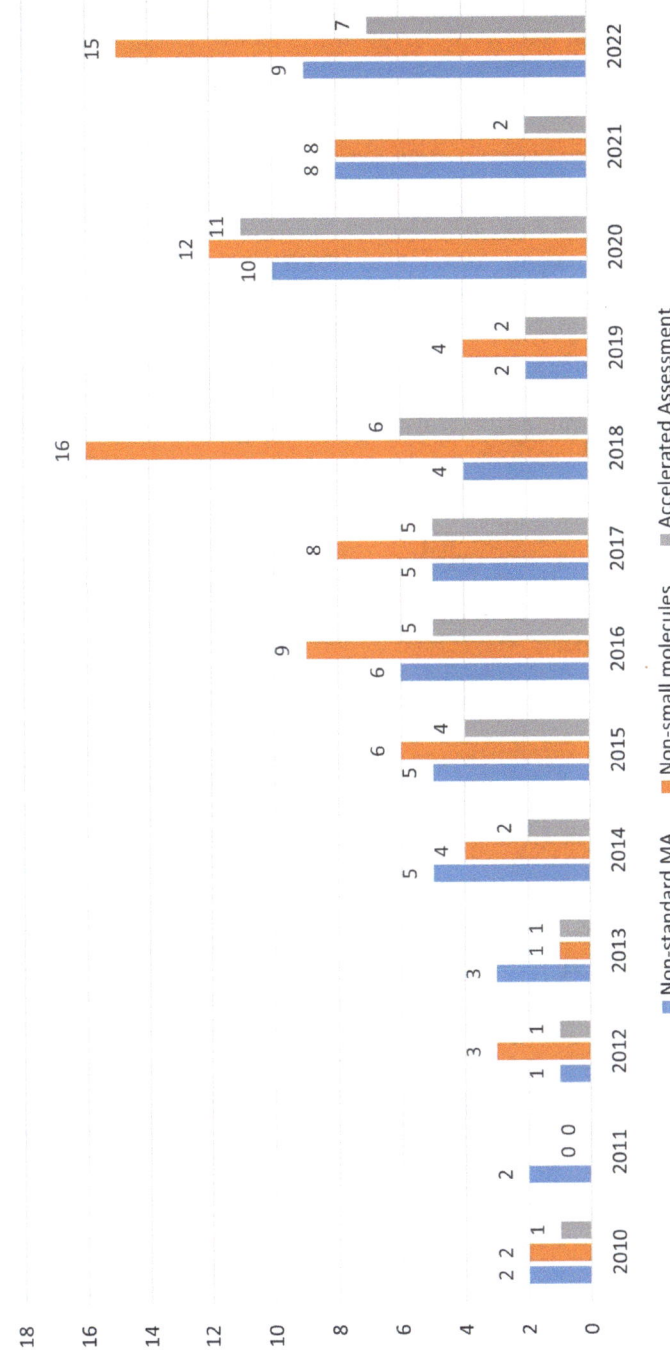

FIGURE 3-6 Evolution of the number of orphan medicinal products that have received a non-standard marketing authorization, are non-small molecules, and have benefited from accelerated assessment.
NOTE: MA = marketing authorization.
SOURCE: Bouwman et al., 2024. CC BY 4.0 https://creativecommons.org/licenses/by/4.0/.

- "the benefit of the medicine's immediate availability to patients is greater than the risk inherent in the fact that additional data are still required" (EMA, n.d.-l).

Process

The request for conditional marketing authorization should be submitted along with the notification of intention to submit a marketing authorization application, about 6 to 7 months before the application. The formal request for conditional marketing authorization is submitted with the marketing authorization application, and the CHMP assesses the request and application together (EMA, n.d.-l). EMA encourages applicants to request a pre-submission meeting in order to discuss plans. If a conditional marketing authorization is granted, the sponsor is required to fulfill specific obligations within a defined time (e.g., collecting additional data). If further data indicate that the benefits do not outweigh the risks or if the sponsor fails to comply with its obligations, conditional authorization may be suspended or revoked. Conditional authorization can be converted to standard marketing authorization once obligations are fulfilled and more complete data confirm that the benefits outweigh the risks (EMA, n.d.-l).

Benefits

If a product is granted a conditional marketing authorization, the review timelines could be accelerated if there is sufficient evidence to meet a positive benefit-risk ratio.

Impact

Between 2010 and 2022 of the 192 OMPs that received marketing authorization, 41 (21 percent) were approved via the conditional approval pathway. Over this time period, there has been an increase in the use of conditional approvals, and OMPs have been approved via the conditional pathway more often than non-orphan medicines. Between 2010 and 2022, 6 of the 192 approved OMPs lost authorization; of these 6, 4 were conditional approvals (Bouwman et al., 2024).

Exceptional Circumstances

A marketing authorization applicant that is unable to provide comprehensive data on safety and efficacy may be eligible for authorization under the exceptional circumstances provision[4] if one of the following is true:

- the indication for which the product is intended is so rare that the applicant cannot reasonably be expected to provide comprehensive data;
- it is not possible to gather comprehensive information due to the present state of scientific knowledge; or
- generally accepted principles of medical ethics preclude the collection of comprehensive data (Prilla, 2018).

Process

An applicant must submit a request for authorization under exceptional circumstances along with the notification of intention to submit a marketing authorization application. In the formal marketing authorization application, the applicant must provide justification for the inability to collect comprehensive data, a listing of the data that cannot be provided, and proposals for the specific procedures and obligations that will be conducted (e.g., conditions on prescribing the product). Unlike a conditional marketing authorization, the applicant is not required or expected to provide comprehensive data after authorization, and the authorization typically cannot be converted to a full authorization. Authorization is reviewed annually to assess the risk-benefit balance (EMA, n.d.-x).

Benefits

A product that is granted authorization under exceptional circumstances receives authorization with fewer data than are normally required, and the applicant is not expected to provide comprehensive data post-authorization (EMA, n.d.-x).

Impact

Exceptional circumstances is the least common type of approval for orphan products: of the 192 OMPs authorized for marketing between 2010 and 2022, 22 (11.5 percent) were approved under exceptional

---

[4] For more information, see https://www.ema.europa.eu/en/glossary/exceptional-circumstances (accessed July 9, 2024).

circumstances (Bouwman et al., 2024). However, orphan products make up the vast majority of approvals under exceptional circumstances; of the products licensed under exceptional circumstances in 2020, 82 percent were designated as orphan products at the time of approval (Marjenberg et al., 2020). Over two-thirds of OMPs approved under exceptional circumstances were biologicals or advanced therapeutic medicinal products (Bouwman et al., 2024).

STAKEHOLDER ENGAGEMENT

Sponsor Engagement

Sponsors will begin to formally work with EMA when submitting for marketing authorization. However, developers are encouraged to reach out to EMA for advice and feedback at any stage of the development of a medical product. The exchange of information between developers and EMA helps to ensure that studies are designed appropriately to generate evidence about safety and efficacy and that no major issues arise during the assessment for marketing authorization. Preparatory meetings are offered early in the process by EMA so that applicants can introduce their proposed plan and receive feedback, identify issues that they may need scientific advice on, ask regulatory questions that are outside the scope of scientific advice, and establish contact with agency staff; these meetings are free-of-charge (EMA, n.d.-z). Applicants shall use EMA's IRIS platform[5] to make requests for scientific advice, share information, and deliver documents. EMA charges a fee for scientific advice; this fee varies by the scope of the advice and fee waivers are available for orphan medicines, SMEs, and products for a public health emergency (EMA, n.d.-z). Individuals from small companies who participated in semi-structured interviews reported some issues with engaging EMA due to the decentralized process (see Appendix E for full methodology and results). They cited difficulties in working with individual countries rather than EMA directly.

Expert Engagement

EMA relies on external experts for a number of tasks. They may serve on committees or steering groups, may provide scientific expertise, or may perform compliance inspections on behalf of EMA. These experts are made available by the national competent authorities of the European Economic Area and must sign a declaration of interests each year. The list of experts

---

[5] For more information, see https://iris.ema.europa.eu/ (accessed July 9, 2024).

is publicly available (EMA, n.d.-n). EMA launched a pilot program in 2020 in which experts are paid by their home institutions but hosted by EMA. The goal of the Collaborating Expert Programme is to provide a mechanism for EMA and external researchers to collaborate on important research questions that address regulatory decision-making (EMA, n.d.-j). Because the Collaborating Expert Programme is still in a pilot phase, the committee cannot comment on its usefulness for rare disease drug development.

Patient Engagement

Organizations, patients, and caregivers interact with EMA in a variety of ways all along the regulatory pathway (EMA, n.d.-q) (see Figure 3-7), a practice that is underpinned by EMA's broader engagement framework for engaging patients and consumers throughout a medical products lifecycle (EMA, 2022a). Depending on the activity, patients may interact as representatives of their community, as representatives of an organization, or as individual experts. Specific opportunities for engagement include serving on EMA's management board,[6] scientific committees, and initiatives, such as the Accelerating Clinical Trials in the EU initiative (EMA, n.d.-b), which aims to further develop innovative clinical research in the European Union; attending consultations and workshops, assisting with providing advice on science and protocols, and involvement in the Patients' and Consumers' Working Party (PCWP) (EMA, n.d.-q). The PCWP was established in 2006 to provide a platform for the exchange of information and discussion of issues between EMA and patients. The group consists of representatives from patient and consumer organizations, representatives of EMA scientific committees, and observers. Organizations currently represented include the European Organisation for Rare Diseases, the Thalassemia International Federation, and the World Duchenne Organization among others (EMA, n.d.-w).

Organizations and individuals can apply to work with EMA if they meet certain requirements. Among other criteria, organizations must be registered in the EU, have a clear mission and objectives, be representative of patients or consumers throughout the EU, and be transparent. Individual patients may also register to have an opportunity to use their real-life experiences to inform EMA's work. EMA maintains a database[7] of patients and

---

[6] EMA's Management Board sets the agency's budget and approves its yearly work plans. For more information, see https://www.ema.europa.eu/en/about-us/who-we-are/management-board (accessed March 18, 2024).

[7] For more information, see https://fmapps.ema.europa.eu/stakeholders/signup.php (accessed March 15, 2024).

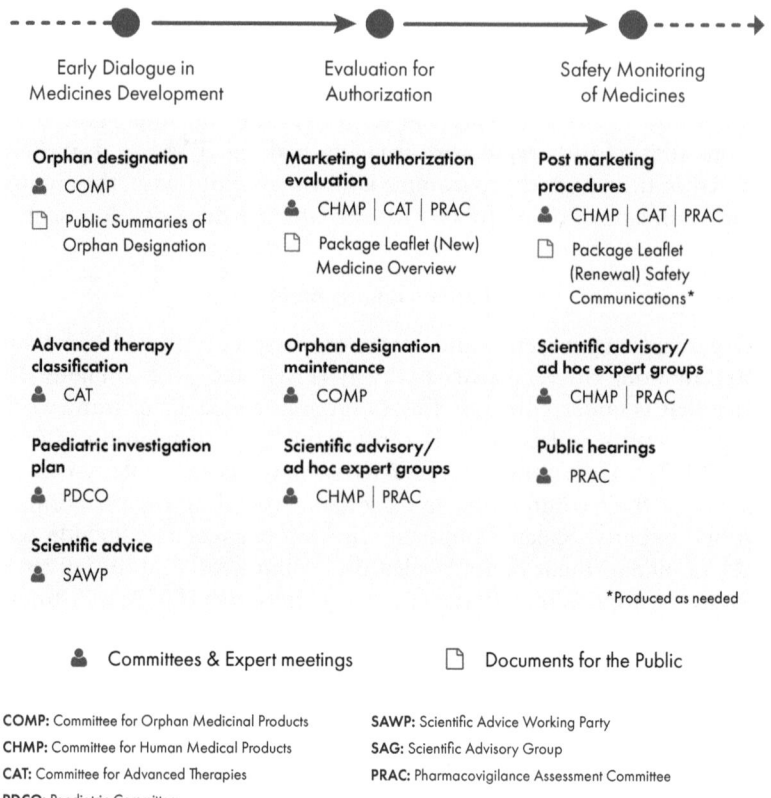

FIGURE 3-7 Patient involvement along the medicines lifecycle at EMA.
SOURCE: Adapted from European Medicines Agency: Getting involved, https://www.ema.europa.eu/en/partners-networks/patients-and-consumers/getting-involved (accessed March 15, 2024).

calls upon them to provide their expertise in various EMA groups and in reviewing EMA documents prepared for the public (EMA, 2022a).

From January 2021 to May 2022, EMA ran a pilot program that explored how patients and organizations could be involved in the early stages of evaluation for orphan product applications. The pilot program included 37 products and involved identifying applications with orphan status; contacting organizations and inviting them to share information about aspects likely to be useful for evaluation (e.g., quality of life, unmet needs); and sharing this information with rapporteurs and product leads. Rapporteurs and product leads assessed whether the information provided added value, whether it was useful for assessing the application, and whether it should be included in the assessment report. An EMA assessment of the pilot program found that patient input highlighted new and valuable information and contributed to interim assessment reports in the marketing authorization process. This pilot program is being expanded to include health care professionals (EMA, 2022b).

RARE DISEASE INITIATIVES

EMA does not currently have programs specific to rare disease drug development. However, one of EMA's stated goals is to encourage and facilitate the use of innovative methods in the development of medicines (EMA, n.d.-ac). To this end, EMA has several initiatives that support the development of innovative methods by fostering collaboration with academia and across the regulatory network. In addition to PRIME (described above), two of these initiatives are particularly relevant to rare diseases: the Innovation Task Force (ITF) and the EU Innovation Network (EU-IN).

Innovation Task Force

ITF[8] is a multidisciplinary group with the task of ensuring coordination across EMA and providing a forum for early dialogue with applicants about innovative aspects of research and development (EMA, n.d.-aa). ITF plays a number of roles, including:

- Establishing early dialogue with applicants, in particular smaller or less-experienced applicants, in order to identify scientific, legal, and regulatory issues that may arise with emerging technologies, and to identify the need for specialized expertise during the development process;
- Exploring the regulatory and scientific implications of emerging therapies and technologies, in particular with respect to EMA's scientific, legal, and regulatory requirements;
- Working with committees and other bodies to provide advice relating to research and development, for example, when there are uncertainties about whether a product fits the definition of a medicinal product;
- Increasing awareness of emerging therapies and technologies at EMA (EMA, 2014).

---

[8] For more information, see https://www.ema.europa.eu/en/human-regulatory-overview/research-and-development/innovation-medicines (accessed July 9, 2024).

ITF holds briefing meetings with developers of innovative medicines, technologies, and methods. These meetings allow for an informal exchange of information in order to ensure that developers are well-informed about the regulatory process and requirements, and that EMA is prepared to assess emerging developments in innovative medicine. ITF is also responsible for overseeing the regulatory acceptance of "new approach methodologies" that are aimed at replacing animals in research (EMA, n.d.-aa).

EU Innovation Network

EU-IN[9] is a group created in 2015 in order to strengthen the collaboration between EMA and regulatory authorities in EU member states, specifically with respect to emerging therapies and associated technologies. The group's aim is to improve regulatory support at both the national and European levels, in order to make investing in innovative medicines more appealing. EU-IN provides training and regulatory support to developers, facilitates collaboration with the European medicines regulatory network, and works to anticipate how emerging therapies may require additional regulatory support. The group identifies emerging trends in science and technology that are relevant to research and development and publishes reports that explore these topics from a regulatory perspective. EU-IN collaborates with the heads of medicines agencies on a pilot project that supports the repurposing of medicines. The goal of this project is to help academics and nonprofit organizations gather or generate evidence on an established medicine for a new indication, with the aim of obtaining marketing authorization for the new indication (EMA, n.d.-m).

TRANSPARENCY

Under EU law and its own regulations, transparency is an important feature of EMA's operations. EMA is required by law[10] to publish an EPAR for each medicine that it approves or denies a marketing authorization. The EPAR is made up of several documents including a "public friendly" overview; information about the marketing authorization holder; details about the product, labeling, and indications; and the history of EMA's assessment (e.g., orphan designation assessment, procedural steps taken) (EMA, n.d.-p). The EPAR also includes information on uncertainties about benefits and risks of the product (EMA, 2009). The EPAR is published after

---

[9] For more information, see https://www.hma.eu/about-hma/working-groups/eu-innovation-network-eu-in.html (accessed July 7, 2024).
[10] Reference (EC) No. 726/2004.

the EC issues a decision on an application as well as whenever product information is updated. Prior to the EC decision and EPAR publication, the relevant EMA committee (CHMP or the Committee for Veterinary Medicinal Products) publishes a "summary of opinion" following their adoption of the scientific opinion. Both the summary of opinion and the EPAR are available on the EMA website, and some components are published in multiple languages (EMA, n.d.-p).

A CHMP report in 2007 made recommendations about how CHMP could improve its methodology and could increase the transparency, consistency, and communication of its benefit–risk assessment (EMA, 2007). In 2009, EMA partnered with experts in decision theory on a 3-year project aimed at identifying decision-making models that could be used to make the agency's work more consistent, transparent, and easier to audit (EMA, n.d.-f). In a 2012 commissioned report, EMA made a recommendation that the agency employ a two-level approach: first, a qualitative analysis using PrOACT-URL (problem formulation, objectives, alternatives, consequences, trade-offs, uncertainties, risk attitude, and linked decisions) along with an MCDA (multiple criteria decision analysis) model for quantitative assessment of more complex situations (EMA, 2012).

Starting in 2016, EMA has published clinical data submitted by sponsors to support marketing applications for human medicines (EMA, n.d.-i). EU law (Article 81 of No 536/2014) mandates that EMA make clinical trial data publicly available while also protecting personal data and commercially confidential information. In accordance with this law, EMA launched the Clinical Trial Information System (CTIS) in January 2022. At the time of the CTIS launch, transparency rules allowed sponsors to apply redactions or defer the publication of certain documents for a certain period of time depending on the type of clinical trial (EMA, 2015; Zhuleku and Preinfalk, 2023). EMA has revised its regulations on clinical data publication through the adoption of EMA/263067/2023 in October 2023. Major changes to the rules include *(See EMA (2023b) for a detailed description)*:

- Selected data will be published using structured data fields that include information on study design, inclusion and exclusion criteria, primary and secondary endpoints, details on the product, and authorization status. These fields were chosen based on relevance for the public and researchers and cannot be redacted.
- The deferral mechanism is removed entirely for every trial category. Timing of document and data publication depends on a number of factors.
- The number of documents published will be rationalized in order to reduce complexity and workload.

In addition to the EPAR and clinical trial data, EMA makes other information available to improve transparency, including dates, agendas, minutes, and outcomes of its scientific committee meetings; information about staff and experts' conflicts of interest; information about manufacturing inspections; pediatric investigation plans; and orphan designations (EMA, n.d.-ab).

Transparency, on the part of regulators, can be an important component in building trust in regulatory processes. At the same time, transparency must be balanced with the protection of personal and commercially confidential information. The introduction of clinical trial publications by EMA was accompanied by public debate (before and around 2016) about potential downsides of transparency, including the risks of damaging industry competitiveness, false health scares (due to publication of safety data that could be misinterpreted), and compromised patient privacy (Bonini et al., 2014; O'Donnell, 2016). As far as can be ascertained by the committee, none of these risks have materialized. Information provided by EMA may help inform drug developers about the successes and failures of past programs and studies, but it is not possible to quantify the benefits for the drug development ecosystem.

REFERENCES

Al-Faruque, F. 2023. *EMA launches stepwise 'PIP' pilot*. https://www.raps.org/news-and-articles/news-articles/2023/2/ema-launches-stepwise-pip-pilot (accessed March 12, 2024).

Bonini, S., H.-G. Eichler, N. Wathion, and G. Rasi. 2014. Transparency and the European Medicines Agency — Sharing of clinical trial data. *New England Journal of Medicine* 371(26):2452-2455.

Bouwman, L., B. Sepodes, H. Leufkens, and C. Torre. 2024. Trends in orphan medicinal products approvals in the European Union between 2010–2022. *Orphanet Journal of Rare Diseases* 19(1):91.

CIRS (Centre for Innovation in Regulatory Science). 2024. Data analysis and summary to help inform the National Academies committee on Processes to Evaluate the Safety and Efficacy of Drugs for Rare Diseases or Conditions in the United States and the European Union. Data analysis commissioned by the Committee on Processes to Evaluate the Safety and Efficacy of Drugs for Rare Diseases or Conditions in the United States and the European Union. National Academies of Sciences, Engineering, and Medicine, Washington, DC.

EMA (European Medicines Agency). 2001. *Points to consider on application with 1. Meta-analyses; 2. One pivotal study*. https://www.ema.europa.eu/en/documents/scientific-guideline/points-consider-application-1meta-analyses-2one-pivotal-study_en.pdf (accessed August 1, 2024).

EMA. 2006. *Guideline on clinical trials in small populations*. https://www.ema.europa.eu/en/documents/scientific-guideline/guideline-clinical-trials-small-populations_en.pdf (accessed August 1, 2024).

EMA. 2007. *Report of the CHMP working group on benefit-risk assessment models and methods.* https://www.ema.europa.eu/en/documents/regulatory-procedural-guideline/report-chmp-working-group-benefit-risk-assessment-models-and-methods_en.pdf (accessed August 1, 2024).

EMA. 2009. *EPAR summaries for the public: A further step for the provision of better information about medicines.* https://www.ema.europa.eu/en/news/epar-summaries-public-further-step-provision-better-information-about-medicines (accessed July 11, 2024).

EMA. 2012. *Benefit-risk methodology project: Work package 4 report: Benefit-risk tools and processes.* https://eprints.lse.ac.uk/64630/1/Wok%20package%204.pdf (accessed August 1, 2024).

EMA. 2014. *Mandate of the EMA Innovation Task Force (ITF).* https://www.ema.europa.eu/en/documents/other/mandate-european-medicines-agency-innovation-task-force-itf_en.pdf (accessed August 1, 2024).

EMA. 2015. *Appendix, on disclosure rules, to the "functional specifications for the EU portal and EU database to be audited - EMA/42176/2014".* https://www.ema.europa.eu/en/documents/other/appendix-disclosure-rules-functional-specifications-eu-portal-and-eu-database-be-audited_en.pdf (accessed August 1, 2024).

EMA. 2016. *Demonstrating significant benefit of orphan medicines: Concepts, methodology and impact on access: Workshop report.* https://www.ema.europa.eu/en/documents/report/workshop-report-demonstrating-significant-benefit-orphan-medicines-concepts-methodology-and-impact-access_en.pdf (accessed August 1, 2024).

EMA. 2021. *Guideline on registry-based studies.* https://www.ema.europa.eu/en/documents/scientific-guideline/guideline-registry-based-studies_en.pdf-0 (accessed August 1, 2024).

EMA. 2022a. *Engagement framework: EMA and patients, consumers and their organizations.* https://www.ema.europa.eu/system/files/documents/other/updated_engagement_framework_-_ema_and_patients_consumers_and_their_organisations_2022-en.pdf (accessed August 1, 2024).

EMA. 2022b. *Pilot on early dialogue with patient organisations for orphan marketing authorisation applications: Outcome Report.* https://www.ema.europa.eu/en/documents/report/pilot-early-dialogue-patient-organisations-orphan-marketing-authorisation-applications-outcome-report_en.pdf (accessed August 1, 2024).

EMA. 2022c. *PRIME: Analysis of the first 5 years' experience.* https://www.ema.europa.eu/system/files/documents/report/2022-03_prime_5_years_report_updated_2022-04-05-en.pdf (accessed August 1, 2024).

EMA. 2023a. *Reflection paper on establishing efficacy based on single arm trials submitted as pivotal evidence in a marketing authorisation.* https://www.ema.europa.eu/en/documents/scientific-guideline/reflection-paper-establishing-efficacy-based-single-arm-trials-submitted-pivotal-evidence-marketing-authorisation_en.pdf (accessed August 1, 2024).

EMA. 2023b. *Revised CTIS transparency rules.* https://www.ema.europa.eu/en/documents/other/revised-ctis-transparency-rules_en.pdf (accessed August 1, 2024).

EMA. 2024. *Reflection paper on use of real-world data in non-interventional studies to generate real-world evidence.* https://www.ema.europa.eu/en/documents/scientific-guideline/reflection-paper-use-real-world-data-non-interventional-studies-generate-real-world-evidence_en.pdf (accessed August 1, 2024).

EMA. n.d.-a. *Accelerated assessment.* https://www.ema.europa.eu/en/human-regulatory-overview/marketing-authorisation/accelerated-assessment (accessed August 15, 2024).

EMA. n.d.-b. *Accelerating Clinical Trials in the EU (ACT EU).* https://www.ema.europa.eu/en/human-regulatory-overview/research-development/clinical-trials-human-medicines/accelerating-clinical-trials-eu-act-eu (accessed August 1, 2024).

EMA. n.d.-c. *Applying for marketing authorisation: Orphan medicines.* https://www.ema.europa.eu/en/human-regulatory-overview/marketing-authorisation/orphan-designation-marketing-authorisation/applying-marketing-authorisation-orphan-medicines (accessed July 10, 2024).

EMA. n.d.-d. *Applying for orphan designation.* https://www.ema.europa.eu/en/human-regulatory-overview/research-development/orphan-designation-research-development/applying-orphan-designation (accessed February 20, 2024).
EMA. n.d.-e. *Authorisation of medicines.* https://www.ema.europa.eu/en/about-us/what-we-do/authorisation-medicines (accessed March 18, 2024).
EMA. n.d.-f. *Benefit-risk methodology.* https://www.ema.europa.eu/en/about-us/what-we-do/regulatory-science-research/benefit-risk-methodology (accessed March 19, 2024).
EMA. n.d.-g. *The centralised procedure at the EMA.* https://www.ema.europa.eu/system/files/documents/presentation/wc500201043_en.pdf (accessed August 1, 2024).
EMA. n.d.-h. *Class waiviers.* https://www.ema.europa.eu/en/human-regulatory-overview/research-and-development/paediatric-medicines-research-and-development/paediatric-investigation-plans/class-waivers (accessed August 15, 2024).
EMA. n.d.-i. *Clinical data publication.* https://www.ema.europa.eu/en/human-regulatory-overview/marketing-authorisation/clinical-data-publication (accessed July 10, 2024).
EMA. n.d.-j. *Collaborating experts.* https://careers.ema.europa.eu/content/Collaborating-Expert/?locale=en_GB (accessed August 15, 2024).
EMA. n.d.-k. *Committee for Medicinal Products for Human Use (CHMP).* https://www.ema.europa.eu/en/committees/committee-medicinal-products-human-use-chmp (accessed August 15, 2024).
EMA. n.d.-l. *Conditional marketing authorization.* https://www.ema.europa.eu/en/human-regulatory-overview/marketing-authorisation/conditional-marketing-authorisation (accessed February 20, 2024).
EMA. n.d.-m. *EU Innovation Network (EU-IN).* https://www.ema.europa.eu/en/committees/working-parties-other-groups/eu-innovation-network-eu (accessed July 10, 2024).
EMA. n.d.-n. *European experts.* https://www.ema.europa.eu/en/about-us/how-we-work/european-medicines-regulatory-network/european-experts (accessed March 15, 2024).
EMA. n.d.-o. *European Medicines Agency (EMA).* https://european-union.europa.eu/institutions-law-budget/institutions-and-bodies/search-all-eu-institutions-and-bodies/european-medicines-agency-ema_en#:~:text=The%20European%20Medicines%20Agency%20(EMA,European%20Economic%20Area%20(EEA (accessed August 15, 2024).
EMA. n.d.-p. *European public assessment reports: Background and context.* https://www.ema.europa.eu/en/medicines/what-we-publish-medicines-and-when/european-public-assessment-reports-background-and-context (accessed March 15, 2024).
EMA. n.d.-q. *Getting involved.* https://www.ema.europa.eu/en/partners-networks/patients-and-consumers/getting-involved (accessed March 15, 2024).
EMA. n.d.-r. *How EMA evaluates medicines for human use.* https://www.ema.europa.eu/en/about-us/what-we-do/authorisation-medicines/how-ema-evaluates-medicines-human-use (accessed August 15, 2024).
EMA. n.d.-s. *Obtaining an EU marketing authorisation, step-by-step.* https://www.ema.europa.eu/en/human-regulatory-overview/marketing-authorisation/obtaining-eu-marketing-authorisation-step-step (accessed August 15, 2024).
EMA. n.d.-t. *Oprhan incentives.* https://www.ema.europa.eu/en/human-regulatory-overview/research-and-development/orphan-designation-research-and-development/orphan-incentives (accessed February 19, 2024).
EMA. n.d.-u. *Orphan designation: Overview.* https://www.ema.europa.eu/en/human-regulatory-overview/orphan-designation-overview (accessed June 25, 2024).
EMA. n.d.-v. *Paediatric investigation plans.* https://www.ema.europa.eu/en/human-regulatory-overview/research-development/paediatric-medicines-research-development/paediatric-investigation-plans (accessed August 15, 2024).

EMA. n.d.-w. *Patients' and Consumers' Working Party.* https://www.ema.europa.eu/en/committees/working-parties-other-groups/comp-working-parties-other-groups/patients-consumers-working-party (accessed August 6, 2024).

EMA. n.d.-x. *Pre-authorization guidance.* https://www.ema.europa.eu/en/human-regulatory-overview/marketing-authorisation/pre-authorisation-guidance (accessed February 10, 2024).

EMA. n.d.-y. *PRIME: Priority Medicines.* https://www.ema.europa.eu/en/human-regulatory-overview/research-development/prime-priority-medicines (accessed August 15, 2024).

EMA. n.d.-z. *Scientific advice and protocol assistance.* https://www.ema.europa.eu/en/human-regulatory-overview/research-development/scientific-advice-protocol-assistance (accessed March 10, 2024).

EMA. n.d.-aa. *Supporting innovation.* https://www.ema.europa.eu/en/human-regulatory-overview/research-development/supporting-innovation (accessed July 10, 2024).

EMA. n.d.-ab. *Transparency.* https://www.ema.europa.eu/en/about-us/how-we-work/transparency (accessed March 5, 2024).

EMA. n.d.-ac. *What we do.* https://www.ema.europa.eu/en/about-us/what-we-do (accessed July 10, 2024).

EMA. n.d.-ad. *Who we are.* https://www.ema.europa.eu/en/about-us/who-we-are (accessed July 9, 2024).

European Commission. 2014a. Commission notice on the application of Articles 3, 5 and 7 of Regulation (EC) No 141/2000 on orphan medicinal products. *Official Journal of the European Union.* https://eur-lex.europa.eu/legal-content/EN/TXT/PDF/?uri=OJ:JOC_2016_424_R_0003 (accessed August 1, 2024).

European Commission. 2014b. *Guideline on the format and content of applications for designation as orphan medicinal products and on the transfer of designations from one sponsor to another.* https://health.ec.europa.eu/system/files/2016-11/2014-03_guideline_rev4_final_0.pdf (accessed August 1, 2024).

European Commission. n.d. *Rare diseases.* https://health.ec.europa.eu/european-reference-networks/rare-diseases_en (accessed August 15, 2024).

European Union. 2004. *Regulation (EC) NO 726/2004 of the European Parliament and of the Council.* https://eur-lex.europa.eu/LexUriServ/LexUriServ.do?uri=OJ:L:2004:136:0001:0033:en:PDF (accessed August 1, 2024).

Marjenberg, Z., R. Teague, and G. Skeldon. 2020. PMU50 a review of exceptional circumstances marketing authorisations granted by the European Medicines Agency. *Value in Health* 23:S611.

O'Donnell, P. 2016. *Will EMA rules calm the disclosure debate?* https://www.appliedclinicaltrialsonline.com/view/will-ema-rules-calm-the-disclosure-debate (accessed August 1, 2024).

Prilla, S. 2018. *Legal basis & types of approvals.* https://www.ema.europa.eu/en/documents/presentation/presentation-legal-basis-and-types-approvals-s-prilla_en.pdf (accessed August 1, 2024).

Thirstrup, S. 2023. Orphan medicines in EU: Processes to Evaluate the Safety and Efficacy of Drugs for Rare Diseases or Conditions in the United States and the European Union (Meeting 2 - Hybrid).

Ungstrup, E., and D. Vanags. 2023. *Aligning global drug development for pediatric populations.* https://www.pharmalex.com/thought-leadership/blogs/aligning-global-drug-development-for-pediatric-populations/ (accessed August 15, 2024).

Zhuleku, E., and F. Preinfalk. 2023. *Clinical trial regulation: Balancing transparency requirements and protection of CCI – new Q&A published.* https://www.allenovery.com/en-gb/global/blogs/life-sciences-talk/clinical-trial-regulation-balancing-transparency-requirements-and-protection-of-cci--new-qa-published (accessed March 10, 2024).

4

Alternative and Confirmatory Data

Conclusion 4-1: The low prevalence of rare diseases and conditions, incomplete understanding of their underlying biology, ethical challenges in giving placebo to patients with rare diseases in double-blind clinical trials, and limitations in the ability to conduct randomized clinical trials (RCTs) for new therapies for them, have necessitated the collection and use of data from sources other than traditional RCTs for marketing authorization applications for rare disease drug products.

In keeping with this reality, the statement of task asked the committee to examine "the consideration and use of supplemental data submitted during review processes in the United States and the European Union, including data associated with open label extension studies and expanded access programs specific to rare diseases or conditions." As described in Chapter 1, given the variety in types and uses of "supplemental" data in marketing authorization submissions, for the purposes of this report, the committee understands "supplemental" data to mean data that are generally collected outside the setting of a traditional randomized controlled clinical trial and used as alternative or confirmatory evidence in support of regulatory submission and review of a drug product.

This chapter is organized based on the following topics: guidance on alternative and confirmatory data (ACD), sources of ACD, trends in regulatory use, novel approaches for study design and data analysis drug review and approval, orphan medicine designation, expedited regulatory programs, biomarkers, and opportunities to enhance innovation. Over time, as new technologies, study designs, and methods for data analysis emerge, additional sources of ACD may be applicable for use in marketing authorization applications for drugs to treat rare diseases and conditions.

GUIDANCE ON ALTERNATIVE AND CONFIRMATORY DATA

As described in Chapter 2, the statutory requirements for drug review and approval for rare diseases and conditions are the same as for non-rare diseases or conditions. The U.S. Food and Drug Administration (FDA) has discretion to accept one adequate and well-controlled clinical investigation in conjunction with alternative and confirmatory data, if FDA determines that, based on relevant science, such data would be sufficient to establish effectiveness.

The Food and Drug Administration Modernization Act of 1997 (Public Law 105–115) made clear that the substantial evidence requirement for effectiveness can be met by a single trial plus confirmatory evidence. A series of FDA guidances for industry[1] elaborates on this thinking, by discussing approaches that can yield evidence that meets the statutory standard for substantial evidence of effectiveness, many of which can be leveraged by rare disease development programs (FDA, 2019b). Examples of types of confirmatory evidence that could be used to supplement one clinical investigation, some of which may be generated during conventional drug development programs, are described in Table 4-1. FDA has used these data sources to make regulatory decisions (see Figure 4-1).

The European Medicines Agency's (EMA's) guidelines on the use of one pivotal trial state that the "fundamental requirement" of Phase 3 studies is that they consist of "adequate and well-controlled data of good quality from a sufficient number of patients, with a sufficient variety of symptoms and disease conditions, collected by a sufficient number of investigators, demonstrating a positive benefit/risk in the intended population at the intended dose and manner of use" (EMA, 2001). The extent of data needed will depend on what is already known about the product and related products; the minimum requirement is generally one study with statistically compelling and clinically relevant results. In applications that rely on only one pivotal study, EMA notes that the study in question will be examined closely for internal validity, external validity, clinical relevance, statistical significance, data quality, internal consistency, center effects, and

---

[1] Providing Clinical Evidence of Effectiveness for Human Drug and Biological Products—FINAL Guidance (FDA, 1998).

Demonstrating Substantial Evidence of Effectiveness for Human Drug and Biological Products—DRAFT Guidance (FDA, 2019b).

Demonstrating Substantial Evidence of Effectiveness with One Adequate and Well-Controlled Clinical Investigation and Confirmatory Evidence—DRAFT Guidance (FDA, 2023d).

TABLE 4-1 Examples of Types of Confirmatory Evidence from FDA Guidance

Evidence Type	Description
Clinical evidence from a related indication	Data from clinical investigation that was used to support a previous approval or data from an adequate and well-controlled study that demonstrated the effectiveness of the drug for a related, unapproved indication
Mechanistic or pharmacodynamic evidence	Data that provide strong mechanistic support (e.g., pharmacokinetic and pharmacodynamic data collected via clinical and/or animal studies) for a treatment effect on a particular disease
Evidence from a relevant animal model	Data (e.g., proof-of-concept, pharmacological, toxicology data) from an established animal model of disease
Evidence from other members of the same pharmacological class	Data from adequate and well-controlled trials of other drugs in the same pharmacological class that have been approved for the same indication
Natural history evidence	Data that can provide confirmatory evidence to support a single adequate and well-controlled clinical trial
Real-world data/evidence	Data related to patient health status or delivery of care that are routinely collected (e.g., electronic health records, medical claims data, registries) and clinical evidence about the use and potential benefits and risks of a drug treatment based on real-world data
Evidence from expanded access use of an investigational drug	Data collected through expanded access that are of sufficient quantity and quality to be considered for use as confirmatory evidence.

NOTE: FDA = U.S. Food and Drug Administration.
SOURCE: FDA, 2023d.

the plausibility of the tested hypotheses (EMA, 2001). EMA also provides guidance on the use of ACD and alternative trial designs as well as on such topics as trials in small populations, real-world evidence, registry-based studies, and single-arm trials (see Table 4-2).

While FDA and EMA have identified some specific types and sources of ACD, as described above, these may change over time as new technologies and methods for data analysis emerge. FDA notes that the list provided in the 2023 guidance is not exhaustive, and each application is considered on a "case-by-case" basis (FDA, 2023d). While this approach could imply that there is no standard approach for considering the use of ACD, examples do provide a helpful basis for how the agency will consider the use of ACD for future marketing authorization applications. Additional context and precedent would give sponsors and patient groups more clarity on how ACD can be incorporated into drug development programs.

TABLE 4-2 EMA Resources on Trial Design, Statistical Methods, and Alternative and Confirmatory Data

Guideline	Source
Complex Clinical Trials—Questions and Answers	EMA (2022a)
Final Concept Paper—E20: Adaptive Clinical Trials	ICH (2019)
Concept Paper on Platform Trials	EMA (2022b)
Design Concept for a Confirmatory Basket Trial	Beckman (2018)
ICH Guideline E17 on General Principles for Planning and Design of Multi-Regional Clinical Trials	EMA (2017)
Points To Consider On Application With 1. Meta-Analyses; 2. One Pivotal Study	EMA (2001)
Guideline on Clinical Trials in Small Populations	EMA (2006)
E10—Choice of Control Group in Clinical Trials (*see sections 1.3 and 2.5 for information on external and historical controls*)	ICH (2001)
Guideline on Registry-Based Studies	EMA (2021a)
A Vision for Use of Real-World Evidence in EU Medicines Regulation	EMA (2021b)
Good Practice Guide for the Use of the Metadata Catalogue of Real-World Data Sources	EMA (2022c)
Real-World Evidence Framework to Support EU Regulatory Decision-Making	EMA (2023b)
Marketing Authorization Applications Made to the European Medicines Agency in 2018–2019: What was the Contribution of Real-World Evidence?	Flynn et al. (2022)

NOTE: EMA = European Medicines Agency.

SOURCES OF ALTERNATIVE AND CONFIRMATORY DATA

Natural History Studies

A natural history study is a preplanned observational study that is designed to capture information about the course of a disease. Information is collected about symptoms and outcomes, as well as about demographic, environmental, genetic, and other variables that may affect the patient's experience with the disease and be associated with the natural history of the disease (FDA, 2023b). Depending on the disease and the availability of treatment, a natural history study may include patients who are untreated, patients receiving the standard of care, or patients receiving an emergent treatment (FDA, 2019c). An example of a common mechanism for acquiring data for natural history studies is a patient or disease registry.

FDA published draft guidance in 2019 on *Rare Diseases: Natural History Studies for Drug Development* which states, "Information obtained from a natural history study can play an important role at every stage of

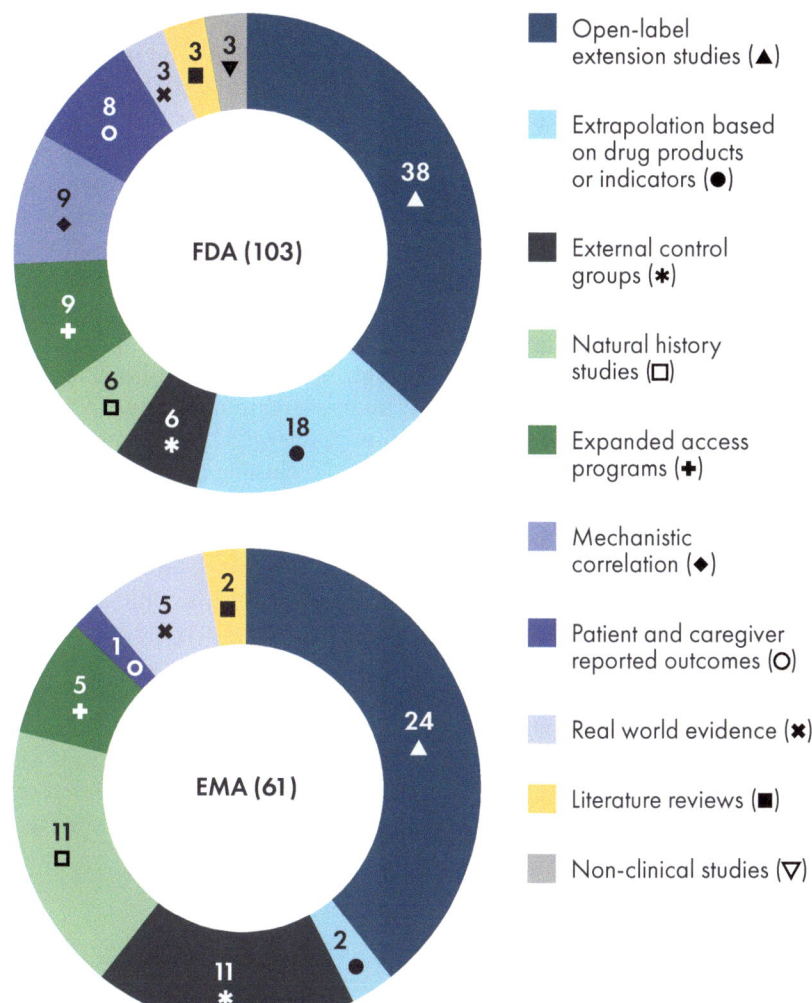

FIGURE 4-1 Distribution of types of alternative and confirmatory data referenced by EMA and FDA for orphan drug products between 2013 and 2022.
NOTES: ACD = alternative and confirmatory data; FDA = U.S. Food and Drug Administration.
SOURCE: CIRS Data Analysis, 2024.

drug development, from drug discovery to the design of clinical studies intended to support marketing approval of a drug and beyond into the post-marketing period" (FDA, 2019c). FDA also notes that natural history studies may have benefits for patients living with rare diseases that go beyond drug development and approval. Natural history studies can establish communication pathways, identify disease-specific centers of excellence, build knowledge about the current standard of care and potential improvements to care, and provide estimates of the prevalence of the disease (FDA, 2019c).

EMA published a guideline in 2021 on the use of registry-based studies to support regulatory decision-making (EMA, 2021a). In the guideline, EMA clarified the differences between a registry-based study and a patient registry: namely, that a registry is an organized system that collects uniform data, and that a registry-based study is an investigation of a research question that uses the infrastructure of such a registry. EMA identified several uses for registries and registry-based studies, including to complement the evidence submitted for marketing authorization. Patient registries can serve as a source of information on standards of care, incidence, prevalence, determinants of disease, and characteristics of the population. In addition, registries can be used for such purposes as recruitment, sample size calculation, and endpoint identification. Patient registries may be particularly valuable for rare disease communities as they serve as a resource to help inform disease characterization and the development and validation of biomarkers and clinical endpoints and, in some cases, may supplement, confirm, or replace information gathered through a traditional randomized clinical trial. EMA emphasized in its guideline that it is recommended that sponsors obtain advice from EMA early on regarding the acceptability of a registry-based study.

Examples

There are several examples that illustrate how natural history studies and patient registries can supplement and augment marketing authorization submissions for drugs to treat rare diseases and conditions. (For further details and references regarding these examples, see Appendix H.) In 2023, after considering confirmatory evidence including natural history data, FDA approved SkyClarys (omaveloxolone) for the treatment of Friedreich's ataxia, a rare, inherited, neurodegenerative disease that typically affects children and teens and gradually worsens over time (see Box 4-1). On the same basis, EMA recommended market approval later in the same year.

Additionally, FDA (in May 2019) and EMA (in March 2020) both approved Zolgensma (onasemnogene abeparvovec-xioi) for spinal muscular atrophy based on a natural history control in comparison to a treatment

BOX 4-1
Use Case: SkyClarys (Friedreich's Ataxia)

On February 28, 2023—Rare Disease Day— the U.S. Food and Drug Administration (FDA) announced approval of SkyClarys (omaveloxolone), the first approved treatment for Friedreich's ataxia (FA), a rare, inherited, neurodegenerative disease that typically affects the nervous system and heart in children, teens, and adults and worsens over time. The sponsor submitted data supplemental to its New Drug Application, including the use of an external control—a cohort of natural history participants who were closely propensity-score matched to the participants in the open-label extension of the single study. Natural history data played a key role in informing regulatory decision-making as FDA's SkyClarys review summary concludes:

> Given the serious and life-threatening nature of FA and the substantial unmet need with no approved treatments, some level of uncertainty is acceptable in this instance and consideration of these results in the context of regulatory flexibility is appropriate. The single adequate and well-controlled study with positive results on a clinically meaningful primary outcome, accompanied by confirmatory evidence from the natural history comparison, in addition to the pharmacodynamic data supporting the biologic plausibility of the treatment effect, are adequate to provide substantial evidence of effectiveness. There are no safety issues that would preclude approval. Additional pharmacovigilance and adequate monitoring for risks of liver injury and cardiac events are warranted in the postmarketing setting. (FDA, 2023h)

Based on the same single-trial results and supplemental data, in December 2023, the European Medicines Agency (EMA) followed with a recommendation for market approval of SkyClarys, and the European Commission approval followed in February 2024. EMA's review summary regarding the confirmatory evidence concludes:

> "This exploratory analysis should be interpreted cautiously given the limitations of data collected outside of a controlled study, which may be subject to confounding" (EMA, 2024d).

This use case demonstrates how Alternative and Confirmatory Data can be used in support of regulatory submission of rare disease drug products provided that (1) it can address regulatory concerns of possible uncertainties, (2) it can provide adequate substantial evidence of effectiveness, and (3) there is no safety issue that would preclude approval.

groups. The increase in survival between treatment groups and the natural history control provided evidence of the treatment's effectiveness. Zolgensma is a directly administered adeno-associated virus (AAV) vector that delivers the survival motor neuron 1 (SMN) gene for the treatment of pediatric patients with spinal muscular atrophy (SMA) who have bi-allelic mutations in the SMN gene. The primary evidence of effectiveness for regulatory approval was based on a single, ongoing, Phase 3, open label, single-arm study of children with infantile onset SMA; natural history data were used as the control, and a completed Phase 1 study provided support of evidence. The primary endpoints in the Phase 3 trial were "alive without permanent ventilation" and "sitting without support." Based on the strong natural history of the disease, no patients meeting the study entry criteria would be expected to attain the ability to sit without support, and only about a quarter of patients would be expected to remain alive without permanent ventilation beyond 14 months of age. Due to this strong knowledge of the natural history and the very significant treatment effect, the Center for Biologics Evaluation and Research (CBER) approved Zolgensma during the ongoing Phase 3 trial and with the natural history control rather than a concurrent control arm (Anatol, 2024).

Programs to Support Natural History and Patient Registries

There are a number of public and private initiatives that are designed to support the development of patient registries and the conduct of natural history studies. A 2016 cooperative agreement between FDA and the National Organization for Rare Disorders (NORD) launched a program that supported 20 rare disease patient groups in the development of natural history studies (NORD, 2016). The groups that were chosen represented diseases with diagnostic challenges, limited or no research, and a broad range of symptoms and systems. Another NORD initiative is called IAMRARE. This registry programs allows patient advocacy groups to build patient registries and collect natural history data (NORD, n.d.). As of 2023, the IAMRARE program has over 50 natural history studies with over 18,000 patients and covers more than 75 rare diseases (NORD, 2023). Similarly, Global Genes, another nonprofit patient advocacy organization, hosts standardized patient-entered natural history data on its RARE-X platform for rare disorders, including 7,700 participants from 90 countries. Many other natural history registries and platforms exist (nonprofit and for-profit) that are designed specifically to collect patient-entered longitudinal natural history data from rare disease groups, such as Simons Searchlight, Across Healthcare's Matrix, Sanford CoRDs, and JEEVA, as well as academic efforts and clinical centers around the country. These natural history projects may or may not be collecting information that is useful or sufficient for submission as natural history controls for drug approvals; thus, pharmaceutical firms often conduct proprietary observational and natural history studies on rare diseases prior to submitting new drug applications.

FDA has supported natural history studies since 2016 for patients with rare diseases. FDA's Office of Orphan Products Development (OOPD) provides sponsors and other entities grants to conduct clinical trials and natural history studies on rare diseases. There are typically 60 to 85 ongoing grant projects every year. OOPD awards approximately five to twelve new grants each year. FDA natural history program funds well-designed, protocol-driven natural history studies that address knowledge gaps, support clinical trials, and advance rare disease medical products. As of the time of writing this report, OOPD has supported more than 15 natural history studies (FDA, 2023b) (see Box 4-2). An FDA study on the clinical trial grant program found that of the 85 grants issued between 2007 and 2011, 9 product approvals were partially supported by grant funding (Miller et al., 2020).

The Rare Disease Cures Accelerator-Data and Analytics Platform (RDCA-DAP®), which is funded by FDA and operated by the Critical Path

---

BOX 4-2
Diseases Studied by Ongoing and Past FDA Office of Orphan Products Development Natural History Grants from 2016 to 2023

- Amyotrophic lateral sclerosis
- Angelman syndrome
- Ataxia–telangiectasia
- Autoimmune pulmonary alveolar proteinosis
- Castleman disease
- Chronic kidney disease
- Duchenne muscular dystrophy
- Friedreich's ataxia
- Hypoparathyroidism
- Medullary thyroid carcinoma
- Myotonic dystrophy Type 1
- Ornithine-δ-aminotransferase
- Osteoporosis
- Pulmonary arterial hypertension
- Sarcoidosis

SOURCE: FDA, 2023b.

Institute in collaboration with NORD, is a centralized database and analytics hub that contains standardized data on a growing number of rare diseases and that allows secure sharing of data collected across multiple sources, including natural history studies/patient registries, control arms of clinical trials, longitudinal observational studies, and real-world data (Critical Path Institute, n.d.). Since RDCA-DAP® was launched in 2021, the platform has enabled access to data from over 30 rare disease areas with more data being added over time (see Box 4-3). Drug developers and other data users can access the platform to better understand disease progression and heterogeneity, to more effectively target therapeutics, and to inform trial design and other aspects of rare disease drug development. The establishment of regulatory-grade fit-for-purpose natural history platforms has the potential to support marketing authorization submissions for drugs to treat rare disease and conditions. RDCA-DAP® offers a trusted and reliable

---

BOX 4-3
Diseases Covered by Critical Path Institute's Rare Disease Cures Accelerator–Data and Analytics Platform

- Angelman syndrome
- Congenital hyperinsulinism
- Desmoid tumor
- Duchenne muscular dystrophy
- Facioscapulohumeral muscular dystrophy (FSHD)
- Friedreich's ataxia
- GNE myopathy
- hnRNP related disorders
- Kidney transplant
- K1F1A associated neurological disorder
- Lennox-Gastaut syndrome
- Mitochondrial disease

- Nectrotizing enterocolitis
- Niemann-Pick disease
- Pemphigus & pemphigoid
- Phenylketonuria (PKU)
- Polycystic kidney disease
- Prader-Willi syndrome*
- Progressive supranuclear palsy*
- Rare epilepsies*
- RYR-1 gene mutation*
- Spinal muscle atrophy with respiratory distress*
- Spinocerebellar ataxias type 1, 2, 3 & 6
- Sturge-Weber syndrome
- Tuberous sclerosis

NOTE: * Indicates disease with datasets that are currently discoverable on the platform.
SOURCE: Critical Path Institute, n.d.

source of standardized ACD that can be used for clinical trial design and effective external controls.[2]

The RDCA-DAP® process (see Figure 4-2) involves aggregating and aligning patient-level data from a variety of trials, observational studies, patient registries, and electronic health records. The Critical Path Institute works with stakeholders to standardize data collection and to curate and standardize data entered into the platform. A number of rare disease consortiums both contribute and use data from the platform; the contribution and use of these data are negotiated between the contributing organization and Critical Path Institute. These data are curated and standardized into databases; researchers can request access for quick analysis. The platform is compliant with European Privacy Regulations (Critical Path Institute, n.d.). On a smaller scale, a data aggregator program called "Linking Angelman and Dup15q Data for Expanded Research" (LADDER) is a database platform that links data on individuals with Angelman or Dup15q syndromes collected from multiple sources, such as research studies, registries, caregiver reports, and clinic visits (Angelman Syndrome Foundation, n.d.).

One goal of RDCA-DAP® is to shorten the timeline for the development of treatments for rare diseases. Prior to LADDER and RDCA-DAP®, existing data on rare diseases tended to be siloed, and data that were available may not have been standardized, digitized, or interoperable (Barrett et al., 2023). Giving researchers and drug developers access to standardized, usable data can lead to new insights about the disease and to improved processes for clinical trials (NORD, 2021). For example, using existing data to develop models of disease can guide the design of clinical trials, potentially making research faster and more cost-effective (NORD, 2021). RDCA-DAP® is designed to make each step of drug development more efficient, including pre-clinical research, clinical research, FDA review, and post-market safety monitoring (NORD, 2021).

Most programs listed above are early on in development, so the committee was unable to assess their impacts on regulatory decision-making. However, the notable success of the approval of SkyClarys for the treatment of Friedreich's ataxia has demonstrated how such tools as RDCA-DAP® can facilitate research and development for rare diseases and conditions (Barrett et al., 2023). Despite the opportunities for using natural history data in regulatory decision-making and efforts on the part of government and nonprofit funders to establish and support natural history registries, most patients living with rare diseases and conditions do not have access to this type of resource.

---

[2] This sentence was edited after release of the prepublication version of the report to correctly specify the type of ACD.

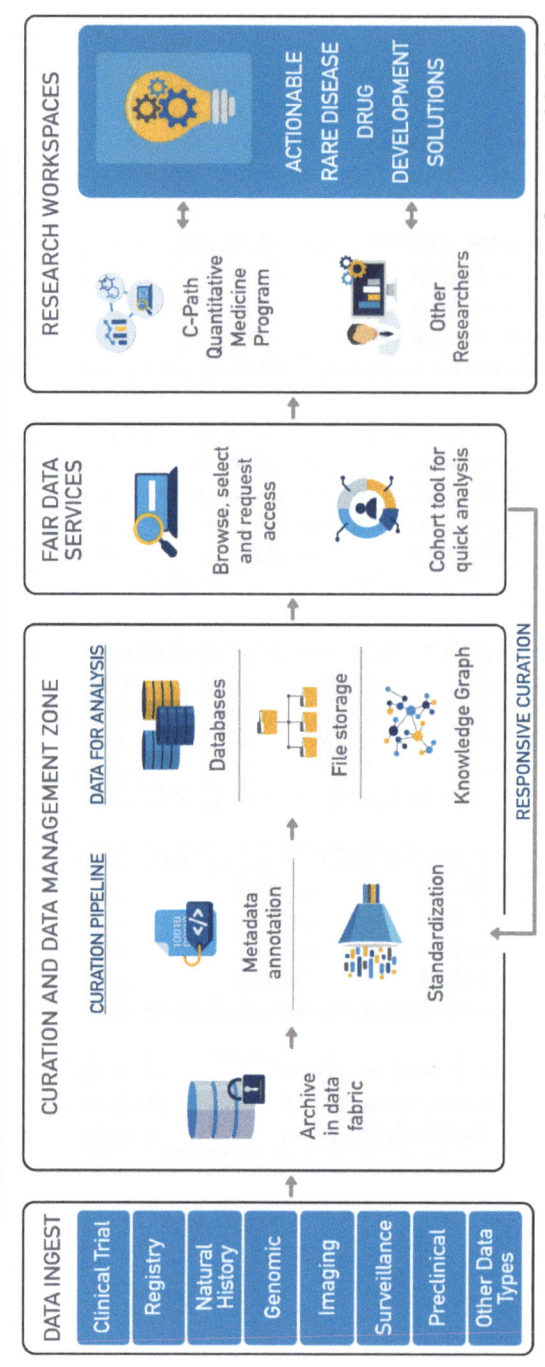

FIGURE 4-2 The Rare Disease Cures Accelerator–Data and Analytics Platform process.
SOURCE: Critical Path Institute, n.d.

Conclusion 4-2: Understanding the natural history of a disease—as well as the factors that affect its progression and outcomes—is important for drug development. However, for most rare diseases and conditions, there is often little information about natural history.

RECOMMENDATION 4-1: The U.S. Food and Drug Administration (FDA) should enable the collection and curation of regulatory-grade natural history data to enhance the quality and accessibility of data for all rare diseases. This should include, but not be limited to:

- Continuation and expansion of support for current rare disease natural history design and data collection programs, such as FDA's Office of Orphan Products Development awarding clinical trial and natural history study grants.
- Continuation and expansion of data aggregation, standardization, and analysis programs, including, but not limited to, Critical Path Institute's Rare Disease Cures Accelerator-Data and Analytics Platform.
- Support, education, training, and access to resources/infrastructure for nascent rare disease advocacy groups to enable the standardization and integration of patient-level data for future regulatory use.
- Continuation and expansion of collaboration with other agencies (e.g., National Institutes of Health Rare Disease Clinical Research Network) to expand natural history design and data collection resources for all rare diseases.
- Periodic assessment regarding the impact and opportunities for improvement of ongoing programs for the collection, curation, and use of natural history data in regulatory decision-making for rare disease drug development programs.

Expanded Access/Compassionate Use

In the United States, expanded access or "compassionate use" allows critically ill patients with a serious or life-threatening disease or condition to receive investigational drugs—products that have not yet been approved for marketing by FDA. In the United States, expanded access may be appropriate when all the following apply:

- "Patient has a serious or immediately life-threatening disease or condition.
- "There is no comparable or satisfactory alternative therapy to diagnose, monitor, or treat the disease or condition.
- "Patient enrollment in a clinical trial is not possible.
- "Potential patient benefit justifies the potential risks of treatment.

- "Providing the investigational medical product will not interfere with investigational trials that could support a medical product's development or marketing approval for the treatment indication" (FDA, 2024b).

Similarly, in the European Union, compassionate use programs can be considered if patients have a "life-threatening, long-lasting, or seriously debilitating illness, which cannot be treated satisfactorily with any currently authorized medicine" (EMA, n.d.). In the case of EMA, the medicine must be in clinical trials or have a submitted marketing authorization application.

Expanded access programs are not designed to collect data for research purposes. However, data collected through these programs could be a source of alternative or confirmatory data that could help supplement clinical trial data in the regulatory review process (Wasser and Greenblatt, 2023). While real-world clinical data about the expanded access use of investigational drugs are not as rigorous or standardized as typical clinical trial data, they may provide insights on safety in real-world settings.

Each year, FDA's Center for Drug Evaluation and Research (CDER) receives over 1,000 requests for expanded access to investigational drugs (Jarow and Moscicki, 2017). A review of expanded access requests over a 10-year period between 2005 and 2014 showed that the number of requests increased over time and that most nonemergency submissions were for anti-infective and oncology products (Jarow et al., 2016). There is the potential for expanded access to help treat rare disease patients and advance drug development. While it is the case that investigational drug products may not be effective and could cause serious side effects, for rare disease patients with unmet medical needs, expanded access may be their only opportunity to receive treatment.

Regulatory Guidance

There is a tension between the primary and original purposes of expanded access—to provide treatment to patients with unmet needs—and the potential for collecting evidence on the safety and effectiveness of these treatments (Polak et al., 2022). While FDA and EMA have both used data from expanded access as part of a regulatory decision (see examples below), neither agency has been explicit about whether and to what extent expanded access data should be collected or used. EMA's 2007 guideline on expanded access states, "Although safety data may be collected during compassionate use programmes, such programmes cannot replace clinical trials for investigational purposes. Compassionate use is not a substitute for properly conducted trials" (EMA, 2007). FDA's guidance on compassionate use distinguishes between expanded access and the use of an investigational drug in a clinical trial by stating that "expanded access uses are not primarily intended to obtain information about the safety or effectiveness of a drug" (FDA, 2022a). Furthermore, FDA expresses concern that expanded access for rare disease treatment has the potential to interfere with clinical trials because the number of potential trial participants is limited; clinical trials should be initiated before expanded access is offered, and expanded access should only be available for patients who are ineligible or unable to participate in a trial (FDA, 2022a).

Despite the use of expanded access data in regulatory submissions, there is no consensus among regulators, bioethicists, or drug developers on the role that these data should play in drug development (Bunnik and Aarts, 2021; Bunnik et al., 2018; Kearns et al., 2021; Polak et al., 2022; Polak et al., 2020; Rozenberg and Greenbaum, 2020; Sarp et al., 2022).

Examples

There are some examples of new drug applications that have included expanded access data, such as:

- "vestronidase to treat mucopolysaccharidosis VII, a rare genetic enzyme deficiency;
- "lutetium 177 dotatate injection, a radiolabeled drug for rare gastroenteropancreatic neuroendocrine tumors;
- "cannabidiol, an adjunctive treatment for seizures associated with two rare conditions;
- "combined sodium phenylacetate and sodium benzoate to treat acute hyperammonaemia in patients with a rare urea cycle disorder; and
- "nitisinone to treat hereditary tyrosinaemia type 1" (Wasser and Greenblatt, 2023).

However, streamlining the use of expanded use data in marketing authorization submissions, would likely require that data collection be standardized and align with the regulatory review process.

As of 2018, FDA and EMA had collectively approved 49 drug-indication pairs based in whole or in part on data from expanded access; of these, 63 percent were designated as orphan medicines (Polak et al., 2022). The treatment for gastroenteropancreatic neuroendocrine tumors was approved based on a small randomized controlled trial (RCT) that was supplemented with data from 558 patients treated under expanded access (Polak et al., 2022). In another case, a treatment was approved by both FDA and EMA based solely on expanded access data; a treatment for rare disorders in bile acid metabolism was approved based on data from two expanded access programs with a total of 85 patients (Polak et al., 2022).

Open-Label Extension Studies

After the completion of Phase 3 of a clinical trial, participants may be offered the opportunity to enroll in an extension study. Unlike a controlled, blinded trial, all participants in an open-label extension study are given the investigational drug with no blinding. The objective of open-label extension studies is generally to gather information about safety and tolerability in the long-term use of the product, which can be useful in the marketing application (Taylor and Wainwright, 2005). In some cases, open-label extension studies can provide longer-term efficacy data as well (Wang et al., 2022).

Relevance to Rare Disease

Patients with rare diseases may be hesitant to participate in a trial with a placebo arm, particularly if there is no existing treatment or the disease is severe or rapidly progressing (Brown and Ekangaki, 2023). In addition, there may be ethical concerns related to giving only some patients the intervention when there is no alternative treatment. Adding an extension study can make participation in a RCT more appealing because all participants will eventually have a chance to take the investigational drug. In a survey of patients with progressive ataxias, a placebo arm in a trial was seen as a disincentive to participation, and many patients reported that they would be more likely to participate in a trial if an open-label extension study was offered (Thomas-Black et al., 2022). Among other examples, open-label extension data were used in the authorization of Relyvrio for amyotrophic lateral sclerosis (ALS) (see Box 4-4).

Regulatory Guidance

FDA does not have guidance specifically on open-label extension studies, but these studies are mentioned in a number of other guidance documents. For example, in the Agency's guidance *Enhancing the Diversity of Clinical Trial Populations* (FDA, 2020b), FDA suggests three approaches for addressing the challenges in recruiting and enrolling participants in clinical trials for rare diseases; one of these is "Make available an open-label extension study with broader inclusion criteria after early-phase studies to encourage participation by ensuring that all study participants, including those who received placebo, will ultimately have access to the investigational treatment" (FDA, 2020b). Additionally, a poster from the 2023 FDA Science Forum provides recommendations on conducting an open-label trial when fully blinding the trial is not possible (Higgens and Levin, n.d.).

> **BOX 4-4**
> **Use Case: Relyvrio (Amyotrophic Lateral Sclerosis)**
>
> Relyvrio (sodium phenylbutyrate and taurursodiol) for amyotrophic lateral sclerosis (ALS)—known as Albrioza in Europe—was approved by the U.S. Food and Drug Administration (FDA) in September 2022 (FDA, 2022c) and received a negative opinion from the European Medicines Agency (EMA) in December of 2023 (EMA, 2024a). At the time of approval and opinion, there were only two available treatments in the United States (FDA, 2022c) and one available treatment in Europe (EMA, 2023a). Both FDA and EMA reviewed the same clinical study along with open label extension data (EMA, 2023a; FDA, 2022c). FDA granted Relyvrio approval because the serious nature of the disease along with the unmet medical need warranted the use of regulatory flexibility. As a result, FDA determined the benefits outweighed the risk (FDA, 2022c). In contrast, EMA provided a negative opinion because the data was found to be "neither robust nor statistically compelling" (EMA, 2023a). In 2024, Relyvrio failed the confirmatory clinical trial with no evidence of clinical benefit in the primary or any of the secondary or exploratory endpoints. The company has withdrawn the drug from the U.S. market (Amylyx Pharmaceuticals, 2024).
>
> ---
>
> NOTE: See Appendix H for more information on Relyvrio.

External Control Groups (Concurrent and Historical)

FDA regulatory standards for substantial evidence of effectiveness from adequate and well-controlled trials typically include the use of a control group that is randomized and evaluated at the same time as the intervention group. However, a concurrent internal control group may not always be feasible or ethical when studying rare diseases, so an external control group may be constructed as a comparator (Jahanshahi et al., 2021). An external control group can be based on data collected at an earlier time (i.e., historical control) or on data that is being collected at the same time as the clinical trial, but in another setting (i.e., concurrent control). For example, if a trial on an investigative drug has already been conducted and included a randomized control group, the data from this group could be compared to new data from a trial with no control group. An external control group must closely resemble the intervention group to ensure an apples-to-apples comparison. One approach for establishing a close match is the use of a statistical method called propensity score matching, which matches the characteristics of individuals in the external control group to group participants' characteristics in the intervention group (Jahanshahi et al., 2021).

Relevance to Rare Disease

For many drug trials for rare diseases and conditions, an internal control may not be feasible or ethical to use due to limited numbers of patients or the unmet medical need of patients or both. Single-arm or non-randomized trials, in which all participants receive the experimental therapy, are often used in rare disease drug development, generally for serious or life-threatening disorders for which there is a poor prognosis, standard of care therapies are inadequate, and there is promising evidence of the therapeutic candidate's potential benefit (e.g., pharmacologic data). In these circumstances, an external control group may be used; data from the intervention group is compared with data from an external group that received a placebo (or standard-of-care) in order to determine the true effect of the intervention (Burcu et al., 2020; Jahanshahi et al., 2021).

Regulatory Guidance

In 2023 FDA published the draft guidance *Considerations for the Design and Conduct of Externally Controlled Trials for Drug and Biological Products* (FDA, 2023c). This guidance provides recommendations to sponsors and investigators on the design and analysis of trials that use external control data; the guidance acknowledges that external controls may come from many sources of data but focuses specifically on patient-level data from other clinical trials or real-world data sources, including from electronic health records or medical claims.[3] In addition, FDA's 2023 guidance *Rare Diseases: Considerations for the Development of Drugs and Biological Products* contains a section on the use of external controls in rare disease trials (FDA, 2023f). FDA notes the limitations of external controls, including the lack of blinding and inability to eliminate systematic differences between groups, and states that trial designs that use an external control group should be "reserved for specific circumstances, such as clinical investigations where the drug effect can be demonstrated in diseases with well-understood and -characterized natural history, high and predictable mortality or progressive and predictable morbidity, and clinical investigations in which the drug effect is large and self-evident" (FDA, 2023f). FDA recommends that sponsors engage in early discussion with the relevant review division if considering such a design.

In 2023, EMA published a reflection paper on establishing efficacy based on single arm trials, which acknowledged that in exceptional cases, external controls could serve as a direct comparison, but also noted that it was beyond the scope of the paper. EMA stated, "While methods that

---

[3] This sentence was updated after release of the prepublication version of the report to specify use of data from external controls.

directly incorporate external data into the analysis come with a promise to provide useful insights and potentially reduce bias, they add complexity to pre-specification and rely on additional assumptions that are often not transparent. Consequently, approaches that directly incorporate external data should be carefully evaluated on a case-by-case basis" (EMA, 2023c).

Examples

External controls have successfully been used in several new drug applications for rare disease products (Khachatryan et al., 2023). For example, Cerliponase alfa (Brineura) was approved by both FDA and EMA in 2017 for the treatment of a rare pediatric neurological disease; the approval was based on data from 23 patients in an open-label single arm trial, with a historical control group derived from a registry database (Khachatryan et al., 2023).

Extrapolation from Existing Studies

In some cases, the safety or efficacy of a drug product, or both, can be supported or demonstrated by extrapolating data from other studies. Extrapolation is often used when a drug was studied in a narrow group of trial participants; the positive results from the trial are extrapolated to a broader population of patients, and the drug is approved with the broader indication (Feldman et al., 2022). For example, a drug may be studied in adults 18–59 who have a mild or moderate version of the disease, but results are extrapolated to grant an indication that includes all adult patients with any level of severity. Extrapolation may also be used to approve a drug approved for adult use for use in the pediatric population if the course of the disease and the expected response to the drug are sufficiently similar between the adult and pediatric patient populations (ICH, 2022).

Relevance to Rare Disease

Some rare diseases may affect only a handful of patients but are closely related to other rare diseases and collectively these variations affect a significant number of patients. For example, cancers can be classified by both location and biomarker profile. In cancers where the location and biomarker profile are rare, there may be too few patients to conduct an RCT. In this case, data from a trial that tested an intervention for a cancer with a specific biomarker and a specific location may be extrapolated to approve an indication for a cancer with the same biomarker but a different location (Cho et al., 2022). Given that rare diseases often present in childhood, extrapolation may also be useful in applying data from adult to pediatric populations.

Regulatory Guidance

In 2022, EMA and FDA, along with other regulatory agencies, adopted the draft *International Council for Harmonisation of Technical Requirements for Pharmaceuticals for Human Use (ICH) Harmonized Guideline: Pediatric Extrapolation* (ICH, 2022). This guidance identifies factors to consider when using extrapolation for pediatric populations and notes that if extrapolation is used for approval, additional data may need to be collected post-approval. The guidance notes special safety considerations when the drug is a new molecular entity, when there are known age-related safety concerns, when there are safety findings that would be of particular importance in children, and when the drug has a narrow therapeutic index (ICH, 2022).

Examples

An analysis of 105 novel FDA approvals between 2015 and 2017 found that extrapolation was used in 23 approvals (Feldman et al., 2022). Extrapolation was most common for disease severity (n=14), followed by disease subtype (n=6) and concomitant medication use (n=3) (Feldman et al., 2022). The study did not note whether any of the approvals were for orphan medicines. In the area of rare disease, the 2017 approval of vemurafenib for a rare cancer called Erdheim-Chester disease (ECD) is an example of the use of extrapolation for regulatory decision-making (Cho et al., 2022). Clinical trials with patients with BRAFV600 mutated metastatic melanoma had found that treatment with vemurafenib, a BRAF-inhibitor, led to improved survival. The BRAFV600 mutation is also present in ECD, for which there are only 800 reported cases in the literature. A "basket trial" of 208 patients in seven cohorts enrolled 22 patients with ECD with BRAF V600 mutation. Results from the group of 22 patients provided evidence that the treatment was associated with improved function and symptoms. The approval of vemurafenib for the treatment of ECD was based on this efficacy data, along with supportive safety data from 3,378 non-ECD patients who were treated with the same dose and schedule (Oneal et al., 2018).

Patient and Caregiver Reported Outcomes

A patient-reported outcome (PRO) is information that is reported directly by the patient, rather than information reported by a clinician or researcher. PROs may include information about symptoms, day-to-day functioning, and mental and emotional well-being (FDA, 2009). As discussed elsewhere in this report, many rare diseases have heterogenous clinical manifestations. Different patients and their caregivers experience the same disease in different ways and may value different types of outcomes. Furthermore, health care professionals and researchers may place emphasis on certain outcomes that are less important to patients and caregivers, and vice versa. For example, a patient may care more about his or her day-to-day function, whereas a researcher is looking at overall survival rates. For these reasons, PROs are a particularly relevant measure in the assessment of products for rare disease. Using PROs to supplement other data on safety and efficacy can provide a fuller picture of whether the benefits of a treatment outweigh the risks and can be used to support marketing authorization applications (FDA, 2009).

Real-World Evidence Studies

Real-world data (RWD) and real-world evidence (RWE) are related but separate terms that are defined by both FDA and EMA. FDA defines RWD as "data relating to patient health status and/or the delivery of health care routinely collected from a variety of sources" (FDA, 2023g). EMA defines RWD as "routinely collected data relating to a patient's health status or the delivery of health care from a variety of sources other than traditional clinical trials" (EMA, 2024c). RWD can come from many sources including electronic health records, claims and billing data, data from patient registries, patient-generated data, and data from wearable technologies (Liu et al., 2022). RWE is defined by FDA as "clinical evidence about the usage and potential benefits or risks of a medical product derived from an analysis of RWD" and by EMA as "information derived from an analysis of RWD" (Cave et al., 2019; FDA, 2023g). Hybrid and pragmatic trial designs, as well as observational studies, can generate RWE (Liu et al., 2022). Due to the lack of information on many rare diseases, and the challenges involved in conducting RCTs, RWD and RWE can serve as a rich source of information about disease progression, patient experiences, treatment effects, and relevant endpoints. In addition, RWD can be used as control data in trials where randomizing patients to a placebo or standard-of-care group may be infeasible or unethical (Liu et al., 2022).

TRENDS IN REGULATORY USE

While there is some evidence that the approval processes for the treatment of several rare diseases have leveraged different approaches to establish efficacy—e.g., single-arm trials, the use of external control data, surrogate endpoints and supplemental data—data on the phenomenon were generally lacking. A study comparing characteristics of orphan cancer drugs and their pivotal clinical trials versus non-orphan drugs, using publicly available data from FDA, found that pivotal trials for recently approved orphan cancer drugs were more likely to have been smaller and to have used surrogate endpoints to assess efficacy (Kesselheim et al., 2011).

In Europe, a study assessing regulatory evidence supporting orphan medicinal product authorizations found uncertainties, including the use of intermediate variables without validation, highlighting opportunities for improvement (Pontes et al., 2018).

To better understand current trends in the regulatory use of ACD, the committee commissioned an analysis of EMA and FDA marketing authorization approvals for orphan drug products to examine trends in the use of these types of data for informing regulatory decision-making. ACD was defined as data deriving from natural history studies (e.g., patient registries), expanded access programs, open-label extension studies, external control arms (concurrent and historical), case reports, extrapolation based on data from related drug products or indications, mechanistic correlation (e.g., pharmacokinetics, pharmacodynamics), nonclinical studies (e.g., stability and quality control data), passive data collection, patient and caregiver reported outcomes (e.g., preference data), real-world evidence, and literature reviews. The committee only reviewed ACD that supported orphan product approval and were articulated in a public assessment report from the following year ranges: 2013–2014, 2017–2018, 2021–2022 (see Appendix D for full methodology).

An examination of the types of accepted ACD referenced by FDA and EMA between 2013 and 2022, while limited in scope based on the selected keywords and fields, indicates that both agencies are willing consider a variety of alternative and confirmatory data sources in their regulatory decision-making for orphan drugs (see Figures 4-1 and 4-3). In 2021–2022, the proportion of orphan drug approvals that included the use of alternative and confirmatory data were similar between FDA (59 percent or 30/51 products) and EMA (63 percent or 24/38 products) (see Figure 4-3). During the time period included in this analysis (2013–2022), the committee observed that both agencies included alternative and confirmatory data in approval packages across therapeutic areas, with an increase noted in the inclusion of ACD in public assessment reports for anti-cancer and immunomodulator drug products (see Figure 4-4).

Expanding the Use of Alternative and Confirmatory Data

While the committee was able to gather some evidence that ACD has been used to support a determination of substantial evidence of effectiveness, data were limited and not easily accessible. In addition to information that had to be obtained directly from FDA (see Chapter 2), the committee used a proprietary database curated by the Centre for Innovation in

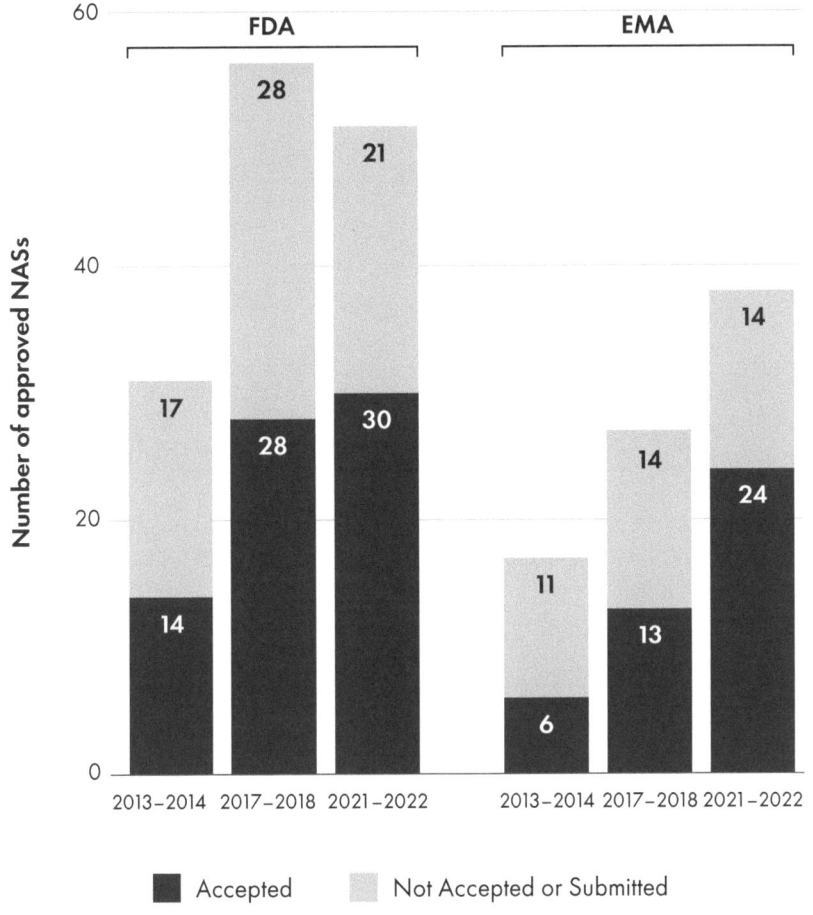

FIGURE 4-3 Use of alternative and confirmatory data by FDA and EMA in marketing authorization approvals for orphan drug products from 2013 to 2022.
NOTES: EMA = European Medicines Agency; FDA = U.S. Food and Drug Administration; NASs = new active substances.
SOURCE: CIRS Data Analysis, 2024.

Regulatory Science from public domain sources such as agency public assessment reports (see Appendix D for full methodology). The addition of context-specific information on whether ACD did or did not meet criteria for informing regulatory decision-making would have enabled the committee to carry out a more informed assessment of how EMA and FDA are considering the types and sources of alternative and confirmatory data for rare disease drug products.

Qualitative interviews with industry representatives suggested that there are mixed perceptions regarding the degree to which EMA and FDA

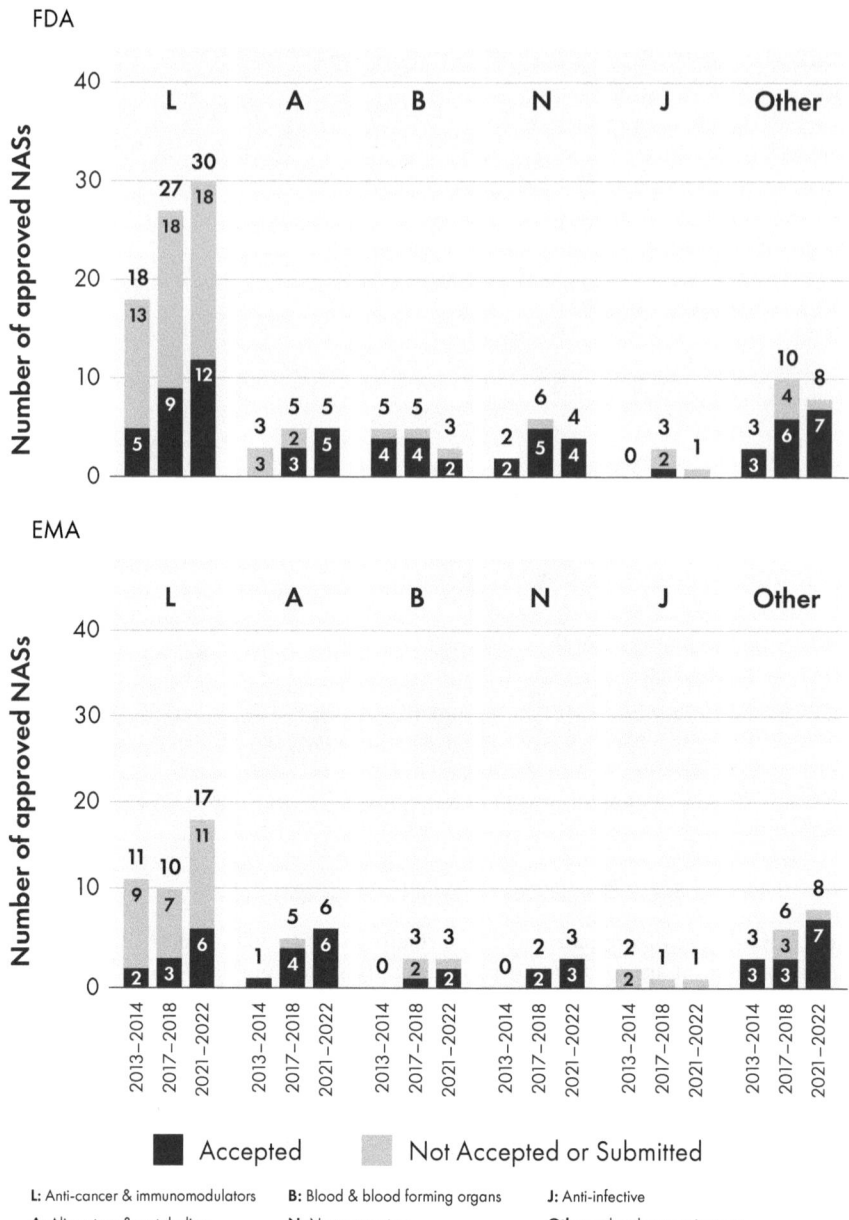

FIGURE 4-4 Accepted alternative and confirmatory data for orphan drug products approved by FDA and EMA from 2013 to 2022 by therapeutic area.
NOTES: EMA = European Medicines Agency; FDA = U.S. Food and Drug Administration; NASs = new active substances; Other = other therapeutic areas not described in the top five therapeutic indications list.
SOURCE: CIRS Data Analysis, 2024.

consider the use of alternative and confirmatory data in regulatory decision-making, and conflicting viewpoints about whether or not there is variability in the acceptance of these data within a given agency or between reviewers (see Appendix E for full methodology and results).

Given proven examples of success, the evolution in regulatory thinking, and advances in new trial designs and methods for data analysis, there is a growing impetus to apply and expand available opportunities for collecting and using ACD to inform researchers, sponsors, regulators, and patient groups on when and how alternative and confirmatory data have informed regulatory decision-making to ensure the integration of lessons learned from past successes and failures.

EMA and FDA can play a critical role in facilitating the use of these types of data in marketing submission applications by standardizing, documenting, and publicly sharing information to enable stakeholders to track over time how ACD have successfully and unsuccessfully informed regulatory decision-making for rare disease drug products. A publicly available and easily accessible (indexed and searchable) listing of products, coupled with standardized information on the types and sources of ACD that were considered as part of a marketing authorization application, would enable drug sponsors, patient and disease advocates, researchers, and regulators to improve the collection and use of these data for rare disease drug development going forward.

As an example, FDA's Center for Devices and Radiological Health (CDRH) reviewed a sample of past regulatory decisions from across CDRH offices to identify examples of how real-world evidence had been used by the agency to inform premarket and postmarket decision making. CDRH then issued a publicly available report (FDA, 2021a), which lays out 90 examples of submissions organized by type of device and summarizes the ways that real-world evidence has been used to inform regulatory decision-making, areas of innovation, and sources of real-world data. This resource builds on FDA guidances and provides stakeholders with concrete examples of how real-world evidence has been and can be applied for supporting FDA regulatory decision-making for medical devices.

An understanding of the opportunities as well as the gaps and inadequacies in alternative and confirmatory data would help guide data collection strategies on the part of patients, caregivers, sponsors, and researchers, and ensure that the data gathered are both relevant and robust enough to support regulatory needs.

RECOMMENDATION 4-2: The U.S. Food and Drug Administration (FDA) should invite the European Medicines Agency (EMA) to jointly conduct systematic reviews of submitted and approved marketing authorization applications to treat rare diseases and conditions that

document cases for which alternative and confirmatory data have contributed to regulatory decision-making. The systematic reviews should include relevant information on the context for whether these data were:
- found to be adequate, and why they were found to be adequate
- found to be inadequate, and why they were found to be inadequate
- found to be useful in supporting decision making and to what extent

Findings from the systematic reviews should be made publicly available and accessible for sponsors, researchers, patients, and their caregivers through public reporting or publication of the results. EMA and FDA should establish a public database for these findings that is continuously updated to ensure that progress over time is captured, opportunities to clarify agency thinking over time are identified, and information on the use of alternative and confirmatory data to inform regulatory decision-making is publicly shared to inform the rare disease drug development community.

FDA draft guidance, *Demonstrating Substantial Evidence of Effectiveness With One Adequate and Well-Controlled Clinical Investigation and Confirmatory Evidence Guidance for Industry*, states that "considerations for a safety evaluation, a benefit-risk analysis, and their impact on the acceptability of one trial with confirmatory evidence to support approval are beyond the scope of this guidance" (FDA, 2023d), suggesting that follow-on guidance on the use of alternative and confirmatory data to establish safety as well as efficacy could help further the work of the agency and provide additional clarity for drug sponsors and patient groups seeking to use these types of data for rare disease drug development. Given that draft guidances can signal agency thinking on a topic, but are not for implementation, the finalization of the 2023 draft guidance would provide much-needed assurance for FDA reviewers, drug sponsors, and patient and disease advocacy groups about FDA's current thinking on the sources and use of alternative and confirmatory data for demonstrating substantial evidence of effectiveness.

Given the urgent need to facilitate development and approval of therapies for rare diseases and conditions, finalizing the draft guidance in a timely manner is incredibly important. Draft guidance documents need to be finalized more quickly to better facilitate and guide drug development, especially for rare diseases.

NOVEL APPROACHES FOR DATA ANALYSIS

There are several novel methods for analyzing relevant data on drug safety and efficacy that can make it possible to generate useful information for regulatory decision-making based on limited data. Further acceptance of these methods on the part of regulatory agencies and sponsors would better enable the use of alternative and confirmatory data as well as data collected through traditional randomized clinical trials for rare diseases and conditions.

Successful drug development relies on evidence that can demonstrate causality—that is, showing that there is a cause-and-effect relationship between a drug treatment and a clinical outcome. Approaches to identifying the causal effects (both safety and efficacy) of a drug treatment are based on a combination of prior knowledge, hypothesis, and correlations observed in the data (Michoel and Zhang, 2023). A major challenge for rare disease drug development is that the evidence needed to demonstrate causality may be based on limited information (e.g., data from very small clinical trials). In practice, it is often difficult to discern, based only on data acquired through traditional randomized clinical trials, whether an observed outcome is due to the drug treatment or some other factor, such as fluctuation in disease severity or other external influences. For this reason, ACD can play a critical role in informing regulatory decision-making.

At the same time, it is important to recognize that causal inferences based on observational studies or other sources of ACD are subject to bias and could produce misleading conclusions. For this reason, validating the reliability and relevance of ACD is critical for making appropriate causal inferences that can inform regulatory decision-making. Additionally, the use of various methodologies, such as Bayesian approaches, can help integrate ACD, incorporate prior knowledge and biases, consider other factors that may affect the outcome, and address confounding variables—factors that are associated with both the treatment/intervention and the outcome. For situations in which traditional randomized clinical trials are not feasible or sufficient to generate adequate evidence to inform regulatory decision-making, there are innovative approaches that can leverage information from randomized clinical trials and sources of ACD (Eichler et al., 2016).

Both FDA and EMA have issued guidance and guidelines on statistical considerations for the interpretation of superiority, non-inferiority, and equivalence trials (EMA, 2000; FDA, 2016). Generally speaking, statistical approaches involve a single-stage superiority test (weighted for effect size of the treatment and risk-benefit calculation of non-treatment) for evaluating the safety and efficacy of a test treatment under investigation. In practice, this single stage process can be viewed as a two-stage process. At the first stage, non-inferiority can be demonstrated through "not ineffectiveness" using data collected from an RCT (or ACD or ACD plus an RCT). Once the non-inferiority of the test treatment has been established, a second test for superiority (i.e., effectiveness) of the test treatment under investigation can be carried out based on any combination of the datasets (Chow, 2020; Chow et al., 2024).

For example, this two-stage process can be implemented by combining two trials—an RCT and a real-world study—into one, which has the advantage of addressing the issue of small patient population and insufficient power in rare disease drug development. In addition, the use of ACD (instead of, or in addition to RCT data) could help maximize statistical power, could provide more accurate and reliable assessment of the treatment effect, and most importantly may shorten the development process and increase the probability of success for rare disease drug development.

For many rare diseases, there can be several competing endpoints of interest, and there are limited historical data to inform the selection of one specific primary endpoint for a specific trial. Novel methods such as Win ratio test and desirability of outcome ranking may be used to integrate evidence from multiple endpoints and address challenges associated with different types of endpoints (e.g., clinical event, functional assessment, biomarker, and patient-reported outcomes) (Pocock et al., 2012; Sandoval, 2023). For diseases that affect multiple organs and tissues and have heterogeneous clinical presentations, global tests for multiple endpoints may improve study power and provide a broad efficacy assessment for novel trials that use different endpoints for different patient subpopulations (Ramchandani et al., 2016). These tests may also allow for varying endpoints among different subsets of patients to accommodate heterogeneous clinical manifestation.

A number of novel approaches can be applied toward data analyses for rare disease drug development, a few of which are briefly described below. Such methods could be adapted for use in rare disease drug trials but require consideration and assessment for when and how such tools could be applied to inform regulatory decision-making.

Bayesian Statistical Methods

Bayesian statistical methods—an approach for learning from evidence as is accumulated—has been increasingly applied in clinical research and may be particularly well suited for certain types of clinical trials for rare diseases and conditions. Perhaps one of the more useful applications of Bayesian statistical methods for rare diseases is in the incorporation of external or Bayesian statistical methods control data (Psioda and Ibrahim, 2019). A Bayesian approach can offer a way of synthesizing alternative and confirmatory data from multiple sources (e.g., historical and external data) into a holistic analysis to evaluate the veracity of the null or alternative hypothesis as part of the inference for the current clinical trial (Ruberg et al., 2023). Methods may also be applied to enable continuous learning throughout the course of a clinical trial and help investigators determine when to make modifications (e.g., dosing, treatment-switching, adding or dropping a treatment arm) under an adaptive trial design.

Unlike traditional frequentist statistics—a well-established approach based on statistical hypothesis testing and confidence intervals, Bayesian statistical methods are used to answer a research question by determining how likely the specified hypothesis is to be true given prior evidence about the hypothesis combined with the accumulated data from the current experiment (Berry, 2006; Ruberg et al., 2023). Bayesian statistical methods can be an effective tool for rare disease drug development as they can help reduce the number of trial participants required to demonstrate the safety and efficacy of a new therapy.

The first step in a Bayesian analysis plan is the selection of a prior probability distribution of the parameter (e.g., mean response, the variability associated with the mean response, or treatment effect size) for which one wishes to make an inference based on the observed data. Once a prior distribution is defined, another key component of the subsequent Bayesian analysis is the weight given to that prior (see Figure 4-5). A posterior probability, which described a range of likely treatment effect values as a result of current experiment, is then derived by combining information from the prior probability distribution and the newly collected data.

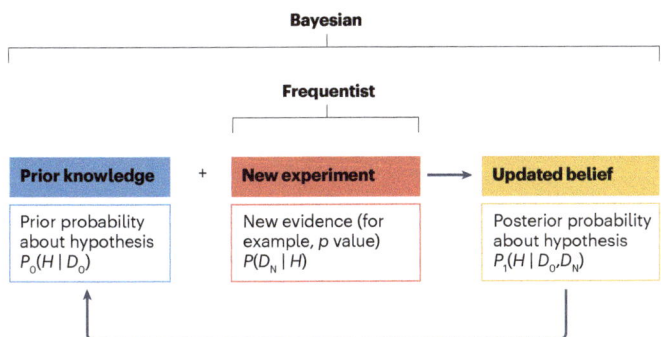

FIGURE 4-5 Comparison between Bayesian and frequentist approaches.
NOTES: A Bayesian approach defines prior knowledge (D_0) about a hypothesis (H) as a prior probability (P_0), which is then combined with evidence from a new experiment (D_N) to determine a posterior probability (P_1) of H being true.
SOURCE: Ruberg et al., Application of Bayesian approaches in drug development: starting a virtuous cycle, *Nature Reviews Drug Discovery*, 22, 235–250, 2023, Springer Nature.

For rare disease drug development, in practice, it is often difficult, if not impossible, to verify the appropriateness of the selected prior distribution due to the unavailability of existing or historical data. Results obtained from a posterior distribution with a wrong prior could be biased and hence misleading in decision making regarding the review and approval of the test treatment under investigation (Ruberg et al., 2023). See Box 4-5 for a use case that applied multiple priors from historical data. Some trials have used non-informative priors to avoid the difficulties in specifying a prior distribution for the treatment effect or other parameter. One example was the PREVAIL II trial of ZMapp conducted during the 2015 Ebola outbreak in West Africa (The PREVAIL II Writing Group, 2016). Bayesian methods were applied in PREVAIL II to accommodate the data monitoring plan. After 20 patients were enrolled, data were analyzed after every 2 patients randomized to see if the trial could stop early, because of difficulties in recruiting, trial conduct, and drug shortages. The issues of prior distribution selection were thereby avoided. There are other applications of Bayesian methods that minimize the difficulties of prior selection, which could be considered for use in rare disease drug trials.

In rare disease drug development, a hybrid two-stage design can consist of an RCT or a single-arm study at the first stage and a real-world evidence study at the second stage. The first stage is used to demonstrate that the test treatment is not-ineffective with a small, but reasonable sample size,

---

BOX 4-5
Application of Bayesian Method: Hypoxic Ischaemic Encephalopathy

Hypoxic ischemic encephalopathy is a rare condition that occurs in newborns in which the brain does not receive enough oxygen or blood flow for a period of time, which can lead to potential organ damage. Multiple randomized clinical trials had demonstrated the benefit of therapeutic hypothermia within 6 hours of birth, but there were practical challenges with implementing such a rapid intervention. To address the question of whether therapeutic hypothermia could be effective at later time points, a Bayesian approach was applied that borrowed from historical data by considering three priors: a skeptical prior, an enthusiastic prior, and a neutral prior. The results of the study indicated that therapeutic hypothermia initiated 6–24 hours after birth reduced mortality and disability compared with the non-cooling standard of care.

SOURCE: Laptook et al., 2017.

while the second stage uses the Bayesian approach in conjunction with the technique of propensity score matching to demonstrate that the test treatment is effective by borrowing information from supplemental data (Chow et al., 2024).

The use of Bayesian methods in clinical trials offers potential benefits, particular for rare disease drug development, but they remain relatively underused, perhaps due to a lack of acceptance and familiarity on the part of regulators and sponsors (Ruberg et al., 2023). There are already in place the regulatory flexibilities for EMA and FDA to consider the use of ACD. Additional flexibilities on the part of EMA and FDA in allowing a two-stage process for demonstrating effectiveness (demonstrating no ineffectiveness first and then demonstrating effectiveness at the second stage) would likely help expand the use of these tools in drug development.

FDA held a public workshop in March 2024, "Advancing the Use of Complex Innovative Designs in Clinical Trials: From Pilot to Practice," and plans to publish draft guidance on the use of Bayesian methodology in clinical trials by the end of 2025 (FDA, 2023i). The workshop focused on the use of external data sources, Bayesian statistical methods, and simulations in complex innovative trial designs as well as on trial implementation (FDA, 2024a). In an FDA newsletter, the agency notes that Bayesian methods can be particularly useful for ultra-rare diseases because they allow for incorporating prior information and adapting the design more easily (FDA, 2023i). In addition, Bayesian methods can be helpful in using information from an adult population and applying it to a pediatric population (FDA, 2023i).

Network Meta-Analysis

Network meta-analysis (NMA) is a statistical approach that enables the simultaneous comparison of multiple interventions by combining evidence from direct and indirect treatment comparisons across trials (Rouse et al., 2017). This approach may be particularly valuable in the context of rare diseases for which limited patient populations often make traditional head-to-head RCTs impractical or unfeasible.

Drug development for rare diseases presents unique challenges, notably the difficulty of assembling large and diverse patient populations for RCTs, which is considered the best available standard for assessing treatment efficacy. The scarcity of patients often results in insufficient statistical power and may preclude the use of traditional RCTs altogether (Pizzamiglio et al., 2022). NMA addresses these challenges by efficiently pooling data from multiple smaller studies. This allows for the consolidation of evidence from diverse sources, thereby enhancing the statistical power and potentially reducing the time and cost associated with drug development (Tonin et al., 2017).

Furthermore, NMAs can help address the issue of comparing multiple treatments in situations where some treatments have never been directly compared in a clinical trial. By synthesizing both direct and indirect treatment comparisons, NMAs provide a more comprehensive view of the treatment landscape (Rouse et al., 2017; Tonin et al., 2017). This is crucial for rare diseases where limited patient numbers make it unfeasible to conduct multiple direct comparison trials. NMAs thus facilitate a better understanding of the relative effectiveness and safety of various treatments, guiding health care professionals in making informed decisions for patient care (Tonin et al., 2017).

To strengthen the reliability of NMAs, particularly when RCT data are sparse or absent, ACD collected through patient registries, observational studies, historical trial data, and non-randomized studies are often integrated to provide a fuller picture of treatment effects. The integration of these data requires robust statistical methods to adjust for potential biases and differences among data sources and to construct a more complete and nuanced analysis. For example, in the case of Friedreich's ataxia, NMAs were instrumental in aggregating data from numerous small-scale studies to provide a more comprehensive understanding of the disease progression and the potential cognitive impact of various interventions. By pooling evidence from multiple sources, these analyses have helped to overcome the limitations of individual studies with small sample sizes (Harding et al., 2021; Naeije, 2022). The insights gained from NMAs have informed the development of treatment guidelines and have been considered by FDA when evaluating new therapies targeting neurological outcomes in this rare disease. This approach has facilitated a more evidence-based decision-making process, ensuring that patients with Friedreich's ataxia have access to the most promising and well-studied treatments.

NMAs that incorporate evidence from case reports and small observational studies have also been pivotal in supporting drug approvals for specific subtypes of congenital myasthenic syndrome (CMS) (Della Marina et al., 2020; Huang et al., 2021). Given the extremely rare nature of these conditions, conducting traditional clinical trials is often not feasible. In such cases, FDA has relied on NMAs to assess the safety and efficacy of treatments like eculizumab for specific CMS subtypes where conventional clinical trial data is scarce. NMAs have enabled regulators to make informed decisions about the approval of targeted therapies for these rare conditions, ultimately improving patient outcomes and quality of life. By synthesizing evidence from diverse sources, NMAs provide a more comprehensive understanding of treatment effects, enabling regulators to make more informed decisions about whether innovative therapies make a meaningful difference in improving patient outcomes and quality of life.

FDA and EMA both use NMAs to inform regulatory decisions, yet their approaches exhibit some differences. FDA has developed draft guidance focusing on the use of RCT meta-analyses in evaluating drug safety, emphasizing the importance of selecting candidate trials that are of high quality (FDA, 2018b). This reflects a more cautious stance toward ensuring trial quality and similarity for indirect comparisons. Conversely, while specific EMA guidelines on NMAs were not highlighted in the search results, participants of qualitative interviews noted that real-world evidence and historical data may be more commonly considered in the European context, especially for rare diseases (see Appendix E for full methodology and results). Both agencies grapple with the challenge of defining the threshold of evidence quality needed for drug approvals without RCTs, but direct comparisons of their use of NMA results in decision making are not readily available. While FDA's guidance is more explicit in its focus on RCT data for safety NMAs, EMA's approach may implicitly encompass a broader spectrum of evidence sources. Further exploration is warranted to clarify these differences and how they may affect the evaluation of NMA evidence in the regulatory context.

Randomization-Based Inference

Randomization-based inference (RBI) is an analytical framework for clinical trials that accounts for any variation that might be intrinsic to the process of randomization or treatment allocation itself (i.e. it assesses the treatment effect on outcome under all possible randomization assignments) (Berger et al., 2021; Li and Izem, 2022). The various approaches include re-randomization and permutation methods. Although less pervasive and more computationally intense than traditional approaches, it is particularly useful in the context of the limited patient populations found with rare diseases (Ravichandran et al., 2024).

For rare disease trials, confounding may appear in the presence of linear time trends due to a long study duration or use of non-random approaches, such as minimization, wherein unspecified covariates are also subject to temporal trends (Li and Izem, 2022). More importantly, most conventional trials are built on a population-based inference assumption or a random sampling from a population of interest that is frequently inappropriate or infeasible for rare diseases. An advantage of RBI is that it does not require any distributional assumptions about the outcome and allows for control and an exact test of type 1 error rate. RBI reliably increases a trial's statistical power and ability to discern average treatment effect in the absence of model-based assumptions (Carter et al., 2023; Chipman, 2023).

A central tenet of RBI approaches is that the randomization approach is itself a key driver of statistical inference, and this underlies a growing recognition of its utility as supplemental data to trials based on likelihood-based testing (Berger et al., 2021). Furthermore, RBI is applicable to any randomization approach and underlying data type (e.g. categorial or continuous). It often leverages Monte Carlo simulation and tests a null hypothesis that an orphan drug has no effect on the treatment and control groups. Procedurally, the data are fixed at the observed values and re-randomization is performed using the original treatment assignment approach wherein each new assignment is treated independently. This process is repeated a significant number of times (> 10,000), and the p-value is estimated by the proportion of re-randomized trials wherein the treatment effect attributable to the placebo was larger than the originally observed treatment effect (The World Bank Group and DIME Analytics, n.d.).

RBI has been a successful method for study design. For example, the study of Nexviazyme for Pompe disease used novel randomization methods for a trial that led to marketing authorization (see Box 4-6).

In a 2015 guideline from EMA, recommendations against deterministic treatment allocation approaches were put forward, and randomization tests were strongly encouraged to mitigate Type 1 error (EMA, 2015). On the other hand, FDA's 2019 guidance on adaptive trial design includes the following language: "Covariate-adaptive treatment assignment techniques do not directly increase the Type I error probability when analyzed with the appropriate methodologies (generally randomization or permutation tests)" (FDA, 2019a).

Quantitative Systems Pharmacology

Quantitative systems pharmacology (QSP) is a type of drug and disease computational modeling that integrates drug features (e.g., dose, regimen, potency) with cellular, molecular, and pathophysiological data. A fundamental advantage of QSP for rare disease drug development programs is the potential to magnify insights based on multiple sources of alternative and confirmatory data which can be used to inform research and development programs from early-stage drug discovery through marketing authorization application. QSP can help mitigate risks to patients by virtually modeling variance or uncertainty and also has applications for identifying, interrogating, and validating biomarkers.

For example, a QSP model has been applied to predict treatment response for people living with Gaucher disease type 1 (GD1), a rare inherited disorder. Based on a virtual population of patients with varying severity of disease, QSP was shown to simulate the effectiveness of eliglustat, a first-line treatment for GD1 (Abrams et al., 2020). The GD1 QSP model provided a causally informed means for measuring response to experimental treatments, given the variability within the GD1 population, and could

BOX 4-6
Use Case: Nexviazyme® (Pompe Disease)

On August 6, 2021, the U.S. Food and Drug Administration (FDA) approved Nexviazyme® (avalglucosidase alfa-ngpt) for the treatment of late-onset Pompe disease, a rare genetic disorder that is characterized by progressive and irreversible weakness of cardiac and skeletal muscles which can lead to dependence on a wheelchair, ventilator support, and death. Nexviazyme received FDA breakthrough therapy, fast track, and orphan designations for the treatment of people with Pompe disease (FDA, 2021b). The European Medicines Agency (EMA) adopted a positive opinion of the drug on November 11, 2021, and the European Commission issued marketing authorization on June 24, 2022 (EMA, 2024b). Nexviazyme had originally received an orphan designation in EMA. However, at the time of authorization, the drug was not found to provide a significant benefit over an existing treatment (EMA, 2022d). Thus, the orphan designation was removed (EMA, 2022d).

For the marketing authorization application, the sponsor submitted results from a double-blinded, placebo-controlled randomized clinical trial along with a supplementary analysis (Proschan et al., 2011; van der Ploeg et al., 2010). The supplementary analysis served as an alternative to conventional randomization and included two features: (1) unequal allocation in which two patients were assigned to treatment for each one person assigned to placebo; and (2) the use of minimization rather than conventional randomization to assign participants to each arm. Minimization is an approach in which trial participants are placed in the treatment or placebo group based on existing imbalances in baseline data between groups.

The sponsor used a re-randomization test to validate the results of their supplementary analysis (Proschan et al., 2011). Re-randomization is an analytics method that simulates different participant randomization possibilities to show that the study result was not biased by the particular randomization used (Proschan et al., 2011). The re-randomization showed a *p*-value of 0.06, which might be considered only marginally significant. In comparison, another supportive test using analysis of covariance showed a standard *p*-value of 0.035. The sponsor argued that the re-randomization test had introduced bias (Proschan et al., 2011).

While the product was approved based on an assessment of the totality of evidence, this use case highlights the potential for confounding results due to the non-random treatment assignments commonly deployed in rare disease trials, especially under conditions of unequal allocation. An argument was made for avoiding the use of minimization that did not include a random element (Carter et al., 2023; Proschan et al., 2011).

be tuned to replicate clinically observed trends in biomarkers and organ volume. The study authors suggest that this model could help predict clinical response in real-world patient populations living with GD1.

Despite the lack of regulatory guidance for applying QSP modeling approaches, there has been a steady increase in the use of QSP models in FDA submissions (see Figure 4-6) (Cucurull-Sanchez, 2024). This has included QSP submissions for rare diseases (Bai et al., 2021).

The expansion and refinement of QSP modeling approaches will continue as the availability and uptake of high-quality alternative and confirmatory data increases. However, additional clarity from regulatory agencies is needed regarding data standards, nomenclature and definitions, and calibration and validation of QSP models (e.g., considerations for the variables, parameters, and virtual patient study cohorts). The potential for QSP models to enable extrapolation from computational prediction models to support clinical studies could mitigate risk for patients and enable the review and approval of much-needed drugs for rare disease patients.

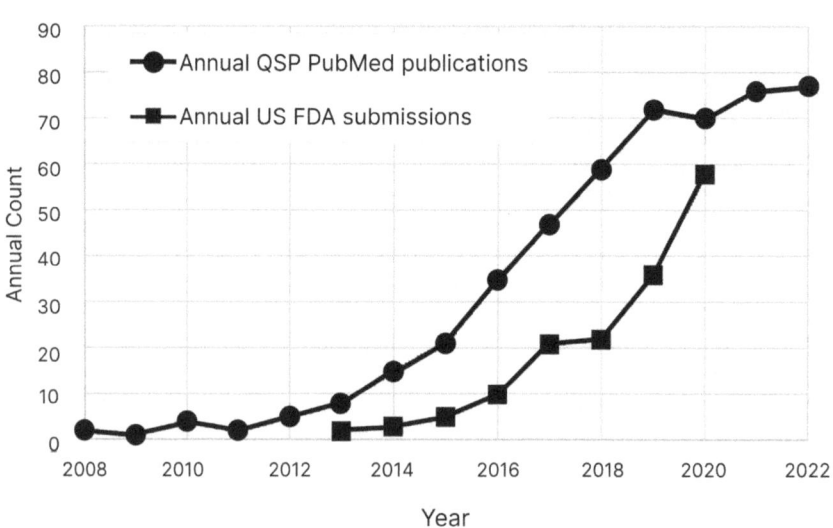

FIGURE 4-6 The number of annual QSP publications deposited to PubMed vs. QSP-based regulatory submissions reported by FDA from 2008 to 2022.
NOTE: QSP = quantitative systems pharmacology.
SOURCE: Adapted from Cucurull-Sanchez, 2024. CC BY 4.0 http://creativecommons.org/licenses/by/4.0/.

BIOMARKERS

Biomarkers used for regulatory decision-making are expected to provide "a clear and objective description of the anticipated benefits and risks of the biomarker for the proposed context of use, as well as any potential risk mitigation strategies" (FDA, 2018a). The use of biomarkers or a panel of biomarkers can help alleviate diagnostic challenges and facilitate clinical trials based on smaller sample sizes and shorter duration (Menkovic et al., 2020). However, as described in Chapters 1 and 2, limited populations and the heterogeneity in clinical presentation combined with a lack of information about disease emergence and progression, make it difficult to identify and validate biomarkers for regulatory decision-making. Additionally, there may be a "lack of readily measurable, recognized clinical endpoints due to unusual clinical disease biology" (Kakkis et al., 2015).

Biomarkers have been used to support orphan designated drug approvals: Among 233 drugs with orphan designations approved in 2001–2021, the primary efficacy endpoint was a pharmacodynamic or response biomarker for 136 (58 percent) (Kubota and Narukawa, 2023). For example, approval of sapropterin for the treatment of phenylketonuria was based on a primary efficacy endpoint (mean change in blood phenylalanine from baseline to 6 weeks) (CDER, 2007). Support for using blood phenylalanine as an endpoint was based on prior clinical experience from dietary restriction and a meta-analysis of previously published data (Kakkis et al., 2016; Waisbren et al., 2007).

While there are some examples of success, well-characterized endpoints are unavailable for many rare diseases (FDA, 2023f). Natural history studies can provide information about potential endpoints and the relationship between disease severity/progression and biomarker changes (FDA, 2019c; Vickers, 2013), as well as about clinical outcome assessments—measures that describe or reflect how a patient feels, functions, or survives (FDA, 2020a; Garrard, 2019). FDA guidance for industry, *Rare Diseases: Considerations for the Development of Drugs and Biological Products*, notes that "genetic, in vitro, animal model, and clinical data in patients with the disease as well as clinical pharmacodynamic data from early clinical investigations with the drug, can contribute to substantiate the use of the proposed biomarker as a surrogate" (FDA, 2023a). As emerging platform technologies, such as organ chips and microphysiological systems, continue to advance, it will be crucial to consider their potential role in supporting rare disease drug development and approval processes, necessitating further guidance on their application and contribution to these efforts.

Technological advancements in recent years (e.g. whole genome sequencing, bioinformatics, metabolomics, proteomics) have led to detection platforms and the growing identification of candidate biomarkers for rare diseases, although the validation of many is still pending (Bax, 2021). This is particularly important for rare diseases that progress more slowly. FDA and EMA have provided some guidance and guidelines for biomarker development (see Box 4-7).

Because of the small number of patients with rare diseases, an inherent challenge is accruing study sample sizes large enough to adequately power all endpoints. This commonly translates to a disproportionate focus on the primary endpoint and concomitant emphasis on the population most relevant for that endpoint. Criteria that focus on power to detect a difference for the study primary endpoint may obfuscate statistical efficacy measurement on important secondary endpoints. Conversely, using study eligibility criteria designed to enroll patients for all endpoints often slows accrual. For these reasons, endpoint selection and the use of biomarkers are particularly crucial in rare disease treatment development where small sample sizes affect statistical power for efficacy and safety determinations. Clinical outcome assessments may be used as endpoints for treatments for rare diseases.

BOX 4-7
Regulatory Guidance and Guidelines on Biomarkers

- The U.S. Food and Drug Administration guidance acknowledges that, given limited sample size, flexibility may be needed in qualifying biomarkers (FDA, 2018a) and that such strategies as exit interviews or surveys may be needed for Clinical Outcome Assessments (FDA, 2023e) to add greater depth to data for rare diseases (FDA, 2022b).
- The European Medicines Agency's (EMA's) 2006 *Guideline on Clinical Trials in Small Populations* has several pertinent statements related to the choice of endpoints that indicate regulatory flexibility (EMA, 2006):
  - Recognition that there may be too few patients to validate endpoints and test treatments.
  - Adequate follow-up in time to progression or time to remission can be obtained in open-label extension studies.
  - Given that the mode of action of the treatment may not be sufficiently well known, EMA states that "the usual approach of prespecifying the primary endpoint may be too conservative, and more knowledge may be gained from collecting all sensible/possible endpoints and then presenting all the data in the final study report. Still, every effort should be made to identify an appropriate hierarchy in the endpoints. If, collectively, the data look compelling, then a Marketing Authorisation may be grantable" (EMA, 2006).

For example, the multi-domain responder index (MDRI) approach was developed as a method to measure the impact of a treatment across multiple clinically relevant independent domains. The MDRI captures the aggregate benefit or decline across an array of pre-specified functional domains in order to evaluate clinically important changes by combining the results of independent domain endpoint responder analyses, each evaluated based on minimally important difference, into an overall responder score. This is proposed as an approach that mitigates the deleterious impact of heterogeneity on endpoint measurement. This sets the stage for less restrictive eligibility criteria to enroll a broader range of study patients and faster study accrual with the goal of increasing the number and speed of rare disease efficacy and safety studies (Tandon and Kakkis, 2021).

A digital biomarker is a characteristic or set of characteristics obtained from a digital health device that can be quantified as an indicator of biological process as well as response to a treatment. This definition includes deriving a digital biomarker sourced from multiple digital technologies simultaneously. The goals are an enhanced representation of population values, baseline study values at the patient level, and broader capture of changes in health status over time that can be particularly beneficial in rare disease populations with limited sample sizes and associated challenges in endpoint assessment. In order to be able to carry out objective, repeated measurement for status assessment in Huntington's disease beyond the existing Unified Huntington's Disease Rating Scale, a group developed a digital biomarker based on an accelerometer device that collected digital data on chest and limb movements in order to measure gait. The wearable sensors used both in clinic and at home were determined to be feasible and to appropriately capture differences in gait between Huntington's disease patients and controls (Andrzejewski et al., 2016).

As described earlier, in the context of rare disease, it is often valuable to use multiple assessment dimensions in determining treatment benefit. In these clinical scenarios, it may be important to establish co-primary endpoints for efficacy or safety determinations. However, this approach is particularly challenging in the rare disease space with limited study power due to small sample sizes if efficacy may only be claimed if each endpoint reaches statistical significance. This traditional strategy controls for type I error, and it is statistically highly conservative. Hence, the traditional method does not support inference when only one of the co-primary endpoints reaches significance. Fall-back tests for evaluation of co-primary endpoints provide for rejection of the null hypothesis in the same way as classical tests, with the benefit of providing inference when only a portion of the co-primary endpoints demonstrates statistically significant difference. Fall-back tests for co-primary endpoints make it possible to continue testing for inference, even in scenarios where the primary objective of the trial was not achieved which is much more likely in rare disease scenarios with small sample sizes (Ristl et al., 2016).

In 2024, the Reagan–Udall Foundation convened a workshop titled "Qualifying Biomarkers to Support Rare Disease Regulatory Pathways" The purpose of the workshop was to explore primary disease activity biomarkers for rare diseases. The workshop focused on neuronopathic lysosomal storage diseases using heparan sulfate as a case study for a biomarker to support accelerated approval. Participants included FDA representatives, patient advocates, researchers, and representatives from regulated industry (Reagan-Udall Foundation, 2024).

OPPORTUNITIES TO ENHANCE INNOVATION

As discussed above, there are well-described innovative methods for data analysis that do not jeopardize the integrity, quality, and scientific validity of rare disease drug development.

Conclusion 4-3: Given the variable and often longtime horizons for rare disease progression, gaps in the knowledge of disease etiology, ethical concerns, the severity of disease, small sample sizes, and unmet medical need, rare diseases require additional methods of demonstrating substantial evidence of effectiveness. New approaches in study design and data analysis need not require lower regulatory standards, but rather they enable the consideration of alternative and confirmatory data and a nuanced interpretation of the benefit–risk assessments that take into account limited availability of data, limited treatment availability, and the risk acceptance threshold in these unique patient populations.

Clinical development programs for rare disease products are often limited by the number of patients and ethical considerations, so, when possible, EMA and FDA are obligated to rely on the same evidence to assess effectiveness and safety of a rare disease treatment. However, in situations of limited evidence or when supporting evidence is not well defined, the interpretation of this evidence can vary between agencies. For example, FDA approved Relyvrio/Albrioza (sodium phenylbutyrate and taurursodiol) based on a study along with an open label extension study while EMA provided a negative opinion of the drug based on the same data (see Box 4-4 and Appendix H). There is an impetus for the agencies to identify areas for collaboration and better harmonization on the collection and use of alternative and confirmatory data. Additionally, there are opportunities for collaborative efforts between the agencies to prospectively validate the use of these data and analytical methodologies for incorporating them into marketing authorization applications for rare disease drug products.

Conclusion 4-4: There is an obligation on the part of regulators and drug sponsors to improve transparency about when and how alternative and confirmatory data have been considered in regulatory decision-making to ensure that there are no missed opportunities to integrate lessons learned from past successes and failures. An understanding of the opportunities as well as the gaps and inadequacies in alternative and confirmatory data would help guide future evidence generation strategies on the part of patients, caregivers, sponsors, and researchers, and ensure that the data gathered are both relevant and robust enough to support regulatory decision-making.

The lack of publicly shared information on the consideration and use of alternative and confirmatory data as well as the innovative study designs and methods restricts the evolution and harmonization of innovative regulatory strategies and methods for data analysis, limiting opportunities for setting robust standards akin to those established for RCTs.

RECOMMENDATION 4-3: The U.S. Food and Drug Administration (FDA) should collect and disseminate information on how state-of-the art regulatory science; innovative study designs and methods; tools, including biomarkers and surrogate endpoints; and effective applications of alternative and confirmatory data inform regulatory decision-making for rare disease drug products by:
- Annually convening the European Medicines Agency, National Institutes of Health (NIH) National Center for Advancing Translational Sciences, industry, patient groups, and the broad stakeholder community to review new advances in regulatory science (pre-clinical, clinical, and platform technologies), iterate on innovative study design and methods, and consider other uses of alternative and confirmatory data for regulatory decision-making. Following each meeting, FDA and NIH should publish a publicly accessible summary of key themes and issues discussed;
- Publishing innovative methods for data analysis that have been used to support regulatory approval of drugs for a rare disease or condition, including information about how the methods were used or considered by the agency;
- Collaborating on the validation of clinical and pre-clinical drug development tools for drugs to treat rare diseases and conditions.

SUMMARY OF CONCLUSIONS AND RECOMMENDATIONS

Conclusion 4-1: The low prevalence of rare diseases and conditions, incomplete understanding of their underlying biology, ethical challenges in giving placebo to patients with rare diseases in double-blind clinical trials, and limitations in the ability to conduct randomized clinical trials (RCTs) for new therapies for them, have necessitated the collection and use of data from sources other than traditional RCTs for marketing authorization applications for rare disease drug products.

Conclusion 4-2: Understanding the natural history of a disease—as well as the factors that affect its progression and outcomes—is important for drug development. However, for most rare diseases and conditions, there is often little information about natural history.

Conclusion 4-3: Given the variable and often longtime horizons for rare disease progression, gaps in the knowledge of disease etiology, ethical concerns, severity of disease, small sample sizes, and unmet medical need, rare diseases require additional methods of demonstrating substantial evidence of effectiveness. New approaches in study design and data analysis need not require lower regulatory standards, but rather they enable the consideration of alternative and confirmatory data and a nuanced interpretation of the benefit–risk assessments that take into account the limited availability of data, limited treatment availability, and the risk acceptance threshold in these unique patient populations.

Conclusion 4-4: There is an obligation on the part of regulators and drug sponsors to improve transparency about when and how alternative and confirmatory data have been considered in regulatory decision-making to ensure that there are no missed opportunities to integrate lessons learned from past successes and failures. An understanding of the opportunities as well as the gaps and inadequacies in alternative and confirmatory data would help guide future evidence generation strategies on the part of patients, caregivers, sponsors, and researchers, and ensure that the data gathered are both relevant and robust enough to support regulatory decision-making.

RECOMMENDATION 4-1: The U.S. Food and Drug Administration (FDA) should enable the collection and curation of regulatory-grade natural history data to enhance the quality and accessibility of data for all rare diseases. This should include, but not be limited to:

- Continuation and expansion of support for current rare disease natural history design and data collection programs, such as FDA's Office of Orphan Products Development awarding clinical trial and natural history study grants
- Continuation and expansion of data aggregation, standardization, and analysis programs, including, but not limited to Critical Path Institute's Rare Disease Cures Accelerator-Data and Analytics Platform
- Support, education, training, and access to resources/infrastructure for nascent rare disease advocacy groups to enable the standardization and integration of patient-level data for future regulatory use.
- Continuation and expansion of collaboration with other agencies (e.g., National Institutes of Health Rare Disease Clinical Research Network) to expand natural history design and data collection resources for all rare diseases.
- Periodic assessment regarding the impact and opportunities for improvement of ongoing programs for the collection, curation, and use of natural history data in regulatory decision-making for rare disease drug development programs.

RECOMMENDATION 4-2: The U.S. Food and Drug Administration (FDA) should invite the European Medicines Agency (EMA) to jointly conduct systematic reviews of submitted and approved marketing authorization applications to treat rare diseases and conditions that document cases for which alternative and confirmatory data have contributed to regulatory decision-making. The systematic reviews should include relevant information on the context for whether these data were:
- found to be adequate, and why they were found to be adequate
- found to be inadequate, and why they were found to be inadequate
- found to be useful in supporting decision making and to what extent

Findings from the systematic reviews should be made publicly available and accessible for sponsors, researchers, patients, and their caregivers through public reporting or publication of the results. EMA and FDA should establish a public database for these findings that is continuously updated to ensure that progress over time is captured, opportunities to clarify agency thinking over time are identified, and information on the use of ACD to inform regulatory decision-making is publicly shared to inform the rare disease drug development community.

RECOMMENDATION 4-3: The U.S. Food and Drug Administration (FDA) should collect and disseminate information on how state-of-the art regulatory science; innovative study designs and methods; tools, including biomarkers and surrogate endpoints; and effective applications of alternative and confirmatory data inform regulatory decision-making for rare disease drug products by:

- Annually convening the European Medicines Agency, National Institutes of Health (NIH) National Center for Advancing Translational Sciences, industry, patient groups, and the broad stakeholder community to review new advances in regulatory science (pre-clinical, clinical, and platform technologies), iterate on innovative study design and methods, and consider other uses of alternative and confirmatory data for regulatory decision-making. Following each meeting, FDA and NIH should publish a publicly accessible summary of key themes and issues discussed;
- Publishing innovative methods for data analysis that have been used to support regulatory approval of drugs for a rare disease or condition, including information about how the methods were used or considered by the agency;
- Collaborating on the validation of clinical and pre-clinical drug development tools for drugs to treat rare diseases and conditions.

REFERENCES

Abrams, R., C. D. Kaddi, M. Tao, R. J. Leiser, G. Simoni, F. Reali, J. Tolsma, P. Jasper, Z. van Rijn, J. Li, B. Niesner, J. S. Barrett, L. Marchetti, M. J. Peterschmitt, K. Azer, and S. Neves-Zaph. 2020. A quantitative systems pharmacology model of Gaucher disease type 1 provides mechanistic insight into the response to substrate reduction therapy with Eliglustat. *CPT: Pharmacometrics & Systems Pharmacology* 9(7):374-383.

Amylyx Pharmaceuticals. 2024. *Amylyx pharmaceuticals announces formal intention to remove Relyvrio®/Albrioza™ from the market; provides updates on access to therapy, pipeline, corporate restructuring, and strategy.* https://www.amylyx.com/news/amylyx-pharmaceuticals-announces-formal-intention-to-remove-relyvrior/albriozatm-from-the-market-provides-updates-on-access-to-therapy-pipeline-corporate-restructuring-and-strategy (accessed August 15, 2024).

Anatol, R. 2024. Regulatory flexibilities for cell and gene therapies for rare diseases. *Processes to Evaluate the Safety and Efficacy of Drugs for Rare Diseases or Conditions in the United States and the European Union* (Meeting 3 - Virtual).

Andrzejewski, K. L., A. V. Dowling, D. Stamler, T. J. Felong, D. A. Harris, C. Wong, H. Cai, R. Reilmann, M. A. Little, J. T. Gwin, K. M. Biglan, and E. R. Dorsey. 2016. Wearable sensors in huntington disease: A pilot study. *Journal of Huntington's Disease* 5(2):199-206.

Angelman Syndrome Foundation. n.d. *LADDER.* https://www.angelman.org/as-research/ladder/ (accessed August 15, 2024).

Bai, J. P. F., J. C. Earp, J. Florian, R. Madabushi, D. G. Strauss, Y. Wang, and H. Zhu. 2021. Quantitative systems pharmacology: Landscape analysis of regulatory submissions to the US Food and Drug Administration. *CPT: Pharmacometrics & Systems Pharmacology* 10(12):1479-1484.

Barrett, J. S., A. Betourne, R. L. Walls, K. Lasater, S. Russell, A. Borens, S. Rohatagi, and W. Roddy. 2023. The future of rare disease drug development: The rare disease cures accelerator data analytics platform (RDCA-DAP). *Journal of Pharmacokinetics and Pharmacodynamics* 50(6):507-519.

Bax, B. E. 2021. Biomarkers in rare diseases. *International Journal of Molecular Sciences* 22(2).

Beckman, R. A. 2018. *Design concept for a confirmatory basket trial.* https://www.ema.europa.eu/en/documents/presentation/presentation-session-5-design-concept-confirmatory-basket-trial-robert-beckman_en.pdf (accessed August 15, 2024).

Berger, V. W., L. J. Bour, K. Carter, J. J. Chipman, C. C. Everett, N. Heussen, C. Hewitt, R.-D. Hilgers, Y. A. Luo, J. Renteria, Y. Ryeznik, O. Sverdlov, D. Uschner, and Randomization Innovative Design Scientific Working Group. 2021. A roadmap to using randomization in clinical trials. *BMC Medical Research Methodology* 21(1).

Berry, D. A. 2006. Bayesian clinical trials. *Nature Reviews Drug Discovery* 5(1).

Brown, J., and A. Ekangaki. 2023. *To placebo or not to placebo? The great debate in rare disease trials.* https://premier-research.com/blog-to-placebo-or-not-to-placebo-the-great-debate-in-rare-disease-trials/ (accessed August 1, 2024).

Bunnik, E. M., and N. Aarts. 2021. The role of physicians in expanded access to investigational drugs: A mixed-methods study of physicians' views and experiences in the Netherlands. *Journal of Bioethical Inquiry* 18(2):319-334.

Bunnik, E. M., N. Aarts, and S. van de Vathorst. 2018. Little to lose and no other options: Ethical issues in efforts to facilitate expanded access to investigational drugs. *Health Policy* 122(9):977-983.

Burcu, M., N. A. Dreyer, J. M. Franklin, M. D. Blum, C. W. Critchlow, E. M. Perfetto, and W. Zhou. 2020. Real-world evidence to support regulatory decision-making for medicines: Considerations for external control arms. *Pharmacoepidemiology and Drug Safety* 29(10):1228-1235.

Carter, K., A. Scheffold, J. Renteria, V. Berger, Y. A. Luo, J. Chipman, and O. Sverdlov. 2023. Regulatory guidance on randomization and the use of randomization tests in clinical trials: A systematic review. *Statistics in Biopharmaceutical Research*, 1–13.

Cave, A., X. Kurz, and P. Arlett. 2019. Real-world data for regulatory decision making: Challenges and possible solutions for Europe. *Clinical Pharmacology and Therapeutics* 106(1):36-39.

CDER (Center for Drug Evaluation and Research). 2007. *Summary Review - Application 22-181.* https://www.accessdata.fda.gov/drugsatfda_docs/nda/2007/022181s000_SumR.pdf (accessed August 1, 2024).

Chipman, J. J., L. Mayberry, and R. A. Greevy Jr., 2023. Rematching on-the-fly: Sequential matched randomization and a case for covariate-adjusted randomization. *Statistics in Medicine* 42(22).

Cho, D., S. Cheyne, S. J. Lord, J. Simes, and C. K. Lee. 2022. Extrapolating evidence for molecularly targeted therapies from common to rare cancers: A scoping review of methodological guidance. *BMJ Open* 12(7):e058350.

Chow, S.-C. 2020. *Innovative methods for rare disease drug development.* 1st ed. Chapman and Hall/CRC.

Chow, S. C., A. Pong, and S. S. Chow. 2024. Novel design and analysis for rare disease drug development. *Mathematics* 12(5):631.

CIRS (Centre for Innovation in Regulatory Science). 2024. Data analysis and summary to help inform the National Academies committee on Processes to Evaluate the Safety and Efficacy of Drugs for Rare Diseases or Conditions in the United States and the European Union. Data analysis commissioned by the Committee on Processes to Evaluate the Safety and Efficacy of Drugs for Rare Diseases or Conditions in the United States and the European Union. National Academies of Sciences, Engineering, and Medicine, Washington, DC.

Critical Path Institute. n.d. *Rare Disease Cures Accelerator-Data and Analytics Platform.* https://c-path.org/program/rare-disease-cures-accelerators-data-and-analytics-platform/ (accessed March 7, 2024).

Cucurull-Sanchez, L. 2024. An industry perspective on current QSP trends in drug development. *Journal of Pharmacokinetics and Pharmacodynamics.* https://doi.org/10.1007/s10928-024-09905-y.

Della Marina, A., E. Wibbeler, A. Abicht, H. Kölbel, H. Lochmüller, A. Roos, and U. Schara. 2020. Long term follow-up on pediatric cases with congenital myasthenic syndromes—A retrospective single centre cohort study. *Frontiers in Human Neuroscience* 14.

Eichler, H.-G., B. Bloechl-Daum, P. Bauer, F. Bretz, J. Brown, L. Hampson, P. Honig, M. Krams, H. Leufkens, R. Lim, M. Lumpkin, M. Murphy, F. Pignatti, M. Posch, S. Schneeweiss, M. Trusheim, and F. Koenig. 2016. "Threshold-crossing": A useful way to establish the counterfactual in clinical trials? *Clinical Pharmacology & Therapeutics* 100(6):699-712.

EMA (European Medicines Agency). 2000. *Points to consider on switching between superiority and non-inferiority.* https://www.ema.europa.eu/en/documents/scientific-guideline/points-consider-switching-between-superiority-and-non-inferiority_en.pdf (accessed August 1, 2024).

EMA. 2001. *Points to consider on application with 1. Meta-analyses; 2. One pivotal study.* https://www.ema.europa.eu/en/documents/scientific-guideline/points-consider-application-1meta-analyses-2one-pivotal-study_en.pdf (accessed August 1, 2024).

EMA. 2006. *Guideline on clinical trials in small populations.* https://www.ema.europa.eu/en/documents/scientific-guideline/guideline-clinical-trials-small-populations_en.pdf (accessed August 1, 2024).

EMA. 2007. *Guideline on compassionate use of medicinal peoducts, pursuant to article 83 of regulation (EC) No 7216/2004.* https://www.ema.europa.eu/en/documents/regulatory-procedural-guideline/guideline-compassionate-use-medicinal-products-pursuant-article-83-regulation-ec-no-7262004_en.pdf (accessed August 1, 2024).

EMA. 2015. *Guideline on adjustment for baseline covariates in clinical trials.* https://www.ema.europa.eu/en/documents/scientific-guideline/guideline-adjustment-baseline-covariates-clinical-trials_en.pdf (accessed August 1, 2024).

EMA. 2017. *ICH guideline E17 on general principles for planning and design of multi-regional clinical trials.* https://www.ema.europa.eu/en/documents/scientific-guideline/ich-guideline-e17-general-principles-planning-design-multi-regional-clinical-trials-step-5-first-version_en.pdf (accessed August 1, 2024).

EMA. 2021a. *Guideline on registry-based studies.* https://www.ema.europa.eu/en/documents/scientific-guideline/guideline-registry-based-studies_en.pdf-0 (accessed August 1, 2024).

EMA. 2021b. *A vision for use of real-world evidence in EU medicines regulation.* https://www.ema.europa.eu/en/news/vision-use-real-world-evidence-eu-medicines-regulation (accessed August 15, 2024).

EMA. 2022a. *Complex clinical trials—Questions and answers.* https://health.ec.europa.eu/system/files/2022-06/medicinal_qa_complex_clinical-trials_en.pdf (accessed August 1, 2024).

EMA. 2022b. *Concept paper on platform trials.* https://www.ema.europa.eu/en/documents/scientific-guideline/concept-paper-platform-trials_en.pdf (accessed August 1, 2024).

EMA. 2022c. *Good practice guide for the use of the metadata catalogue of real-world data sources.* https://www.ema.europa.eu/en/documents/regulatory-procedural-guideline/good-practice-guide-use-metadata-catalogue-real-world-data-sources_en.pdf (accessed August 1, 2024).

EMA. 2022d. *Nexviadyme: Orphan maintenance assessment report.* https://www.ema.europa.eu/system/files/documents/orphan-maintenance-report/nexviadyme_-_orphan_maintenance_assessment_report_en.pdf (accessed August 1, 2024).

EMA. 2023a. *Albrioza: Assessment report.* https://www.ema.europa.eu/en/documents/assessment-report/albrioza-epar-refusal-public-assessment-report_en.pdf (accessed August 1, 2024).

EMA. 2023b. *Real-world evidence framework to support EU regulatory decision-making.* https://www.ema.europa.eu/system/files/documents/report/real-world-evidence-framework-support-eu-regulatory-decision-making-report-experience-gained_en.pdf (accessed August 1, 2024).

EMA. 2023c. *Reflection paper on establishing efficacy based on single arm trials submitted as pivotal evidence in a marketing authorisation.* https://www.ema.europa.eu/en/documents/scientific-guideline/reflection-paper-establishing-efficacy-based-single-arm-trials-submitted-pivotal-evidence-marketing-authorisation_en.pdf (accessed August 1, 2024).

EMA. 2024a. *Albrioza: EPAR.* https://www.ema.europa.eu/en/medicines/human/EPAR/albrioza (accessed August 15, 2024).

EMA. 2024b. *Nexviadyme.* https://www.ema.europa.eu/en/medicines/human/EPAR/nexviadyme (accessed August 15, 2024).

EMA. 2024c. *Real-world evidence provided by EMA.* https://www.ema.europa.eu/en/documents/other/guidance-real-world-evidence-provided-ema-support-regulatory-decision-making_en.pdf (accessed August 1, 2024).

EMA. 2024d. *SkyClarys: EPAR.* https://www.ema.europa.eu/en/medicines/human/EPAR/skyclarys (accessed August 15, 2024).

EMA. n.d. *Compassionate use.* https://www.ema.europa.eu/en/human-regulatory-overview/research-development/compassionate-use (accessed August 15, 2024).

FDA (U.S. Food and Drug Administration). 1998. *Providing clinical evidence of effectiveness for human drug and biological product: Guidance for industry.* https://www.fda.gov/media/71655/download (accessed August 1, 2024).

FDA. 2009. *Patient-reported outcome measures: Use in medical product development to support labeling claims: Guidance for industry.* https://www.fda.gov/media/77832/download (accessed August 1, 2024).

FDA. 2016. *Non-inferiority clinical trials to establish effectiveness: Guidance for industry.* https://www.fda.gov/media/78504/download (accessed August 1, 2024).

FDA. 2018a. *Biomarker qualification: Evidentiary framework: Guidance for industry and FDA staff* https://www.fda.gov/media/122319/download (accessed August 1, 2024).

FDA. 2018b. *Meta-analyses of randomized controlled clinical trials to evaluate the safety of human drugs or biological products: Guidance for industry.* https://www.fda.gov/media/117976/download (accessed August 1, 2024).

FDA. 2019a. *Adaptive designs for clinical trials of drugs and biologics: Guidance for industry.* https://www.fda.gov/media/78495/download (accessed August 1, 2024).

FDA. 2019b. *Demonstrating substantial evidence of effectiveness for human drug and biological products: Guidance for industry.* https://www.fda.gov/media/133660/download (accessed August 1, 2024).

FDA. 2019c. *Rare diseases: Natural history studies for drug development: Guidance for industry.* https://www.fda.gov/media/122425/download (accessed August 1, 2024).

FDA. 2020a. *Clinical outcome assessment (COA): Frequently asked questions.* https://www.fda.gov/about-fda/clinical-outcome-assessment-coa-frequently-asked-questions (accessed August 15, 2024).

FDA. 2020b. *Enhancing the diversity of clinical trial populations—Eligibility criteria, enrollment practices, and trial designs: Guidance for industry.* https://www.fda.gov/media/127712/download (accessed August 1, 2024).

FDA. 2021a. *Examples of real-world evidence (RWE) used in medical device regulatory decisions.* https://www.fda.gov/media/146258/download (accessed August 1, 2024).

FDA. 2021b. *Nexviazyme: Integrated assessment.* https://www.accessdata.fda.gov/drugsatfda_docs/nda/2021/761194Orig1s000IntegratedR.pdf (accessed August 1, 2024).

FDA. 2022a. *Expanded access to investigational drugs for treatment use: Questions and answers: Guidance for industry.* https://www.fda.gov/media/162793/download (accessed August 1, 2024).

FDA. 2022b. *Patient-focused drug development: Methods to identify what is important to patients: Guidance for industry, Food and Drug Administration staff, and other stakeholders.* https://www.fda.gov/media/131230/download (accessed August 1, 2024).

FDA. 2022c. *Relyvrio: Summary review.* https://www.accessdata.fda.gov/drugsatfda_docs/nda/2022/216660Orig1s000SumR.pdf (accessed August 1, 2024).

FDA. 2023a. *Benefit-risk assessment for new drug and biological products: Guidance for industry.* https://www.fda.gov/media/152544/download (accessed August 1, 2024).

FDA. 2023b. *Clinical trial and natural history study grants.* https://www.fda.gov/industry/clinical-trial-and-natural-history-study-grants (accessed March 15, 2024).

FDA. 2023c. *Considerations for the design and conduct of externally controlled trials for drug and biological products: Guidance for industry.* https://www.fda.gov/media/164960/download (accessed August 1, 2024).

FDA. 2023d. *Demonstrating substantial evidence of effectiveness with one adequate and well-controlled clinical investigation and confirmatory evidence: Guidance for industry.* https://www.fda.gov/media/172166/download (accessed August 1, 2024).

FDA. 2023e. *Patient-focused drug development: Incorporating clinical outcome assessments into endpoints for regulatory decision-making: Guidance for industry, food and drug administration staff, and other stakeholders.* https://www.fda.gov/media/166830/download (accessed August 1, 2024).

FDA. 2023f. *Rare diseases: Considerations for the development of drugs and biological products: Guidance for industry.* https://www.fda.gov/media/119757/download (accessed August 1, 2024).

FDA. 2023g. *Real-world evidence.* https://www.fda.gov/science-research/science-and-research-special-topics/real-world-evidence (accessed June 25, 2024).

FDA. 2023h. *SkyClarys: Summary review.* https://www.accessdata.fda.gov/drugsatfda_docs/nda/2023/216718Orig1s000SumR.pdf (accessed August 1, 2024).

FDA. 2023i. *Using Bayesian statistical approaches to advance our ability to evaluate drug products.* https://www.fda.gov/drugs/cder-small-business-industry-assistance-sbia/using-bayesian-statistical-approaches-advance-our-ability-evaluate-drug-products (accessed August 1, 2024).

FDA. 2024a. *Advancing the use of complex innovative designs in clinical trials: From pilot to practice.* https://www.fda.gov/news-events/advancing-use-complex-innovative-designs-clinical-trials-pilot-practice-03052024 (accessed August 15, 2024).

FDA. 2024b. *Expanded access.* https://www.fda.gov/news-events/public-health-focus/expanded-access (accessed August 15, 2024).

Feldman, D., J. Avorn, and A. S. Kesselheim. 2022. Use of extrapolation in new drug approvals by the US Food and Drug Administration. *JAMA Netw Open* 5(4):e227958.

Flynn, R., K. Plueschke, C. Quinten, V. Strassmann, R. G. Duijnhoven, M. Gordillo-Maranon, M. Rueckbeil, C. Cohet, and X. Kurz. 2022. Marketing authorization applications made to the European Medicines Agency in 2018-2019: What was the contribution of real-world evidence? *Clinical Pharmacology & Therapeutics* 111(1):90-97.

Garrard, L. 2019. *Endpoint selection and use of clinical outcome assessments (COAs) in rare disease and pediatric trials.* https://www.fda.gov/media/133752/download (accessed August 1, 2024).

Harding, I. H., S. Chopra, F. Arrigoni, S. Boesch, A. Brunetti, S. Cocozza, L. A. Corben, A. Deistung, M. Delatycki, S. Diciotti, I. Dogan, S. Evangelisti, M. C. França, Jr., S. L. Göricke, N. Georgiou-Karistianis, L. L. Gramegna, P. G. Henry, C. R. Hernandez-Castillo, D. Hutter, N. Jahanshad, J. M. Joers, C. Lenglet, R. Lodi, D. N. Manners, A. R. M. Martinez, A. Martinuzzi, C. Marzi, M. Mascalchi, W. Nachbauer, C. Pane, D. Peruzzo, P. K. Pisharady, G. Pontillo, K. Reetz, T. J. R. Rezende, S. Romanzetti, F. Saccà, C. Scherfler, J. B. Schulz, A. Stefani, C. Testa, S. I. Thomopoulos, D. Timmann, S. Tirelli, C. Tonon, M. Vavla, G. F. Egan, and P. M. Thompson. 2021. Brain structure and degeneration staging in Friedreich Ataxia: Magnetic resonance imaging volumetrics from the ENIGMA-Ataxia Working Group. *Annals of Neurology* 90(4):570-583.

Higgens, K. M., and G. Levin. n.d. *Considerations for open-label clinical trials: Design, conduct, and analysis.* https://www.fda.gov/media/168664/download (accessed August 1, 2024).

Huang, K., Y.-B. Luo, F.-F. Bi, and H. Yang. 2021. Pharmacological strategy for congenital myasthenic syndrome with CHRNE mutations: A meta-analysis of case reports. *Current Neuropharmacology* 19(5).

ICH (International Council for Harmonisation of Technical Requirements for Pharmaceuticals for Human Use). 2001. *E10 choice of control group and related issues in clinical trials: Guidance for industry.* https://www.ema.europa.eu/en/documents/scientific-guideline/ich-e-10-choice-control-group-clinical-trials-step-5_en.pdf (accessed August 1, 2024).

ICH. 2019. *Final concept paper - E20: Adaptive clinical trials.* https://database.ich.org/sites/default/files/E20_FinalConceptPaper_2019_1107_0.pdf (accessed August 1, 2024).

ICH. 2022. *Pediatric extrapolation - E11A.* https://www.fda.gov/media/161190/download (accessed August 1, 2024).

Jahanshahi, M., K. Gregg, G. Davis, A. Ndu, V. Miller, J. Vockley, C. Ollivier, T. Franolic, and S. Sakai. 2021. The use of external controls in FDA regulatory decision making. *Therapeutic Innovation & Regulatory Science* 55(5).

Jarow, J. P., and R. Moscicki. 2017. Impact of expanded access on FDA regulatory action and product labeling. *Therapeutic Innovation & Regulatory Science* 51(6):787-789.

Jarow, J. P., S. Lemery, K. Bugin, S. Khozin, and R. Moscicki. 2016. Expanded access of investigational drugs: The experience of the Center for Drug Evaluation and Research over a 10-year period. *Therapeutic Innovation & Regulatory Science* 50(6):705-709.

Kakkis, E. D., M. O'Donovan, G. Cox, M. Hayes, F. Goodsaid, P. K. Tandon, P. Furlong, S. Boynton, M. Bozic, M. Orfali, and M. Thornton. 2015. Recommendations for the development of rare disease drugs using the accelerated approval pathway and for qualifying biomarkers as primary endpoints. *Orphanet Journal of Rare Diseases* 10:16.

Kakkis, E. D., S. Kowalcyk, M. G. Bronstein, E. D. Kakkis, S. Kowalcyk, and M. G. Bronstein. 2016. Accessing the accelerated approval pathway for rare disease therapeutics. *Nature Biotechnology* 34(4).

Kearns, L., C. R. Chapman, K. I. Moch, A. L. Caplan, T. Watson, A. McFadyen, P. Furlong, and A. Bateman-House. 2021. Gene therapy companies have an ethical obligation to develop expanded access policies. *Molecular Therapy* 29(4):1367-1369.

Kesselheim, A. S., J. A. Myers, and J. Avorn. 2011. Characteristics of clinical trials to support approval of orphan vs nonorphan drugs for cancer. *JAMA* 305(22):2320-2326.

Khachatryan, A., S. H. Read, and T. Madison. 2023. External control arms for rare diseases: Building a body of supporting evidence. *Journal of Pharmacokinetics and Pharmacodynamics* 50(6):501-506.

Kubota, Y., and M. Narukawa. 2023. Randomized controlled trial data for successful new drug application for rare diseases in the United States. *Orphanet Journal of Rare Diseases* 18(1):89.

Laptook, A., S. Shankaran, J. Tyson, B. Munoz, E. Bell, R. Goldberg, N. Parikh, N. Ambalavanan, C. Pedroza, A. Pappas, A. Das, A. Chaudhary, R. Ehrenkranz, A. Hensman, K. Van Meurs, L. Chalak, A. Khan, S. Hamrick, G. Sokol, M. Walsh, B. Poindexter, R. Faix, K. Watterberg, I. I. Frantz, R. Guillet, U. Devaskar, W. Truog, V. Chock, M. Wyckoff, E. McGowan, D. Carlton, H. Harmon, J. Brumbaugh, C. Cotten, P. Sánchez, A. Hibbs, and R. Higgins. 2017. Effect of therapeutic hypothermia initiated after 6 hours of age on death or disability among newborns with hypoxic-ischemic encephalopathy: A randomized clinical trial. *JAMA* 318(16).

Li, Y., and R. Izem. 2022. Novel clinical trial design and analytic methods to tackle challenges in therapeutic development in rare diseases. *Annals of Translational Medicine* 10(18).

Liu, J., J. S. Barrett, E. T. Leonardi, L. Lee, S. Roychoudhury, Y. Chen, and P. Trifillis. 2022. Natural history and real-world data in rare diseases: Applications, limitations, and future perspectives. *Journal of Clinical Pharmacology* 62 Suppl 2(Suppl 2):S38-S55.

Menkovic, I., M. Boutin, A. Alayoubi, F. E. Mercier, G.-É. Rivard, and C. Auray-Blais. 2020. Identification of a reliable biomarker profile for the diagnosis of Gaucher disease type 1 patients using a mass spectrometry-based metabolomic approach. *International Journal of Molecular Sciences* 21(21):7869.

Michael, T., and J. D. Zhang. 2023. Causal inference in drug discovery and development. *Drug Discovery Today* 28(10).

Miller, K. L., C. Mueller, G. Liu, K. I. Miller Needleman, and J. Maynard. 2020. FDA orphan products clinical trial grants: assessment of outcomes and impact on rare disease product development. *Orphanet Journal of Rare Diseases* 15(1):234.

Naeije, G., J. B. Schulz, and L. A. Corben. 2022. The cognitive profile of Friedreich ataxia: A systematic review and meta-analysis. *BMC Neurology* 22(1).

NORD (National Organization for Rare Disorders). 2016. *NORD announces 20 rare disease patient groups selected to develop natural history studies as part of FDA cooperative agreement.* https://rarediseases.org/nord-announces-20-rare-disease-patient-groups-selected-to-develop-natural-history-studies-as-part-of-fda-cooperative-agreement/ (accessed March 12, 2024).

NORD. 2021. *RDCA-DAP: Shortening the timeline for developing new treatments for rare diseases.* https://www.youtube.com/watch?v=CKxrZH4HAs0 (accessed August 1, 2024).

NORD. 2023. *IAMRARE program overview.* https://rarediseases.org/wp-content/uploads/2023/12/IAMRARE-Overview.pdf (accessed August 1, 2024).

NORD. n.d. *IAMRARE program powered by NORD.* https://iamrare.org/?utm_source=rarediseases_org&utm_medium=website&utm_campaign=IAMRARE+Referral&utm_id=Rare+Disease+Org+Referral (accessed August 1, 2024).

Oneal, P. A., V. Kwitkowski, L. Luo, Y. L. Shen, S. Subramaniam, S. Shord, K. B. Goldberg, A. E. McKee, E. Kaminskas, A. Farrell, and R. Pazdur. 2018. FDA approval summary: Vemurafenib for the treatment of patients with Erdheim-Chester Disease with the BRAFV600 mutation. *Oncologist* 23(12):1520-1524.

Pizzamiglio, C., H. J. Vernon, M. G. Hanna, and R. D. S. Pitceathly. 2022. Designing clinical trials for rare diseases: Unique challenges and opportunities. *Nature Reviews Methods Primers* 2(1):13.

Pocock, S. J., C. A. Ariti, T. J. Collier, and D. Wang. 2012. The WIN ratio: A new approach to the analysis of composite endpoints in clinical trials based on clinical priorities. *European Heart Journal* 33(2):176-182.

Polak, T. B., J. van Rosmalen, and C. A. Uyl-De Groot. 2020. Response to open peer commentary "Making it count: Extracting real world data from compassionate use and expanded access programs." *The American Journal of Bioethics* 20(11):W4-W5.

Polak, T. B., D. G. J. Cucchi, J. van Rosmalen, C. A. Uyl-de Groot, and J. J. Darrow. 2022. Generating evidence from expanded access use of rare disease medicines: Challenges and recommendations. *Frontiers in Pharmacology* 13:913567.

Pontes, C., J. M. Fontanet, R. Vives, A. Sancho, M. Gómez-Valent, J. Ríos, R. Morros, J. Martinalbo, M. Posch, A. Koch, K. Roes, K. Oude Rengerink, J. Torrent-Farnell, F. Torres, C. Pontes, J. M. Fontanet, R. Vives, A. Sancho, M. Gómez-Valent, J. Ríos, R. Morros, J. Martinalbo, M. Posch, A. Koch, K. Roes, K. Oude Rengerink, J. Torrent-Farnell, and F. Torres. 2018. Evidence supporting regulatory-decision making on orphan medicinal products authorisation in Europe: Methodological uncertainties. *Orphanet Journal of Rare Diseases* 13(1).

Proschan, M., E. Brittain, and L. Kammerman. 2011. Minimize the use of minimization with unequal allocation. *Biometrics* 67(3).

Psioda, M. A., and J. G. Ibrahim. 2019. Bayesian clinical trial design using historical data that inform the treatment effect. *Biostatistics* 20(3):400-415.

Ramchandani, R., D. A. Schoenfeld, and D. M. Finkelstein. 2016. Global rank tests for multiple, possibly censored, outcomes. *Biometrics* 72(3):926-935.

Ravichandran, A., N. E. Pashley, B. Libgober, and T. Dasgupta. 2024. Optimal allocation of sample size for randomization-based inference from 2K factorial designs—DOAJ. *Journal of Causal Inference* 12(1).

Reagan-Udall Foundation. 2024. *Qualifying biomarkers to support rare disease regulatory pathways case example: Heparan sulfate in neuronopathic lysosomal storage diseases.* https://reaganudall.org/news-and-events/events/qualifying-biomarkers-support-rare-disease-regulatory-pathways (accessed August 15, 2024).

Ristl, R., F. Frommlet, A. Koch, and M. Posch. 2016. Fallback tests for co-primary endpoints. *Statistics in Medicine* 35(16):2669-2686.

Rouse, B., A. Chaimani, and T. Li. 2017. Network meta-analysis: an introduction for clinicians. *Internal and Emergency Medicine* 12(1):103-111.

Rozenberg, O., and D. Greenbaum. 2020. Making it count: Extracting real world data from compassionate use and expanded access programs. *The American Journal of Bioethics* 20(7):89-92.

Ruberg, S. J., F. Beckers, R. Hemmings, P. Honig, T. Irony, L. LaVange, G. Lieberman, J. Mayne, and R. Moscicki. 2023. Application of Bayesian approaches in drug development: Starting a virtuous cycle. *Nature Review Drug Discovery* 22(3):235-250.

Sandoval, G. J. 2023. Desirability of outcome ranking (DOOR) methodology applied to a trial of induction versus expectant management. *American Journal of Obstetrics & Gynecology* 228(1):S315-S316.

Sarp, S., R. Reichenbach, and P. Aliu. 2022. An approach to data collection in compassionate use/managed access. *Frontiers in Pharmacology* 13:1095860.

Tandon, P. K., and E. D. Kakkis. 2021. The multi-domain responder index: a novel analysis tool to capture a broader assessment of clinical benefit in heterogeneous complex rare diseases. *Orphanet Journal of Rare Diseases* 16(1):183.

Taylor, G. J., and P. Wainwright. 2005. Open label extension studies: Research or marketing? *BMJ* 331(7516):572-574.

The PREVAIL II Writing Group. 2016. A randomized, controlled trial of ZMapp for Ebola virus infection. *New England Journal of Medicine* 375(15):1448-1456.

The World Bank Group and DIME Analytics. n.d. *Randomization inference.* https://dimewiki.worldbank.org/Randomization_Inference (accessed August 15, 2024).

Thomas-Black, G., A. Dumitrascu, H. Garcia-Moreno, J. Vallortigara, J. Greenfield, B. Hunt, S. Walther, M. Wells, D. R. Lynch, H. Montgomery, and P. Giunti. 2022. The attitude of patients with progressive ataxias towards clinical trials. *Orphanet Journal of Rare Diseases* 17(1):1.

Tonin, F. S., I. Rotta, A. M. Mendes, and R. Pontarolo. 2017. Network meta-analysis: a technique to gather evidence from direct and indirect comparisons. *Pharmacy Practice (Granada)* 15(1):943.

van der Ploeg, A. T., D. C. Paula, R Clemens, D. M. Escolar, J. Florence, G. J. Groeneveld, S. Herson, P. S. Kishnani, P. Laforet, S. L. Lake, D. J. Lange, R. T. Leshner, J. E. Mayhew, C. Morgan, K. Nozaki, D. J. Park, A. Pestronk, B. Rosenbloom, A. Skrinar, C. I. van Capelle, N. A. van der Beek, M. Wasserstein, and S. A. Zivkovic. 2010. A randomized study of alglucosidase alfa in late-onset Pompe's disease. *The New England Journal of Medicine* 362(15).

Vickers, P. J. 2013. *Challenges and opportunities in the treatment of rare diseases.* https://www.ddw-online.com/media/32/challenges-and-opportunities-in-the-treatment-of-rare-diseases.pdf (accessed August 1, 2024).

Waisbren, S. E., K. Noel, K. Fahrbach, C. Cella, D. Frame, A. Dorenbaum, and H. Levy. 2007. Phenylalanine blood levels and clinical outcomes in phenylketonuria: A systematic literature review and meta-analysis. *Molecular Genetics and Metabolism* 92(1-2).

Wang, C.-Y., J. A. Berlin, B. Gertz, K. Davis, J. Li, N. A. Dreyer, W. Zhou, J. D. Seeger, N. Santanello, and A. G. Winterstein. 2022. Uncontrolled extensions of clinical trials and the use of external controls—Scoping opportunities and methods. *Clinical Pharmacology & Therapeutics* 111(1):187-199.

Wasser, J. S., and D. J. Greenblatt. 2023. Applying real-world data from expanded-access ("compassionate use") patients to drug development. *Journal of Clinical and Translational Science* 7(1):e181.

5

FDA and EMA Collaboration

A common understanding of how to develop a facilitating ecosystem would create a rising tide that would raise all boats in the pursuit of effective treatment and cures for rare diseases.

Robert Califf,
Commissioner of Food and Drugs, 2022
(FDA, 2022b)

Over the past several decades, drug development has grown increasingly complex and global. To gain access to the U.S. and European markets, drug sponsors must submit marketing applications to both the European Medicines Agency (EMA) and the U.S. Food and Drug Administration (FDA), which have different organizational structures, applicable laws, risk management procedures, and regulations. While both agencies generally align on evidence-based approaches and have similar programs in place to expedite the review and approval of drugs to treat rare disease and conditions, the differences between them can lead to variation in marketing authorization applications.

Once sponsors decide that they will be seeking regulatory approval and marketing of their product in both the United States and European Union (EU), they typically seek early regulatory advice from both jurisdictions. The results of these meetings may result in changes to sponsor decisions relating to the sequencing of submissions because one authority may present a more expedited pathway to approval. The types of studies and data required by each agency may not be the same. Without an established set of common requirements between FDA and EMA, sponsors may opt to submit a marketing authorization application to the agency perceived as offering the shortest time to approval. Additionally, market sizes and pricing considerations play a critical role in sponsor decisions about regulatory submission, given that the anticipated lifetime global revenues of a new drug are one of the primary factors impacting company decisions. The real and perceived concerns about EMA and FDA parallel scientific advice—a process that is often perceived as cumbersome and inefficient—is another barrier to use and may put smaller companies with fewer resources and capacity at a disadvantage. There is no required process for regulators to jointly discuss a potential product together. This can lead to an arbitrage-like process that is disconnected from considerations about patient needs and may result in sponsors choosing the path of least resistance rather than the path that is the most efficient way to demonstrate effectiveness and get the product to patients in both jurisdictions.

The complex regulatory landscape and the differences between regulatory agencies can have an outsized impact on patients with rare diseases and conditions. Due to the nature of rare disease drug development (e.g., small patient populations, high rates of morbidity and mortality), sponsors may only get "one bite at the apple" when it comes to designing and executing studies for regulatory decision-making (Lee et al., 2023). Early collaboration and information exchange between the agencies to coordinate on study design and align on data requirements could help reduce duplication of clinical testing, streamline the regulatory process for sponsors submitting marketing authorization applications to both agencies, and reduce incentives for regulatory arbitrage.

The agencies share a reliance on the best available data, including alternative and confirmatory data and novel approaches for data analysis, to reduce uncertainty regarding potential risks and benefits, and both agencies are committed to international collaborative efforts around best practices. However, both agencies have limited capacity to take advantage of these opportunities. Nevertheless, FDA, EMA, and other regulatory authorities have responded to pressure from patient groups, drug sponsors, and other key stakeholders by working collaboratively to better harmonize drug regulatory processes. This type of collaboration has the potential to have a significant impact on drug development and the health of patients; for example, FDA and EMA worked together closely during the COVID-19 pandemic to streamline the development of a vaccine and to quickly and efficiently grant approval through regulatory convergence (Marks, 2020). While the two authorities have the capacity to coordinate well under pressure, the usual practice is for them to work separately except under certain circumstances such as parallel reviews, which rarely occur.

This chapter is organized based on the following topics: similarities and differences between FDA and EMA, collaboration between regulatory agencies and opportunities for enhanced collaboration.

SIMILARITIES AND DIFFERENCES BETWEEN FDA AND EMA

While FDA and EMA are considered regulatory counterparts, there are a few key differences in their jurisdiction and authority as well as in how the organizations operate (see Appendix I for a comprehensive comparison between the agencies). FDA is a centralized regulatory body that oversees the evaluation of safety and efficacy of drugs approved in the United States and has a dedicated workforce and authority to issue guidance and make regulatory decisions on medications and medical devices. EMA is an independent agency of the European Union that is responsible for evaluating the safety and efficacy of drugs in Europe (EMA, n.d.-g). However, it does not have the authority to approve medications. Instead, EMA can issue guidance documents, review marketing authorization applications, and make authorization recommendations on medical products, which the European Commission then has the final decision as to whether they will be allowed to be marketed in the European Union (EMA, n.d.-g). Day-to-day operations at EMA are carried out by dedicated staff who rely on a network of experts from across Europe and collaboration with member states to pool resources and coordinate work to regulate medicines for use in humans (EMA, n.d.-q).

FDA and EMA each have regulatory policies in place to support and incentivize drug development for rare diseases and conditions.

Drug Review and Approval Process

The processes of drug evaluation and approval are fairly similar between FDA and EMA, though there are notable differences. FDA evaluates all drugs to be marketed in the United States[1,2] and EMA evaluates almost all new drugs (orphan medicines, products with new active substances, products that are a significant innovation, and products that are in the interest of public health) (EMA, n.d.-b). Prior to the formal application for evaluation—called a new drug application (NDA) for FDA (FDA, 2022a) and a marketing authorization application (MAA) for EMA (EMA, n.d.-k)—a sponsor may request an expedited pathway or specific designation (e.g., orphan designation). Once the formal application is received, FDA assigns an internal review team to evaluate safety and efficacy (FDA,

---

[1] P.L. 75–717. Federal Food, Drug, and Cosmetic Act (June 25, 1938).
[2] P.L. 78–410. Public Health Service Act (July 1, 1944).

2015a), while EMA assigns (co-)rapporteurs from member states to prepare an assessment report (EMA, n.d.-l). The FDA review team consists of staff experts in multiple disciplines (FDA, 2015a); they may also call on external advisory committees to provide opinions and recommendations (FDA, 2024d). EMA rapporteurs can establish multinational assessment teams in order to bring in experts from other member states (EMA, n.d.-j).

At EMA, the Committee for Medicinal Products for Human Use (CHMP), which is made up of experts nominated by EU member states, considers the assessment report that was prepared by the rapporteurs and attempts to reach a consensus opinion; if a consensus cannot be met, a vote is taken (EMA, n.d.-i). The CHMP's opinion is sent to the European Commission, which reaches a final decision on marketing approval (EMA, n.d.-b).

Conclusion 5-1: Despite some key differences, FDA and EMA have similar approaches to the evaluation and approval of drugs for rare diseases. Given these parallel approaches, there are existing mechanisms for close collaboration between the two agencies, as well as opportunities for enhanced collaboration in the future that would allow each agency to retain sovereign authority and accountability in regulatory decision-making.

Standards of Evidence

As discussed in Chapters 2 and 3, FDA and EMA each define standards of evidence in different ways. By statute, FDA approval of a drug product requires a demonstration of substantial evidence of effectiveness, which has generally been interpreted as requiring at least two adequate and well-controlled studies. However, amendments have clarified that substantial effectiveness may be demonstrated with one adequate and well-controlled study along with confirmatory evidence. FDA and EMA approval processes require a risk-benefit assessment that requires consideration of many complex factors (e.g., therapeutic context, seriousness of condition). FDA has published a number of guidance documents that are relevant to rare disease drug development, including *Demonstrating Substantial Evidence of Effectiveness for Human Drug and Biological Products* (2019a), *Rare Diseases: Considerations for the Development of Drugs and Biological Products* (2023d), *Benefit–Risk Assessment for New Drug and Biological Products* (2023a), *Demonstrating Substantial Evidence of Effectiveness with One Adequate and Well-Controlled Clinical Investigation and Confirmatory Evidence* (2023b), and *Rare Diseases: Natural History Studies for Drug Development* (2019b). EMA has not issued general guidance on drug development for rare diseases and conditions, but there are a number of publications that apply to issues involved in rare disease drug development, including trials in small populations, real-world evidence, registry-based studies, single-arm trials, and use of one pivotal study in drug application (EMA, 2001, 2021a, 2021b, 2022b, 2023b).

Despite some of these differences, the two agencies often reach the same decisions regarding orphan products (see Figure 5-1). Of the 33 orphan new active substances (NASs) approved by FDA only, 7 were refused approval or withdrawn by the sponsor, while the rest were not submitted, approved outside the date range, or are still in review (see Figure 5-2). Of the six NASs approved by EMA only, one received a complete response letter, while the rest were not submitted or are still in review (see Appendix G for a full list of discordant decisions).

Designation Programs

Both FDA and EMA offer an orphan designation for drugs that are targeted at rare diseases. The criteria are similar but not identical. FDA offers orphan designation to products that treat conditions affecting fewer

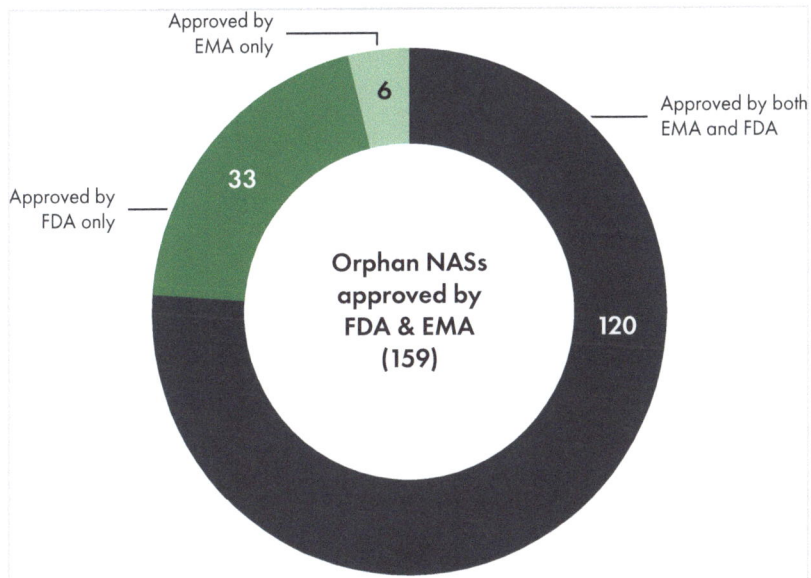

FIGURE 5-1 Number of orphan drugs approved by FDA and EMA from 2018 to 2022.
NOTES: EMA = European Medicines Agency; FDA = U.S. Food and Drug Administration; NASs = new active substances.
SOURCE: CIRS Data Analysis, 2024.

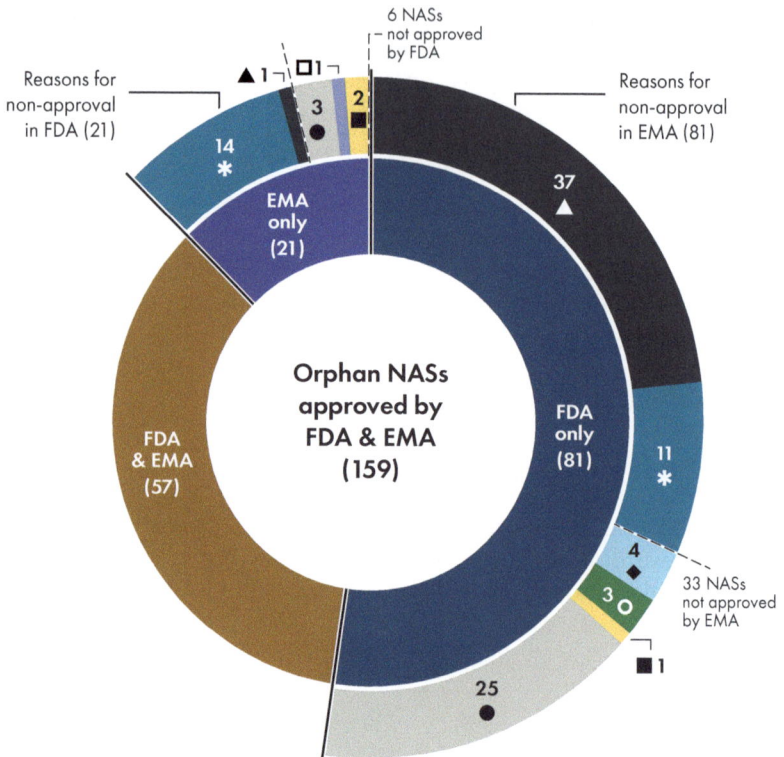
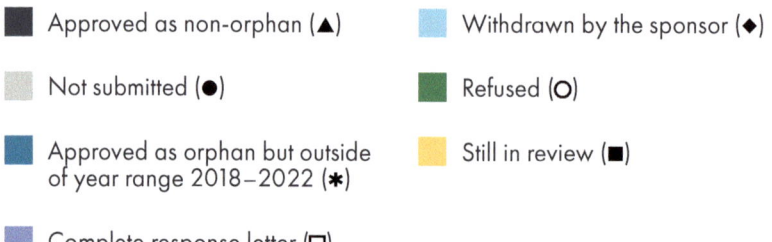

FIGURE 5-2 Discordance on the approval of orphan new active substances approved by FDA and EMA from 2018 to 2022.[a]

[a] This figure was corrected after release of the prepublication version of the report to accurately reflect the orphan status of the drugs and decisions made by FDA and EMA.
NOTES: EMA = European Medicines Agency; FDA = U.S. Food and Drug Administration; NASs = new active substances.
SOURCE: CIRS Data Analysis, 2024.

than 200,000 individuals in the United States or that affect more than 200,000 individuals but there is no reasonable expectation that the cost of developing a drug for the condition would be recovered by sales of the drug.[3] EMA offers orphan designation to products that treat conditions affecting not more than 5 in 10,000 individuals in the European Union or that affect more than 5 in 10,000 individuals but the market is unlikely to generate sufficient return on the investment. EMA further requires that the product targets a condition for which there is either no treatment available, or the product provides a "significant benefit" over available treatments. This significant benefit may be related to either improvements in clinical outcomes or improvements in patient care (e.g., ease of use).[4] FDA also has a program for rare pediatric disease designation,[5] while EMA does not have a designation specifically for rare pediatric conditions.

For the purposes of orphan designation, FDA and EMA define "condition" slightly differently. FDA requires that a product be targeted at a distinct condition, as determined by a variety of factors. A product targeted at a subset of a more common condition may be eligible if the drug itself has properties that make it inappropriate for patients with the more common version of the condition; for example, a drug that is only effective in patients with a specific biomarker may be eligible, given that those without the biomarker or drug-target would not be expected to respond (for example, mutationally-defined cancers).[6] EMA also specifies that the targeted condition must be clearly distinct from other conditions, and states that differences in severity or stages do not make a condition distinct (European Commission, 2014). A treatment targeted at a subtype of the condition may be eligible if the characteristics of the subtype make the treatment ineffective for patients with a more common subtype of the condition, but biomarkers of a subtype are not currently accepted as evidence of a distinct condition (Thirstrup, 2023). For these reasons, it can be more difficult for a drug product to be granted and keep an orphan designation by EMA.

As stated in Chapter 1, orphan designation in the United States qualifies sponsors for incentives (see Box 1-1). Similarly, in the European Union, sponsors may also receive incentives including (EMA, n.d.-m):

- Reduced fees for regulatory activities, which may include reduced fees for protocol assistance, marketing-authorization applications, inspections before authorization, applications for changes to

---

[3] Federal Food, Drug, and Cosmetic Act, SEC. 526(a)(2).
[4] Regulation (EC) 141/2000, 1999.
[5] 21 U.S.C. § 360ff.
[6] 78 FR 35117.

marketing authorizations made after approval, and reduced annual fees; and
- Potential 10 years of market exclusivity after approval.

Approval Rates for Orphan Designated Products

To understand the approval rates for orphan designated products, the committee commissioned work to examine FDA and EMA orphan designated products and marketing authorization applications and approvals of NASs to treat rare diseases (see Appendix D for full data analysis methodology). Between 2015 and 2020, more orphan NASs were submitted to FDA (184) than to EMA (123). Between 2015 and 2020, FDA approval rates for orphan NAS marketing applications were generally high (approaching 90 percent) (see Figure 5-3). EMA approval rates appeared slightly lower (closer to 80 percent). However, these differences could be accounted for differences in the number of granted orphan designations.

When divided by therapeutic area (FDA office was used as a surrogate for therapeutic area), the number of applications was generally low, with the exception of oncology products, so the committee was unable to discern whether there are meaningful differences in approval rates across therapeutic areas by each agency (see Figures 5-4 and 5-5). These similar approval rates, despite the regulatory and other differences are consistent with the common FDA and EMA reliance on a range of data from randomized controlled trials (RCTs) to alternative and confirmatory data.

Expedited Pathways

FDA and EMA both offer a number of expedited pathways that allow products to be approved on a shorter timeline or with preliminary or limited data or both. There are many similarities across the expedited pathways in both agencies (see Figure 5-6). The pathways fall into several categories: approval based on a shortened review timeline, approval based on preliminary data, and approval based on limited data.

Approval on a Shortened Review Timeline

FDA's breakthrough therapy designation and EMA's Priority Medicines (PRIME) scheme are similar programs; they are both designed to assist sponsors of products developed for conditions with an unmet need and offer the potential for shortened review. Breakthrough therapy designation is for products that are intended to treat a serious or life-threatening condition and for which preliminary clinical evidence indicates a substantial

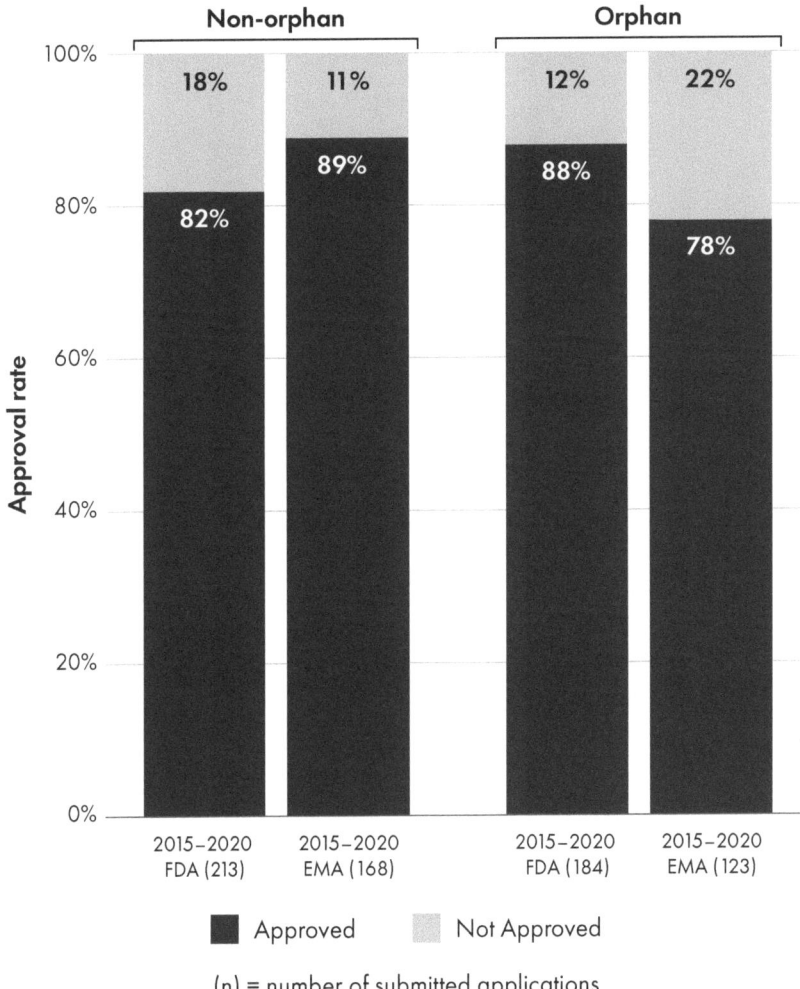

FIGURE 5-3 Approval rates for new active substance applications submitted to FDA and EMA between 2015 and 2020.
NOTES: EMA = European Medicines Agency; FDA = U.S. Food and Drug Administration.
SOURCE: CIRS Data Analysis, 2024.

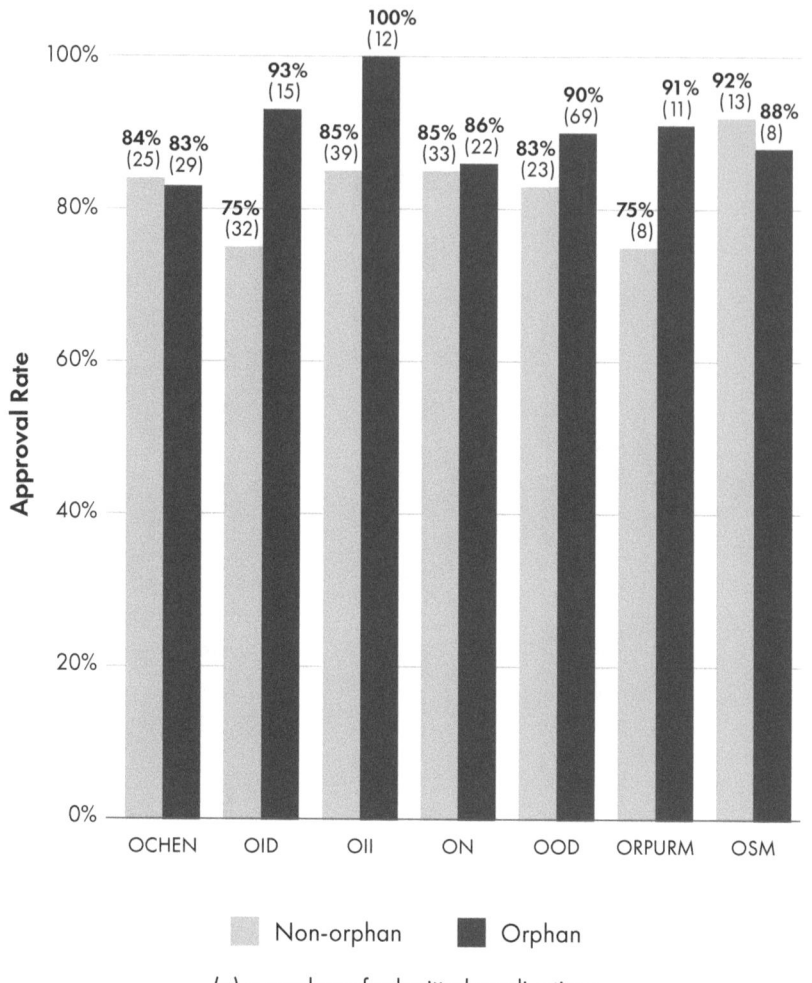

FIGURE 5-4 Novel approval rates for non-orphan and orphan new drug applications submitted to the Center for Drug Evaluation and Research from 2015 to 2020 by office.
NOTES: OCHEN = Office of Cardiology, Hematology, Endocrinology and Nephrology; OID = Office of Infectious Diseases; OII = Office of Immunology and Inflammation; ON = Office of Neuroscience; OOD = Office of Oncologic Diseases; OROURM = Office of Rare Diseases, Pediatrics, Urologic and Reproductive Medicine; OSM = Office of Specialty Medicine.
SOURCE: CIRS Data Analysis, 2024; data directly provided by FDA.

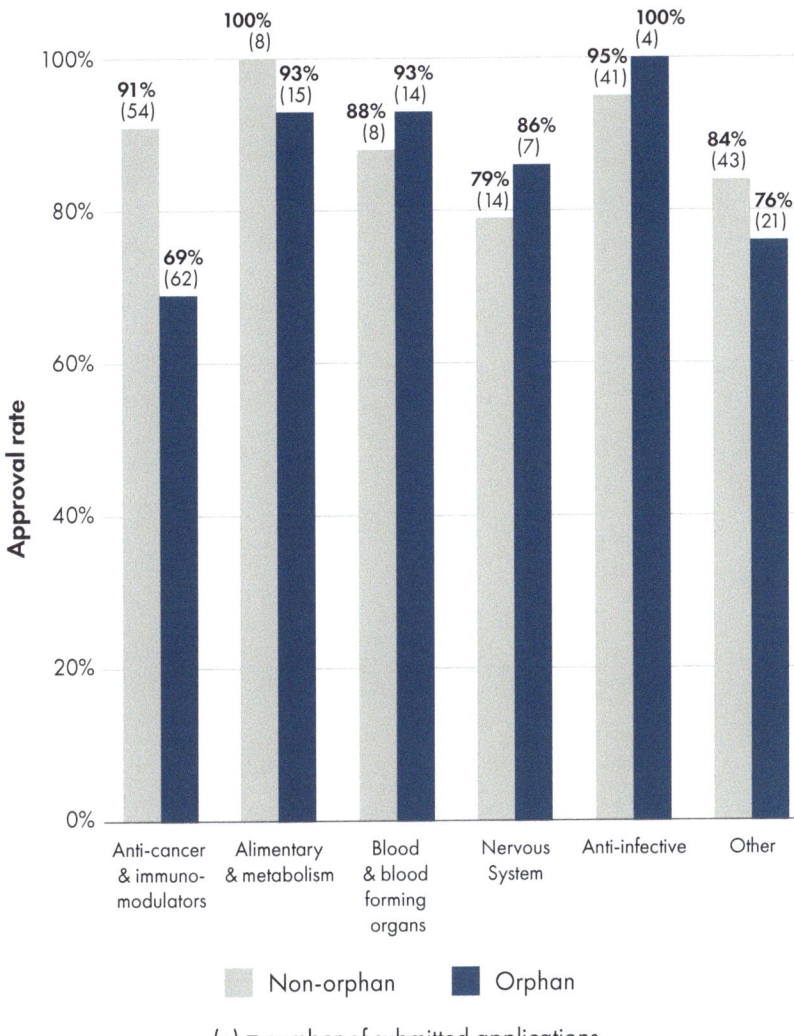

FIGURE 5-5 Approval rates for non-orphan and orphan new active substance applications submitted to European Medicines Agency from 2015 to 2020 per therapeutic area.
NOTE: Other = other therapeutic areas not described in the top five therapeutic indications list.
SOURCE: CIRS Data Analysis, 2024.

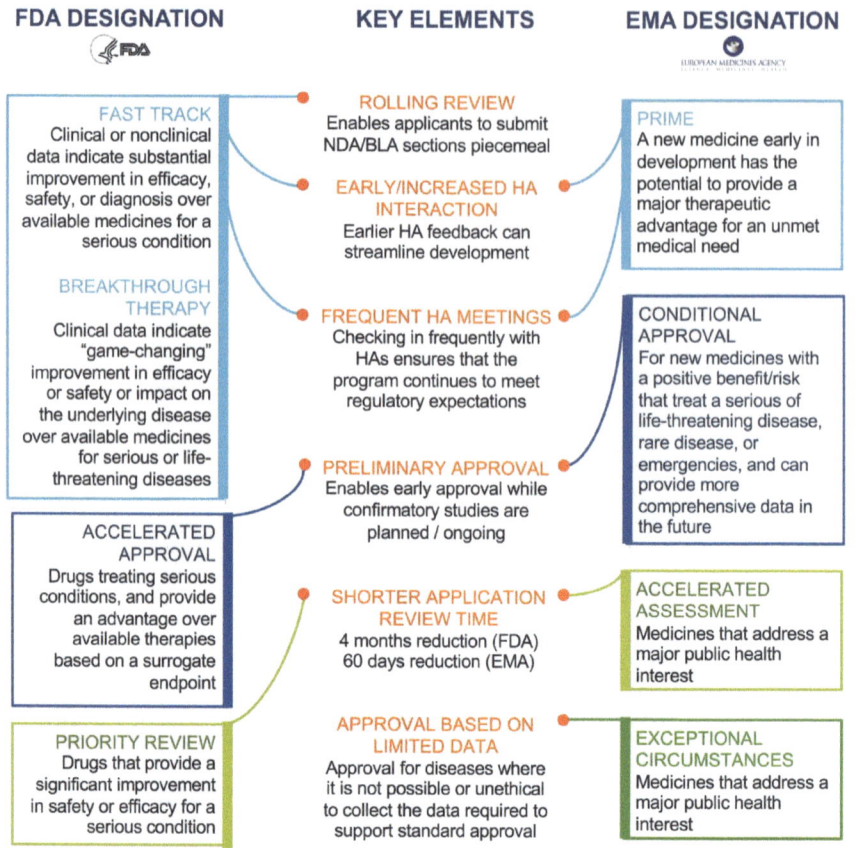

FIGURE 5-6 FDA and EMA expedited programs.
NOTES: Drugs may qualify for more than one expedited program. For U.S. programs, drugs may be eligible for all of these programs, provided they meet the criteria. For EU programs, medicines may be eligible for most of these programs, if criteria are met. The only exception is that drugs pursuing approval under exceptional circumstances are not eligible for conditional approval. BLA = Biologics License Application; EMA = European Medicines Agency; FDA = U.S. Food and Drug Administration; HA = Health Authority; NDA = New Drug Application.
SOURCE: Cox et al., 2020. CC BY 4.0 http://creativecommons.org/licenses/by-nc-nd/4.0/.

improvement on a clinically significant endpoint over available therapies (FDA, 2014). For PRIME designation, an applicant must provide data that demonstrate a meaningful improvement of clinical outcomes (EMA, n.d.-o). Breakthrough therapy designation comes with intensive guidance on drug development, meetings and communication with FDA staff, and the potential for accelerated approval or priority review (FDA, 2014). A PRIME designation offers similar benefits including meetings with EMA experts, iterative and expedited scientific advice, and the potential for accelerated assessment (EMA, n.d.-o).

FDA has one program that shortens review time, called Priority Review. EMA has one program, called Accelerated Assessment. Priority Review, for products aimed at a serious condition that demonstrate a significant improvement in safety or effectiveness, which offers review of the application in 6 months (FDA, 2014). EMA's accelerated assessment is for products that are of "major public health interest," particularly ones that involve innovations or improvements for unmet needs. The program reduces the timeframe for application assessment from 210 days to 150 days (EMA, n.d.-a).

Approval Based on Preliminary Data

Both agencies have a mechanism that allows a product to be approved with preliminary data, with confirmatory data required to be provided after the approval. FDA's accelerated approval pathway can be used when a product has a meaningful advantage over available therapies, and evidence demonstrates an effect on a surrogate or intermediate endpoint that is reasonably likely to predict clinical benefit. This pathway allows for a shorter development timeline and requires sponsors to collect data after approval to confirm the clinical benefit (FDA, 2014). EMA's conditional marketing authorization is used when there is an unmet need and the benefits of making the product available to the public outweigh the risks; sponsors are required to collect additional data after approval to confirm the benefit-risk analysis (EMA, n.d.-e).

Approval Based on Limited Data

Only EMA has a mechanism for approving a product for which comprehensive data on safety and efficacy are not available. Under the exceptional circumstances pathway, EMA may grant approval to a product if it is not possible to collect comprehensive data because the condition is too rare, because of the current state of scientific knowledge, or because it would be unethical (EMA, n.d.-h; Prilla, 2018).

Both agencies have the legal authority to exercise a great degree of flexibility in the amount and type of data necessary for rare disease product approval.

Sponsor Engagement

Both agencies offer sponsors the opportunity to engage throughout the development and approval process. Sponsors may request a meeting with FDA at any time during drug development. In general, communication with the agency is through the regulatory project manager, and sponsors are discouraged from contacting reviewers directly (FDA, 2017). Sponsors may solicit advice on a variety of topics and may also request a formal meeting at critical junctures of development (FDA, 2023c). EMA offers preparatory meetings for sponsors early in the development process in order to avoid major issues, and sponsors are encouraged to reach out at any time for feedback. Scientific advice is available from EMA for a fee; the fee can be waived for orphan medicines, smaller sponsors, and in the case of public emergencies (EMA, n.d.-p).

While the committee found little evidence pointing to systemic differences between the agencies with regard to their capacity to engage with sponsors, in qualitative interviews conducted by National Academies staff, some interviewees noted that the structure of FDA allows for more accessible engagement between regulators and sponsors than EMA (see Appendix E for full methodology and results). Interviewees said that the timeline and structure of advice from FDA was helpful. In comparison, interviewees noted that the European process of engaging national regulatory bodies within the European Union before submitting a marketing authorization application to EMA was a barrier to agency engagement.

Expert Engagement

FDA uses advisory committees and special government employees to engage experts during drug development (FDA, 2016). EMA can also engage with experts, but engagement on the European side usually occurs through its Scientific Committees or Scientific Advisory Groups (EMA, n.d.-f). EMA also has a program in a pilot phase that intends to provide a mechanism for EMA and experts to collaborate (EMA, n.d.-d). Although there are differences in how FDA and EMA engage with scientific experts, there is no evidence that the differences are systematically impactful for rare disease drug sponsors.

Patient Engagement Programs

FDA and EMA both have several mechanisms for engaging with patients, caregivers, and patient groups. FDA uses the Patient-Focused Drug Development program as a systematic approach for incorporating patient perspectives into drug development (FDA, 2024b), while EMA uses the Patients' and Consumers' Working Party to provide a platform for the exchange of information between the agency and patients (EMA, n.d.-n). Individual patients can serve on FDA advisory committees and provide advice to FDA through the Patient Representative Program (FDA, 2024a), while at EMA patients and organizations can apply to be part of a database of patients who can be called on by EMA during the drug evaluation process (EMA, 2022a). Although there are differences in how each agency engages with patients, there is no evidence that one agency's methods are superior.

Rare Disease Programs

The discrepancy between programs in the Unites States and the European Union also presents special challenges for developers. For example, using the Rare Disease Cures Accelerator-Data and Analytics Platform (RDCA-DAP®) in the United States could raise specific new review challenges in the European Union as there may be additional constraints in data usability and differences in data acceptance.

The data gathered by the committee indicate that there is significant overlap between FDA and EMA regulatory decision-making. Discrepancies between the agencies seem to be based on which location a marketing authorization for a rare disease product was first submitted. For the most part, the agencies seem to rely on the same data for marketing authorization applications. Programs, such as RDCA-DAP®, may benefit U.S.- and EU-based drug development programs, but only time will tell.

Receptiveness to Alternative and Confirmatory Data and Novel Methods of Data Analysis

In general, both agencies have demonstrated an openness to the use of alternative and confirmatory data (e.g., natural history studies) as well as novel approaches for data analysis (e.g., Bayesian statistical methods).

Enhancing Regulatory Transparency

EMA publicly shares information on marketing authorization submissions[7] (European Union, 2004); FDA does not. FDA does not share information about unsuccessful sponsor applications; EMA does. These differences appear to stem from different legal frameworks for transparency in the United States and the European Union. Information about the reasons why sponsor applications are unsuccessful or successful would help guide companies in the rare disease space and avoid unnecessary duplication of effort and unnecessary exposure of the small number of patients with rare diseases to unproven drugs in clinical trials. In a worst-case scenario, the transparency of data relating to drug evaluation serves an important public benefit, but sponsors may see transparency as an impediment to their commercial competitiveness or, in the case of corporate sponsors, to their corporate reputation.

It is common that multiple sponsors investigate candidate drugs for the same indication, including some rare disease indications, simultaneously competing on speed to be the first to receive regulatory approval. Data that reveal agency views early on in a drug development program could be used by competitors to their advantage (e.g., modifying a scientific approach for a competitive program). Data may also be used by investigators for different indications, presumably increasing their chance of success. Arguably this improves the efficiency of drug development by allowing companies to avoid the mistakes of their peers, but it also may be seen as providing an unfair advantage to second-place sponsors in a competitive environment.

In both the United States and the European Union, data transparency on the part of regulators relies on complex policy and legal frameworks which are different in each jurisdiction. While the total amount of public data about marketing application review and submission has dramatically improved over time in both jurisdictions, important differences and gaps remain. As of 2024, only EMA posts public assessment reports, which describe the basis for regulatory opinions on how medicines should be used. As a general rule, EMA also publishes clinical reports submitted by sponsors in support of regulatory applications (EMA, n.d.-c). In contrast, FDA does not post complete response letters, which may include information on why a marketing authorization submission was considered by the agency to be inadequate or incomplete. The absence of such information may lead sponsors to repeat the methodological or regulatory missteps of other sponsors to the detriment of patients.

---

[7] Regulation (EC) No 726/2004, Article 13 (3).

Conclusion 5-2: To meet the needs of rare disease patients and their caregivers, there is an ethical obligation on the part of regulatory agencies to share relevant information on the review and approval of drugs to treat rare diseases and conditions. If researchers and sponsors working on rare disease drug development had a better understanding of the reasons for successes and failures of marketing authorization applications, they could better innovate new therapeutics that have a higher likelihood of reaching patients. Additionally, more transparency would enhance public understanding and confidence in the important work carried out by regulatory agencies.

There have been calls for increased transparency at FDA. For example, the 2010 Transparency Initiative Task Force was launched in response to a memo issued by President Obama in 2009 to federal agencies and departments asking them to take steps to create more transparency, public participation, and collaboration (FDA, 2010). The task force published reports in 2010 and 2011 which contained draft proposals and action items, many of which sought to increase disclosure of the elements noted above (FDA, 2015b,c). While many of the task force's recommendations were adopted, none of those covering product applications related to disclosure of applications and regulatory decisions were addressed. Information regarding the submission of drug marketing authorization applications and reasons for regulatory decision-making are generally not publicly disclosed by FDA. In the absence of such disclosure, the public must rely on sponsors to voluntarily share information on why a marketing authorization application was not approved, which is an unreliable source given that sponsors are not required to disclose this information and, as evidenced by the lack of press releases in response to complete response letters, may have strong disincentives for public sharing (Lurie et al., 2015). Third parties that aggregate disclosures by pharmaceutical companies may offer information for those who can pay for the cost of such services.

FDA should follow the early lead of EMA and adopt greater transparency with regard to regulatory rationale for approval or disapproval of marketing authorization submissions for rare disease drug products. Increased transparency at FDA would have multiple benefits:

- Sponsors would have a better understanding of the use of regulatory flexibilities for advancing the review and approval of drugs to treat rare diseases and conditions and of the reasons for the successes and failures of marketing authorization applications, which would enable them to better learn from past experience and develop new therapeutics that have a higher likelihood of reaching patients;

- Patients and patient groups would be better informed about progress in the development of much-needed treatments and could build on regulatory experiences across disease areas; and
- The public would have a better understanding of and increased confidence in the work of the agency.

To this end, the committee identified the following focus areas for which enhanced public disclosure would improve the likelihood of success for rare disease drug development:

- The impact of new and ongoing programs within FDA that support drug development for rare diseases and conditions to improve the regulatory/approval process.
- Lessons learned across therapeutic areas on the use of available regulatory flexibilities.
- Types of information relevant for public understanding of when and how available regulatory policies are applied for rare disease drug products.

Practical Considerations

The committee recognizes there are multiple barriers to achieving greater transparency on the part of FDA, including laws that govern how the agency can or cannot share information. Some have argued that FDA has broad discretion on what is considered confidential.[8] Sharfstein et al. (2017) have suggested that FDA does not require an act of Congress to make progress on publicly sharing information about marketing authorization applications for drug products (see Box 5-1 for a case study on FDA using its discretion to share information with the public). FDA has the ability to incentivize and facilitate pathways for enhancing information sharing, but there are practical and legal considerations, which may require modification of some of the laws that restrict the agency from sharing certain types of information. For these reasons, the committee recognizes the need for more transparency on the part of FDA, but acknowledges that additional consideration, assessment, and legal review are needed to determine how such measures should be implemented.

---

[8] Relevant regulations include: 21 CFR. §312.130(a) (non-disclosure of Investigational New Drug applications for drugs); §601.50 (non-disclosure of Investigational New Drug applications for biological products); §314.430(b)(non-disclosure of New Drug Applications prior to approval); §601.51(b) (non-disclosure of Biologics Licenses Applications prior to approval); §814.9(b) & (c) (non-disclosure of Pre-Market Approval applications prior to approval).

> **BOX 5-1**
> **FDA Demonstration of Discretion about Disclosure:**
> **COVID-19 Pandemic**
>
> Demonstrating the U.S. Food and Drug Administration's (FDA's) discretion to make decisions about sharing information, FDA announced during the COVID-19 pandemic that it would make several types of information publicly available. First, FDA pledged to begin disclosing information from emergency use authorization (EUA) review documents once the process was complete, with redactions as appropriate. In addition, noting that health care providers needed details about products approved under the EUA in make informed decisions about care, FDA posted information including fact sheets for patients and providers, and the letter of authorization sent to the product's developer. The letter of authorization gives details about the medical product, regulatory history, the criteria for issuance of the EUA, the scope of authorization, and the conditions of authorization. In FDA's announcement of these new transparency efforts, the agency stated that transparency provides helpful information to the public, helps inform providers, and ensures public confidence in the FDA review process.
>
> ---
>
> SOURCE: FDA, 2020.

RECOMMENDATION 5-1: The U.S. Food and Drug Administration (FDA) should take steps to make relevant information on marketing authorization submissions, review milestones, approval and negative review decisions (refusal to file, clinical hold, and complete response letters), and the use of regulatory flexibilities for rare disease drug products publicly available and easily accessible to inform sponsors, patients, researchers, and reviewers on decision-making rationales and when and how available policies are applied. While the committee acknowledges the legal challenges surrounding disclosure of information, actions should include, but not be limited to:

- Mirroring the level of information disclosed by the European Medicines Agency (EMA) presented on submissions, review milestones, and review decisions, such that there is parity between what FDA and EMA share publicly;

- Building on the work of the 2010 FDA Transparency Task Force, to implement Phase II product application's disclosure requirements:[9] considerations for product applications (including investigational applications);
- Organizing and structuring the information made public in such a way that the public can identify trends (e.g., increases or decreases in the use of regulatory flexibility by product type or therapeutic area over time and expedited and designation program use);
- Link clinical trials to FDA disclosures by using national clinical trial identifiers[10] to allow the public to better understand the connection between clinical trials and the regulatory process.

COLLABORATION BETWEEN REGULATORY AGENCIES

Despite some key differences, FDA and EMA have similar approaches to the evaluation and approval of drugs for rare diseases. Given this overlap, there are several existing mechanisms for close collaboration between the two agencies as well as opportunities for enhanced collaboration in the future. Since the signing of a confidentiality agreement in 2003, which permits the agencies to share nonpublic information, including confidential commercial information, FDA and EMA have created multiple formalized mechanisms to facilitate communication and collaboration. These collaborations cover a wide range of topics and activities, including scientific advice, orphan designations, marketing authorizations, post-authorization requirements, inspections, pharmacovigilance, guidance documents, and other topics (EMA, 2024d) (see Figure 5-7). In addition to these formal mechanisms, which are further discussed below, there is ongoing informal communication between FDA and EMA, which enables staff to observe each other's scientific meetings, participate in each other's trainings, and share information on an ad hoc basis (Lee et al., 2023).

---

[9] On May 19, 2010, the Transparency Task Force released a report containing 21 draft proposals about expanding the disclosure of information by FDA while maintaining confidentiality for trade secrets and individually identifiable patient information. FDA accepted public comment on the proposals, as well as on which draft proposals should be given priority, on this website from May 19, 2010, through July 20, 2010. https://wayback.archiveit.org/7993/20171105152021/https://www.fda.gov/AboutFDA/Transparency/PublicDisclosure/DraftProposalbyTopicArea/ucm211691.htm (accessed May 14, 2024).

[10] A national clinical trial number is an 8-digit unique identifier assigned to a clinical study when it is registered on ClinicalTrials.gov.

FDA AND EMA COLLABORATION

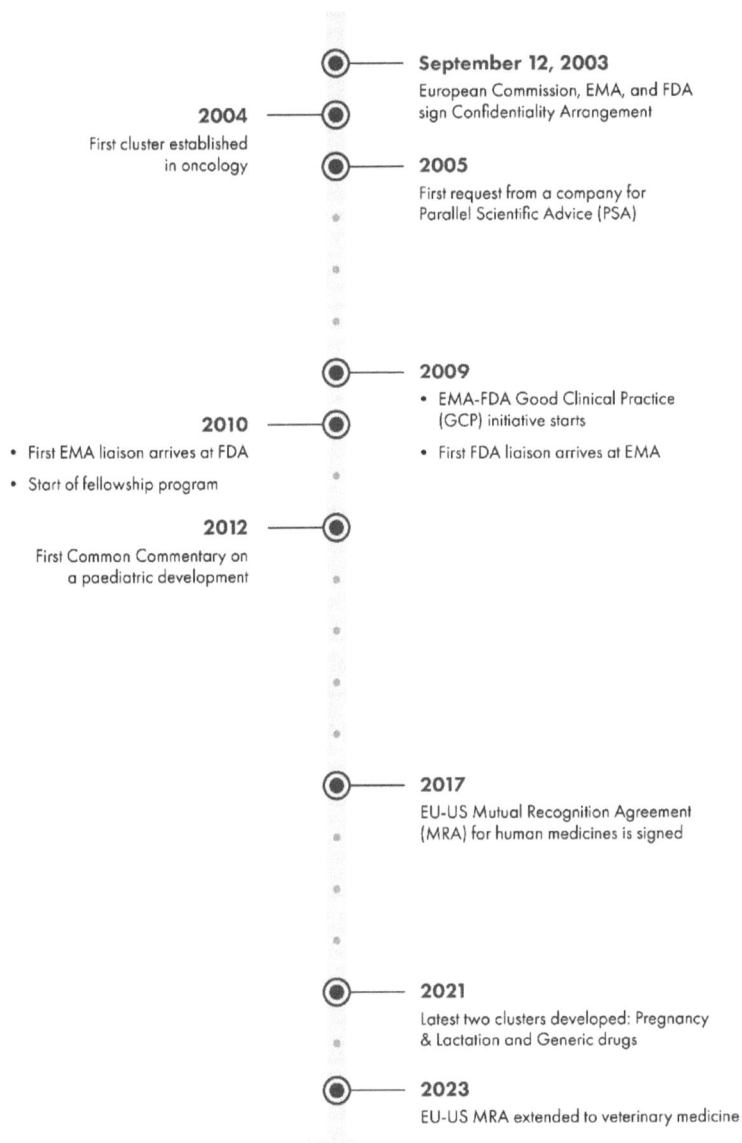

FIGURE 5-7 20 years of EU/U.S. collaboration on medicines regulation.
SOURCE: Adapted from European Medicines Agency: 20 years EU/US collaboration on medicines regulation, https://www.ema.europa.eu/system/files/documents/other/2023-09_ema-fda-20-years-arrangement_en.pdf (accessed March 15, 2024).

Clusters

One of the primary formal mechanisms for collaboration between EMA and FDA is so-called "clusters"—regular virtual meetings between EMA and FDA staff focused on specific topics and therapeutic areas that would benefit from an "intensified exchange of information and collaboration" (EMA, 2024a). Documents exchanged within clusters may include draft guidances/guidelines, assessment reports, review memos, and meeting minutes. The agencies typically set the agenda for what is discussed at a cluster meeting. However, sponsors also have the option of asking that a drug program or topic be discussed. Topics discussed within clusters range from emerging scientific and ethical issues to challenges in product development to issues with the review of marketing authorization applications (see Figure 5-8).

Since the first EMA–FDA cluster on oncology-hematology medicines was established in 2004, clusters have grown in number and size (EMA, 2024a). Clusters were initially designed as a forum for dialogue between FDA and EMA but have since expanded to include other regulators, including those from Canada, Australia, and Japan (EMA, 2024a; Lee et al., 2023). As of 2024, there were 31 clusters that cover a variety of topics and disease areas, including several that are relevant for rare diseases and conditions (see Table 5-1). In addition to regularly scheduled meetings, the relationships that are built through the work of the clusters have facilitated additional ad hoc conversations on time-sensitive issues (Tyner et al., 2023).

Impact of Clusters

While the impact of the clusters on marketing authorization approval rates or regulatory harmonization cannot be easily quantified, discussions do help to disseminate information among regulatory staff and to facilitate better understanding of agency perspectives and approaches and can serve as a form of "peer review" among regulators (Teixeira et al., 2020). EMA and FDA staff have noted that clusters provide opportunities for regulators to discuss challenging issues for rare disease drug review and approval, such as novel endpoints, statistical methodologies, use of regulatory flexibilities, and post-marketing requirements (Tyner et al., 2023).

A 2017 survey conducted by EMA and FDA indicated that cluster participants from across regulatory agencies (EMA; FDA; Health Canada; Ministry of Health, Labour, and Welfare of Japan/Pharmaceuticals and Medical Devices Agency; Therapeutic Goods Administration; Swissmedic; and the European Directorate for the Quality of Medicines & HealthCare) found that this collaborative mechanism helps inform regulatory decision-making (Teixeira et al., 2020). Other reported impacts of the cluster program by the agencies include the establishment of new initiatives, such as the Patient Engagement Collaborative (FDA, 2024e), the FDA–EMA

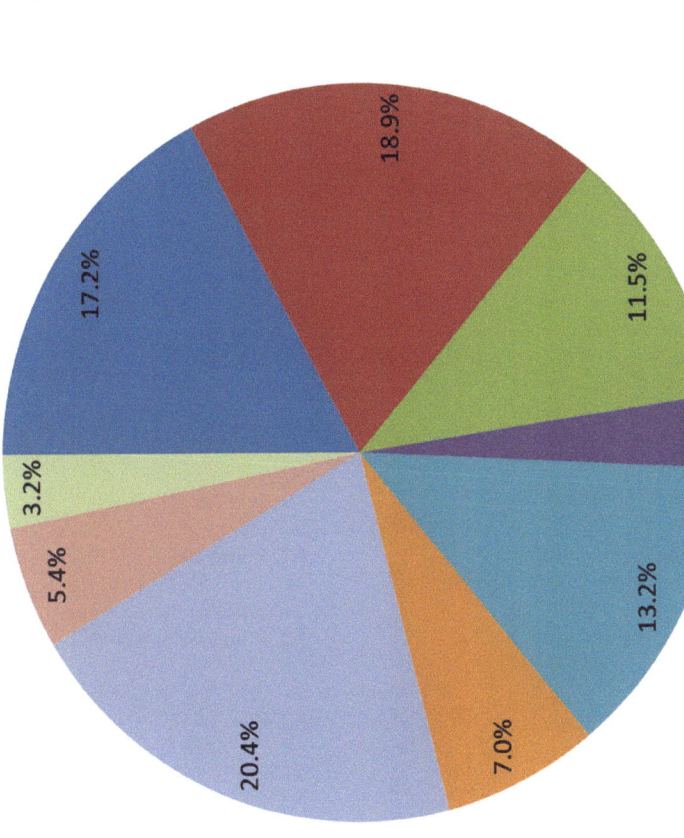

FIGURE 5-8 Top topic areas discussed in clusters.
NOTES: Values shown are from aggregate results from a compiled list of the topic areas identified for all clusters. MAA = marketing authorization application; NDA = new drug application.
SOURCE: Teixeira et al., 2020. CC BY 4.0 http://creativecommons.org/licenses/by/4.0/.

TABLE 5-1 Examples of Clusters Relevant for Rare Diseases[a]

Cluster	Description	Relevance for Rare Diseases
Advanced Therapy Medical Products (ATMP)	Established: 2008 Meeting frequency: several times a year in conjunction with the Committee for Advanced Therapies meetings Participants: EMA, FDA, and HC Objective: to develop a common understanding of the regulatory approaches of each agency for advanced-therapy medicinal products (EMA, 2024a)	Cluster participants share documents, including draft guidance, scientific advice, and assessment reports from IND and marketing applications (EMA, 2024a). Experience has shown that many treatments (and most of the approvals) for rare diseases fall under the definition of ATMP, and this trend is expected to grow in future with the continuing rise of gene therapies underlining the relevance for rare disease of this cluster.
Blood Products	Established: 2010 Meeting frequency: quarterly by teleconference Participants: EMA, FDA, and HC Objective: to discuss issues related to development programs and medicinal products for this therapeutic area (EMA, 2024a)	There are several rare blood conditions including hemophilia and other clotting disorders
Oncology–Hematology Medicinal Products	Established: 2004 Meeting frequency: monthly by teleconference Participants: EMA, FDA, HC, PMDA/MHLW, TGA, Swissmedic Objective: to share clinical review information, with a strong focus on clinical and statistical issues, of medicines to treat cancer under review by both agencies (EMA, 2024a)	Many rare disease fall in the category of oncology-hematology (e.g. childhood cancers)
Orphan Medicinal Products	Established: 2008 Meeting frequency: monthly by teleconference Participants: EMA and FDA Objective: to collaborate on orphan designation, product development, and administrative simplification (EMA, 2024a)	Complements the Rare Disease Cluster and focuses specifically on issues related to orphan designation. Discussions focus on current applications for orphan designation, explore challenging regulatory or scientific issues, and consider divergent opinions on designation. This cluster also discusses draft guidance and legislative approaches for facilitating and regulating the development of orphan products (EMA, 2024a).

TABLE 5-1 Continued

Cluster	Description	Relevance for Rare Diseases
Patient Engagement	Established: 2016 Meeting frequency: quarterly by teleconference Participants: EMA, FDA, and HC Objective: to share best practices on involving patients along the medical product regulatory lifecycle, to further improve and extend both agencies' current activities in this area (EMA, 2024a)	Experience has shown that patients (or caregivers) with rare diseases are very active in the field of treatment advocacy and wish to engage with regulatory agencies
Pediatric	Established: 2007 Meeting frequency: Monthly and ad hoc as needed by teleconference Participants: EMA, FDA, HC, PMDA, and TGA Objective: to help ensure that pediatric studies are conducted in a scientifically rigorous and ethical manner and that pediatric patients are not exposed to unnecessary or duplicative clinical trials (FDA, 2024c)	Agency participants may discuss and share documents on topics including pediatric investigational plans, study design, endpoints, safety issues, reports from each agency's pediatric committee, new drug applications and approvals, and Pediatric Research Equity Act requirements. Drug sponsors who submit plans for pediatric studies may request that their product be discussed at a cluster meeting (Reaman et al., 2020; Ungstrup and Vanags, 2023). For select marketing authorization applications, the Pediatric Cluster may prepare common commentary, which provides informal and non-binding comment on pediatric development plans that have been submitted to both EMA and FDA (EMA, 2024a).
Rare Disease Cluster	Established: 2016 Meeting frequency: three to four times a year by teleconference Participants: EMA and FDA Objective: to exchange information on the development and scientific evaluation of medical products for rare diseases (EMA, 2024a)	Cluster topics include discussion of protocols, marketing applications, and informational topics related to the use of pre-clinical evidence to support rare disease product development, issues and challenges with the conduct and evaluation of clinical trials in small populations, risk management strategies for long-term safety issues in rare disease patient populations, and the design and conduct of post-marketing studies (EMA, 2024a).

continued

TABLE 5-1 Continued

Cluster	Description	Relevance for Rare Diseases
Real-World Evidence	Established: 2018 Meeting frequency: Four times a year Participants: EMA and FDA Objective: to foster consistency of approach, address common challenges, and leverage data, network, and expertise available to facilitate advances in regulatory science (Teixeira et al., 2020)	The constraints of running clinical trials in rare diseases necessitate increased reliance on real world data to generate evidence about safety and efficacy of emerging and older treatments

NOTES: EMA = European Medicines Agency; FDA = U.S. Food and Drug Administration; HC = Health Canada; IND = investigational new drug; MHLW = Ministry of Health, Labour and Welfare of Japan; PMDA = Pharmaceuticals and Medical Devices Agency (Japan); TGA = Therapeutic Goods Administration (Australia).

[a] This table was modified after release of the prepublication report to more accurately reflect cluster meeting frequency and the topics discussed.

pediatric Common Commentaries (FDA, 2024c), a collaborative approach to facilitate pediatric drug development for Gaucher disease (EMA, 2017), joint publications and workshops, resolution of divergences, and professional growth among participants (Teixeira et al., 2020).

Patient Engagement Collaborative

In response to requests from patient communities, the Patient Engagement Collaborative (PEC) was established in 2018 as a joint project of FDA and the Clinical Trials Transformation Initiative (CTTI), a public–private partnership of Duke University and FDA (CTTI, 2023). PEC was modeled after EMA's Patients' and Consumers' Working Party (FDA, 2024e), which facilitates EMA engagement with patients and consumer organizations and provides recommendations to EMA (EMA, n.d.-n). While PEC is not considered an FDA advisory committee and does not discuss specific medical products or treatments, meetings are an opportunity for patient communities to share views, ideas, and experiences with FDA and CTTI in order to inform communication, education, and engagement activities (CTTI, 2023).

Pediatric Common Commentary

In 2012, EMA and FDA began issuing common commentaries to share unofficial high-level summaries of discussions held during Pediatric Cluster meetings. Publicly and confidentially issued common commentaries may highlight scientific, ethical, or regulatory topics related to pediatric product development where EMA and FDA are working toward a harmonized view. Common commentaries might also identify discordant EMA and FDA agency views (FDA, 2024c). Common commentary for pediatric drug development has been critically important given the small patient populations for rare diseases, including childhood cancer.[11]

In 2021, EMA and FDA published a common commentary on pediatric oncology drug development, which lays out common issues requested for discussions by both agencies so that sponsors have an opportunity to address key issues early on and enable simultaneous submission of paediatric investigation plans (PIPs) to EMA and initial pediatric study plans (iPSPs) to FDA (FDA and EMA, 2021). Common commentary has also been issued on other topics relevant to rare disease, including discussions about trial design for Gaucher disease (see Box 5-2).

Opportunities for Clusters

While clusters help inform drug development and approval processes and provide a valuable forum for collaboration between the regulatory agencies, there is substantial unfulfilled potential. The impact of the clusters on the drug development ecosystem may be limited by the fact that cluster discussions are largely *reactive*, focused on specific issues, such as

---

BOX 5-2
Gaucher Disease: A Strategic Collaborative Approach from EMA and FDA

Based on Pediatric Cluster meetings, the European Medicines Agency (EMA) and the U.S. Food and Drug Administration (FDA) published a strategic collaborative approach on Gaucher disease, a rare metabolic disorder that is passed down from parents to their children. Given the number of drugs in the pipeline and based on work of the Pediatric Cluster, EMA and FDA undertook a collaborative approach to lay out the necessary parameters for demonstrating the safety and efficacy of drug products to treat Gaucher disease in pediatric populations. In addition to discussing opportunities for extrapolation of efficacy and use of nonclinical models to strengthen development plans, EMA and FDA explored the possibility of establishing a multi-arm, multi-company development program (EMA, 2017).

This collaborative approach has the potential to streamline the testing of drugs to treat Gaucher disease by avoiding unnecessary pediatric studies and reducing burden on patients. Although developed specifically for Gaucher disease, EMA notes that this type of approach could be applied toward drug development for other rare diseases and conditions (EMA, 2024a).

---

[11] This section was edited after release of the prepublication version of the report to more accurately reflect the content and approach to common commentaries.

an existing development plan or safety concern. With the exception of a handful of targeted activities, such as the collaborative approach for Gaucher disease (see Box 5-2), clusters are not designed to more *prospectively* address challenges for rare disease drug development.

And yet, clusters have the potential to build and expand on current activities. In addition to strategic collaborative approaches for other rare diseases, clusters provide a mechanism for EMA and FDA to address early-stage barriers to successful marketing authorization approval that cut across therapeutic areas. The existing cluster structure could additionally be used to prospectively address common challenges for rare disease drug development, thereby harmonizing and streamlining the orphan designation and drug evaluation process. For example, increased use of EMA and FDA common commentary to include issues related to how drug development tools, extrapolation of efficacy, innovative trial design, new methodologies, and use of alternative and confirmatory data sources, such as patient registries and real-world data sources, could be used to strengthen rare disease development plans across therapeutic areas and would give sponsors more clarity on the regulatory considerations for rare disease drug programs.

An expansion and shift in focus on the part of the clusters to include prospective issues facing rare disease drug development would align with current objectives, build on existing collaborative efforts, and help inform regulatory decision-making. It is also important to note that this type of approach would further enhance scientific exchange and trust building between FDA and EMA staff and could have synergistic and cumulative impact—benefiting interagency cooperation, scientific review, and ultimately public health across therapeutic areas and drug types for disease both rare and common.

There may be concerns on the part of the agencies or sponsors that such an approach could constrain discussions if information were to be made publicly available. However, common commentary is intended to highlight issues where FDA and EMA are working toward a more harmonized view (or to provide clarity for sponsors on areas where the agency may be unable to reach alignment). These documents are not binding and could serve as a valuable source of information for sponsors, researchers, and patient groups. Agencies could use these documents to share common thinking on how they weigh urgency and pragmatic limitations against the need for data to support marketing authorization applications for rare diseases and conditions and considerations for how FDA and EMA might address areas of misalignment, such as on clinical trial endpoints, the determination of non-inferiority (or similarity) margins, use/acceptance of novel statistical methodologies, and totality-of-evidence determinations.

RECOMMENDATION 5-2: To facilitate the efficient global development of orphan drugs, the U.S. Food and Drug Administration (FDA)

and the European Medicines Agency (EMA) should build on the existing clusters relevant for rare diseases by undertaking the following:
- Create a forum, which includes key decision makers within the agencies, for forward-looking discussion of issues and common challenges for rare disease drug development that EMA and FDA could use to achieve a more harmonized approach to rare disease development.
- Devote resources to discuss and resolve misalignment related to rare disease drug development.
- Publicly issue findings on key scientific or regulatory topics related to rare disease drug development.
- Conduct and publicly share an annual review of all orphan drug applications for the agencies to facilitate more immediate sharing of lessons learned and surface issues that cut across rare disease drug development programs.

Parallel Scientific Advice

Established in 2005, the Parallel Scientific Advice (PSA) program is a voluntary mechanism through which FDA and EMA can concurrently provide scientific advice to sponsors during the development of new drugs, biological products, vaccines, or advanced therapies (EMA and FDA, 2021). The goals of the PSA program are to: (1) increase dialogue early on in the product lifecycle, (2) deepen understanding of regulatory decisions, (3) optimize product development, and (4) avoid unnecessary or duplicative testing (Thor et al., 2023). The program does not guarantee alignment between EMA and FDA, but it can offer a number of potential benefits for sponsors, including agency convergence on approaches to development, a better understanding of each agency's concerns and requirements, and the opportunity for sponsors and agencies to ask and answer questions (Thor et al., 2023).

The process is typically requested by the drug sponsor but may also be initiated by EMA or FDA (EMA and FDA, 2021). Acceptance of the request by both agencies is required to proceed. The timelines for PSA are intended to align with what would be expected of similar processes to enable sponsors to predict when advice can be expected from EMA and FDA (see Table 5-2). A 5-year review of PSA indicated that the timelines were comparable to timelines for EMA's Scientific Advice Working Party, which provides scientific advice and protocol assistance for sponsors, and to timelines for FDA Type B meetings (Thor et al., 2023).[12]

---

[12] This section was modified after release of the prepublication version of the report to more accurately reflect Type B meetings.

TABLE 5-2 Timeline for Parallel Scientific Advice

Responsible Party	Action	Timeframe
Sponsor	By email, send FDA and EMA rationale for why PSA would be beneficial, proposed scientific questions, goals for the meeting	Unspecified—depends on sponsor
EMA and FDA	Accept or decline the PSA request	On average, 13 calendar days post-request
Sponsor	Prepare full meeting package according to EMA's Scientific Advice Working Party procedure schedule	Unspecified—depends on sponsor
EMA	Validates the meeting package	PSA begins
EMA and FDA	Hold a bilateral meeting	On average, 35 days post-validation
EMA and FDA	Provide preliminary written feedback to sponsor	
Sponsor, EMA, and FDA	Hold trilateral meeting	65 days post-validation
EMA	Issue final advice letter	10 days post-trilateral meeting
FDA	Issue final meeting minutes	30 days post-trilateral meeting

NOTES: EMA = European Medicines Agency; FDA = U.S. Food and Drug Administration.
SOURCE: Thor et al., 2023.

Products designed for the treatment of rare diseases and conditions, as well as those targeted to address unmet medical need and treat special populations, may be good candidates for PSA due to their potential public health value and because they may be more likely to break new ground in terms of innovative science and treatment modalities (Kweder, 2022). Special consideration is given to products that may offer public health value, such as products that address an unmet medical need or are intended to treat rare diseases or special populations (Kweder, 2022). Products that are selected for PSA fall into a several categories (see Figure 5-9).

Impact of PSA Program

Regulatory staff who have overseen, coordinated, and participated in the PSA program describe it as "remarkably productive and positive for all parties" (Thor et al., 2023, 660). While this experience is difficult to quantify, regulators have said that the discussions between EMA and FDA have helped expand their thinking and given them opportunities to discuss ways to address common challenges, particularly for therapeutic areas for which there is limited experience or difficult scientific questions (Thor et

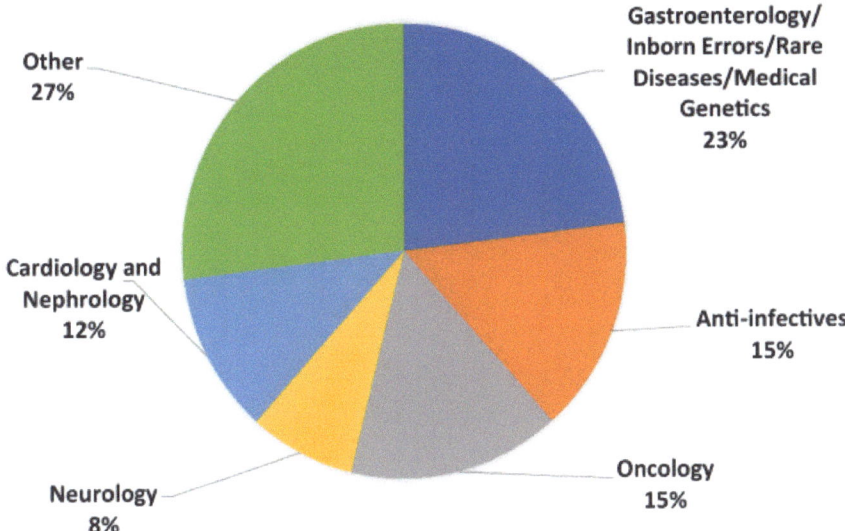

FIGURE 5-9 Accepted Parallel Scientific Advice requests (N=26) by product category from 2017 to 2021.
SOURCE: Thor et al., 2023. CC BY 4.0 http://creativecommons.org/licenses/by/4.0/.

al., 2023). For products that do not have a straightforward regulatory path, discussions between FDA and EMA allow for an exploration of alternative or innovative approaches and can add value to the advice given to the sponsor (Thor et al., 2023).

Despite the potential benefits of the PSA program, only a handful of sponsors apply each year. A review published by FDA and EMA staff showed that between 2017 and 2021, the agencies received 37 PSA requests, of which 26 (70 percent) were accepted (see Figure 5-9). Four of the sponsors withdrew their requests or chose not to proceed. Of the accepted PSA requests, 23 percent were for gastroenterological, inborn errors, rare diseases, and medical genetics[13] (Thor et al., 2023). Compared to the number of marketing applications that are submitted and approved to EMA and FDA each year, few applications use the PSA program. Between 2017 and 2020, the PSA program accepted 19 submissions (see Figure 5-10). Similar to other therapeutic products, the majority of orphan-designated products submitted for marketing authorization do not receive PSA.

When the PSA program was launched in 2005, uptake was so slow that the agencies considered ending the program (Gingery, 2021). Similar

---

[13] Authors combined therapeutic areas into this broad category because FDA reorganized during the period of the cohort analysis and its categorization of submissions changed.

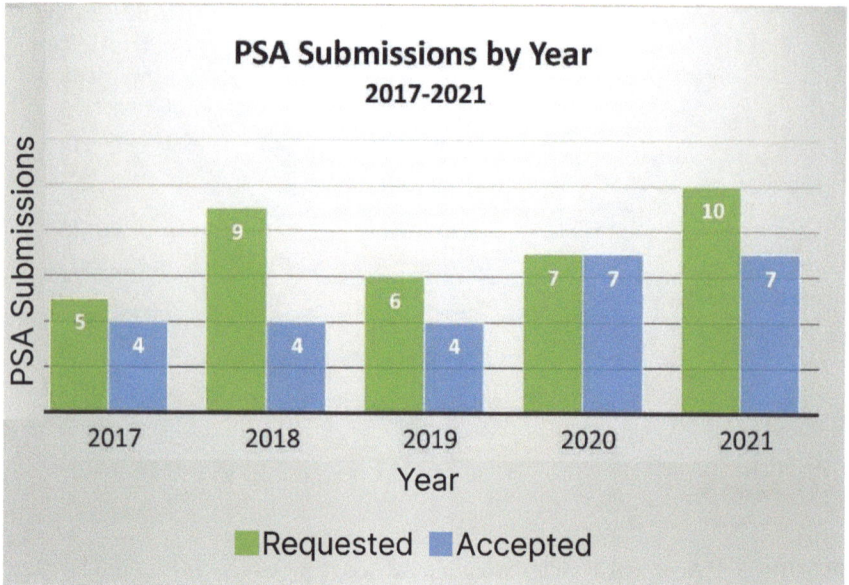

FIGURE 5-10 Parallel Scientific Advice submissions by year from 2017 to 2021.
NOTE: PSA = Parallel Scientific Advice.
SOURCE: Adapted from Thor et al., 2023. CC BY 4.0 http://creativecommons.org/licenses/by/4.0/.

concerns have arisen for a related pilot project that offers PSA for complex generic drugs; FDA reported that some applicants were hesitant to join the program due to misperceptions about the consequences of conflicting advice, questions about the value of the advice because it is non-binding, and concerns about sharing confidential information (Ibrahim, 2024).

To better understand some of the real or perceived concerns that sponsors may have regarding the PSA program, the Committee considered results from a series of qualitative interviews carried out by National Academies staff, which showed that interviewees were aware of the PSA program but had varying opinions about its potential value (see Appendix E for full methodology and results). One interviewee stated, "PSA meetings can be protracted, discordant, and non-binding. Sponsors need them to be rapid, concordant, and binding." Other interviewees listed issues with the PSA program that stem from the non-binding nature of PSA, potential for misaligned advice between EMA and FDA, issues with timing of the program, and concerns that in the event of divergent opinions, the agencies may follow the lead of the agency with the higher evidence threshold.

Discordant scientific advice between FDA and EMA can create confusion or uncertainty on the part of sponsors about how to proceed with a development program and could particularly impact smaller companies that are developing drugs to treat rare diseases and conditions. Smaller companies often have a limited product pipeline and contingent funding. As such, they are more likely to seek direction from a single regulatory agency that they consider most likely to view their development program favorably; and are more likely to disfavor use of PSA.

Another reason for the lack of uptake could be that the logistics of the PSA program—including timing, components of a request, and communicating with both agencies—may be difficult to navigate for companies, particularly those that are smaller or less experienced with regulatory submissions. Applying for PSA requires staff time, resources, and know-how. Additionally, it may be the case that for some companies, early access to the U.S. market is a key factor in decision making and the priority for development programs.

Participants at a public workshop convened by FDA and the Duke-Margolis Center for Health Policy in 2017 suggested that more transparency on the requirements and timelines for the PSA program would help address some of the issues leading to lack of uptake (Richardson et al., 2018). FDA has made efforts to share information on the PSA program, but Thor et al., observed that by 2023, the agencies and pharmaceutical companies still had not widely promoted or publicized the program (Thor et al., 2023).

Despite potential issues with the PSA program, a few orphan drug products have used PSA and received marketing authorization (see Box 5-3).

Opportunities for the PSA Program

There are limited data available on the approval rate of products in the PSA program, but seeking and complying with scientific advice from individual agencies has been positively correlated with the success of an application (Hofer et al., 2015; Regnstrom et al., 2009; Welch, 2015). One study found that two-thirds of applicants who received scientific advice were advised by EMA to alter their trial designs (Hofer et al., 2015). Of the applicants that changed their trial designs, 86 percent received marketing authorization; of those that did not comply with the scientific advice given, only 41 percent received authorization (Hofer et al., 2015).

As discussed above, under the current circumstances there may be pragmatic financial or business reasons that companies do not apply for PSA. In part, this may be due to business priorities within a company or a lack of resources. To overcome the practical hurdles and perceived drawbacks, it may be that sponsors need additional incentives for requesting PSA. An understanding of the resources required for sponsors to apply for PSA and publicly available reporting on the impact of PSA over time would better enable the agencies to identify appropriate mechanisms for increasing

> **BOX 5-3**
> **Select Examples of Drug Products to Treat Rare Diseases and Conditions that Received Parallel Scientific Advice**[a]
>
> **Soliris (eculizumab):** A monoclonal antibody that is used to treat rare blood disorders, such as paroxysmal nocturnal hemoglobinuria and atypical hemolytic uremic syndrome. Soliris was designated an orphan medicine by the European Medicines Agency (EMA) and the U.S. Food and Drug Administration (FDA). It was approved by EMA and FDA in 2007 (EMA, 2023c; FDA, 2007).
>
> **Kalydeco (Ivacaftor):** A medication for the treatment of cystic fibrosis in patients with specific genetic mutations. Kalydeco was designated an orphan medicine by EMA and FDA (EMA, 2012; FDA, 2012). It was approved by EMA and FDA in 2012 (EMA, 2024b; FDA, 2012).
>
> **Tegsedi (Inotersen):** A medication used to treat hereditary transthyretin amyloidosis (hATTR), which is characterized by a buildup of amyloid protein throughout the body, including around nerves. Tegsedi was designated an orphan medicine by EMA and FDA. It was approved by EMA and FDA in 2018 (EMA, 2024c; FDA, 2018).
>
> ---
>
> [a] This box was corrected after release of the prepublication version of the report to accurately reflect orphan designation.

uptake of the use of PSA for companies seeking to develop new therapeutics to treat rare diseases and conditions.

Additionally, there may be ways to integrate the use of PSA more dynamically into the review process, which could help streamline procedures and timelines for rare disease programs. For example, offering PSA to sponsors as an option to consider at the point of orphan drug designation, after completion of Phase 1 and Phase 2 trials, or other key points throughout the drug development process. FDA and EMA discussions with the sponsor would be non-binding for any party but would provide a venue for the parties to prospectively discuss key issues and potential solutions, learn, and evolve in a collaborative and adaptive way.

When different experts discuss the available evidence for a given marketing authorization application, it is not unlikely that some may set the bar higher than others. From the perspective of drug developers, there may be a risk that the more demanding view will prevail given that evidence should be robust, and standards should not be lowered. This tension—whether real or perceived—could be alleviated by increased transparency on the part of FDA and EMA regarding the different agencies' relative positions and the non-binding nature of scientific advice through PSA.

Conclusion 5-3: Despite underuse of the PSA program and lack of available evidence related to its impact, the committee acknowledges and expects that, in principle, concurrent scientific discourse through PSA should better enable more streamlined clinical trials, regulatory review, and approval of drugs to treat rare diseases and conditions.

The committee determined that EMA and FDA should undertake an assessment of the PSA program to include a review of how the types of scientific advice each agency has or would consider providing given the unmet medical need for rare disease patients and what can be accomplished by sponsors within a reasonable period of time. More generally speaking, increased transparency on the part of FDA and EMA on what is commonly held between the agencies regarding the types of questions asked and considerations for study design, data collection and analysis, and use of innovative tools would give sponsors better clarity on the regulatory pathway forward and help ensure that clinical trials are conducted in a scientifically rigorous and ethical manner and that rare disease patients are not exposed to unnecessary or duplicative studies.

RECOMMENDATION 5-3: The U.S. Food and Drug Administration (FDA), along with the European Medicines Agency (EMA) and other key stakeholders, should assess the impact of the Parallel Scientific Advice (PSA) program over the past decade on drug development for rare diseases and conditions, publicly share the results of this assessment, seek sponsor input on approaches to improve and enhance the use and utility of the program, and take action to increase access, use, and impact of the PSA program going forward. This assessment and plan for improvement should include:
- Reasons (real and perceived) for continued underuse of the PSA program and address the issues identified;
- Information-gathering on sponsor experience with PSA regarding the practical considerations (e.g., resources, location) for large and small companies to participate in PSA;
- Incentives that encourage use of the PSA program earlier in development (i.e., prior to enrolling patients in trials);
- Metrics for assessing the impact of the PSA program; and
- Criteria and goals for demonstrating improvement of the PSA program with established timeframes over a 5-year period.

If the actions taken do not lead to an increased use and greater impact of the PSA program within a 5-year period after the assessment and improvement plan has taken place, FDA should implement other mechanisms for parallel advice between FDA and EMA on drug development programs for rare diseases and conditions.

OPPORTUNITIES FOR ENHANCED COLLABORATION

FDA and EMA have the opportunity to serve as enablers of drug development for rare diseases and conditions by providing additional clarity on how alternative and confirmatory data (ACD) can be used to inform regulatory decision-making, reducing uncertainty about how to implement new trial designs and methodologies, and, when permissible, publicly sharing relevant information on marketing authorization submissions and approvals. Additionally, the agencies can work collaboratively with other organizations to proactively consider the use of new trial designs and methodologies in incorporating ACD into rare disease drug marketing applications.

Conclusion 5-4: FDA and EMA have mechanisms in place to coordinate and collaborate in ways that better enable drug review and approval, but more is needed to stimulate innovation and drug development for rare diseases and conditions. There is an opportunity for the agencies to take a more proactive approach when engaging with one another through existing collaborative mechanisms and to more effectively communicate this work with sponsors, patients, and other stakeholders. Collaboration between EMA and FDA can help maximize opportunities for each agency to leverage the other's expertise and experience, share learnings, streamline the review process, and work through scientific and regulatory bottlenecks to help pave the way for new treatments for people living with rare diseases and conditions.[14]

It is not uncommon for innovations in rare disease drug development to be a vanguard for applications across therapeutic areas, so lessons learned in the rare disease space could be considered by the agencies on a broader scale. For example, most rare diseases (roughly 80 percent) have well understood genetic precursors (Nature Genetics, 2022). Gene therapy—an intervention that modifies or manipulates the expression of a person's gene to treat or cure disease—offers promise for the treatment of gene-based conditions. Although the phenotypic presentation varies, advancements in biomedical technologies (e.g., CRISPR), improved understanding of disease etiology and trajectory, and the high cumulative burden (health-related and economic) of rare diseases have led to growing interest in the applicability of gene therapies. Additionally, many rare diseases are not amenable to small molecule therapies although there are some exceptions (e.g., Imatinib

---

[14] This conclusion was modified after release of the prepublication version of the report to more accurately represent coordination and collaborative efforts of FDA and EMA.

for acute lymphoblastic leukemia) (Biondi et al., 2018; Papaioannou et al., 2023). The use of CRISPR (clustered regularly interspaced short palindromic repeats) and adeno-associated viruses in gene therapy is now being pursued by multiple drug sponsors for the treatment of rare and chronic diseases and conditions.

Over the past 20 years, there has been a shift in thinking on the part of FDA and EMA, which were founded to ensure that drug products are safe and effective. In addition to playing a critical role in protecting human health, the agencies serve as enablers by actively promoting scientific and technological innovation for advancing drug development. To meet the future needs of people living with rare diseases and conditions, it is important for the ecosystem that the regulatory agencies have the knowledge and capacity to review and assess the new innovative products they are charged with regulating. This will require thinking ahead to what the future will look like a decade from now—ensuring that there are experts with transversal knowledge across rare diseases and conditions and that people with lived experience are fully integrated throughout the regulatory process, to better enable patient-centered collaboration across and within the agencies.

Conclusion 5-5: Continued and intensified collaboration between FDA and EMA through the clusters, PSA program, and other shared initiatives has the potential to accelerate and scale up drug development for rare diseases and conditions by minimizing the number of trials conducted, improving the quality of trial design (i.e., analytical methods, study endpoints, use of biomarkers, safety mitigation approaches), and providing more clarity for sponsors on the evidence that is necessary for demonstrating that drugs are safe and effective.

EMA and FDA individually and collectively have an opportunity to strengthen their roles as facilitators of drug innovation, sharing insights of lessons learned within and across the agencies, as well as with researchers, drug sponsors, providers, patients, and their caregivers. The committee hopes that through the adoption of the recommendations in this report, the regulatory process for rare diseases will become more transparent, work more smoothly and collaboratively, and ultimately lead to more therapies for patients living with rare diseases and conditions.

SUMMARY OF CONCLUSIONS AND RECOMMENDATIONS

Conclusion 5-1: Despite some key differences, FDA and EMA have similar approaches to the evaluation and approval of drugs for rare diseases. Given these parallel approaches, there are existing mechanisms for close collaboration between the two agencies, as well as opportunities for enhanced collaboration in the future, that would allow each agency to retain sovereign authority and accountability in regulatory decision-making.

Conclusion 5-2: To meet the needs of rare disease patients and their caregivers, there is an ethical obligation on the part of regulatory agencies to share relevant information on the review and approval of drugs to treat rare diseases and conditions. If researchers and sponsors working on rare disease drug development had a better understanding of the reasons for successes and failures of marketing authorization applications, they could better innovate new therapeutics that have a higher likelihood of reaching patients. Additionally, more transparency would enhance public understanding and confidence in the important work carried out by regulatory agencies.

Conclusion 5-3: Despite the underuse of the PSA program and lack of available evidence related to its impact, the committee acknowledges and expects that, in principle, concurrent scientific discourse through PSA should better enable more streamlined clinical trials, regulatory review, and approval of drugs to treat rare diseases and conditions.

Conclusion 5-4: FDA and EMA have mechanisms in place to coordinate and collaborate in ways that better enable drug review and approval, but more is needed to stimulate innovation and drug development for rare diseases and conditions. There is an opportunity for the agencies to take a more proactive approach when engaging with one another through existing collaborative mechanisms and to more effectively communicate this work with sponsors, patients, and other stakeholders. Collaboration between EMA and FDA can help maximize opportunities for each agency to leverage the other's expertise and experience, share learnings, streamline the review process, and work through scientific and regulatory bottlenecks to help pave the way for new treatments for people living with rare diseases and conditions.[15]

Conclusion 5-5: Continued and intensified collaboration between FDA and EMA through the clusters, PSA program, and other shared initiatives has the potential to accelerate and scale up drug development for rare diseases and conditions by minimizing the number of trials conducted, improving the quality of trial design (i.e. analytical methods, study endpoints, use of biomarkers, safety mitigation approaches), and

---

[15] This conclusion was modified after release of the prepublication version of the report to more accurately represent coordination and collaborative efforts of FDA and EMA.

providing more clarity for sponsors on the evidence that is necessary for demonstrating that drugs are safe and effective.

RECOMMENDATION 5-1: The U.S. Food and Drug Administration (FDA) should take steps to make relevant information on marketing authorization submissions, review milestones, approval and negative review decisions (refusal to file, clinical hold, and complete response letters), and the use of regulatory flexibilities for rare disease drug products publicly available and easily accessible to inform sponsors, patients, researchers, and reviewers on decision-making rationales and when and how available policies are applied. While the committee acknowledges the legal challenges surrounding disclosure of information, actions should include, but not be limited to:
- Mirroring the level of information disclosed by the European Medicines Agency (EMA) presented on submissions, review milestones, and review decisions, such that there is parity between what FDA and EMA share publicly;
- Building on the work of the 2010 FDA Transparency Task Force, to implement Phase II product application's disclosure requirements:[16] considerations for product applications (including investigational applications);
- Organizing and structuring the information made public in such a way that the public can identify trends (e.g., increases or decreases in the use of regulatory flexibility by product type or therapeutic area over time and expedited and designation program use);
- Link clinical trials to FDA disclosures by using national clinical trial identifiers[17] to allow the public to better understand the connection between clinical trials and the regulatory process.

RECOMMENDATION 5-2: To facilitate the efficient global development of orphan drugs, the U.S. Food and Drug Administration (FDA) and the European Medicines Agency (EMA) should build on the existing clusters relevant for rare diseases by undertaking the following:

---

[16] On May 19, 2010, the Transparency Task Force released a report containing 21 draft proposals about expanding the disclosure of information by FDA while maintaining confidentiality for trade secrets and individually identifiable patient information. FDA accepted public comment on the proposals, as well as on which draft proposals should be given priority, on this website from May 19, 2010, through July 20, 2010. https://wayback.archiveit.org/7993/20171105152021/https://www.fda.gov/AboutFDA/Transparency/PublicDisclosure/DraftProposalbyTopicArea/ucm211691.htm (accessed May 14, 2024).

[17] A national clinical trial number is an 8-digit unique identifier assigned to a clinical study when it is registered on ClinicalTrials.gov.

- Create a forum, which includes key decision makers within the agencies, for forward-looking discussion of issues and common challenges for rare disease drug development that EMA and FDA could use to achieve a more harmonized approach to rare disease development.
- Devote resources to discuss and resolve misalignment related to rare disease drug development.
- Publicly issue findings on key scientific or regulatory topics related to rare disease drug development.
- Conduct and publicly share an annual review of all orphan drug applications for the agencies to facilitate more immediate sharing of lessons learned and surface issues that cut across rare disease drug development programs.

RECOMMENDATION 5-3: The U.S. Food and Drug Administration (FDA), along with the European Medicines Agency (EMA) and other key stakeholders, should assess the impact of the Parallel Scientific Advice (PSA) program over the past decade on drug development for rare diseases and conditions, publicly share the results of this assessment, seek sponsor input on approaches to improve and enhance the use and utility of the program, and take action to increase access, use, and impact of the PSA program going forward. This assessment and plan for improvement should include:
- Reasons (real and perceived) for continued underuse of the PSA program and address the issues identified;
- Information-gathering on sponsor experience with PSA regarding the practical considerations (e.g., resources, location) for large and small companies to participate in PSA;
- Incentives that encourage use of the PSA program earlier in development (i.e., prior to enrolling patients in trials);
- Metrics for assessing the impact of the PSA program; and
- Criteria and goals for demonstrating improvement of the PSA program with established timeframes over a 5-year period.

If the actions taken do not lead to an increased use and greater impact of the PSA program within a five-year period after the assessment and improvement plan has taken place, FDA should implement other mechanisms for parallel advice between FDA and EMA on drug development programs for rare diseases and conditions.

REFERENCES

Biondi, A., V. Gandemer, P. D. Lorenzo, G. Cario, M. Campbell, A. Castor, R. Pieters, A. Baruchel, A. Vora, V. Leoni, J. Stary, G. Escherich, C.-K. Li, G. Cazzaniga, H. Cavé, J. Bradtke, V. Conter, V. Saha, M. Schrappe, and M. G. Valsecch. 2018. Imatinib treatment of paediatric Philadelphia chromosome-positive acute lymphoblastic leukaemia (EsPhALL2010): A prospective, intergroup, open-label, single-arm clinical trial. *The Lancet. Haematology* 5(12).

CTTI (Clinical Trials Transformation Initative). 2023. *Framework of the FDA/CTTI Patient Engagement Collaborative*. https://ctti-clinicaltrials.org/wp-content/uploads/2023/05/PEC-Framework_Compliant-Apr-10-2023_FINAL.pdf (accessed August 15, 2024).

Cox, E. M., A. V. Edmund, E. Kratz, S. H. Lockwood, and A. Shankar. 2020. Regulatory affairs 101: Introduction to expedited regulatory pathways. *Clinical and Translational Science* 13(3):451-461.

EMA (European Medicines Agency). 2001. *Points to consider on application with 1. Meta-analyses; 2. One pivotal study*. https://www.ema.europa.eu/en/documents/scientific-guideline/points-consider-application-1meta-analyses-2one-pivotal-study_en.pdf (accessed August 1, 2024).

EMA. 2012. *Recommendation for maintenance of orphan designation at the time of marketing authorisation*. https://www.ema.europa.eu/en/documents/orphan-review/recommendation-maintenance-orphan-designation-time-marketing-authorisation-kalydeco-ivacaftor-treatment-cystic-fibrosis_en.pdf (accessed August 1, 2024).

EMA. 2017. *Paediatric Gaucher disease: A strategic collaborative approach from EMA and FDA*. https://www.ema.europa.eu/en/documents/scientific-guideline/gaucher-disease-strategic-collaborative-approach-european-medicines-agency-and-food-and-drug-administration_en.pdf (accessed August 1, 2024).

EMA. 2021a. *Guideline on registry-based studies*. https://www.ema.europa.eu/en/documents/scientific-guideline/guideline-registry-based-studies_en.pdf-0 (accessed August 1, 2024).

EMA. 2021b. *A vision for use of real-world evidence in EU medicines regulation*. https://www.ema.europa.eu/en/news/vision-use-real-world-evidence-eu-medicines-regulation (accessed August 15, 2024).

EMA. 2022a. *Engagement framework: EMA and patients, consumers and their organizations*. https://www.ema.europa.eu/system/files/documents/other/updated_engagement_framework_-_ema_and_patients_consumers_and_their_organisations_2022-en.pdf (accessed August 1, 2024).

EMA. 2022b. *Good practice guide for the use of the metadata catalogue of real-world data sources*. https://www.ema.europa.eu/en/documents/regulatory-procedural-guideline/good-practice-guide-use-metadata-catalogue-real-world-data-sources_en.pdf (accessed August 1, 2024).

EMA. 2023a. *20 years EU/US collaboration on medicines regulation*. https://www.ema.europa.eu/system/files/documents/other/2023-09_ema-fda-20-years-arrangement_en.pdf (accessed August 15, 2024).

EMA. 2023b. *Real-world evidence framework to support EU regulatory decision-making*. https://www.ema.europa.eu/system/files/documents/report/real-world-evidence-framework-support-eu-regulatory-decision-making-report-experience-gained_en.pdf (accessed August 1, 2024).

EMA. 2023c. *Soliris*. https://www.ema.europa.eu/en/medicines/human/EPAR/soliris (accessed August 15, 2024).

EMA. 2024a. *Cluster activities*. https://www.ema.europa.eu/en/partners-networks/international-activities/cluster-activities (accessed August 15, 2024).

EMA. 2024b. *Kalydeco*. https://www.ema.europa.eu/en/medicines/human/EPAR/kalydeco (accessed August 15, 2024).

EMA. 2024c. *Tegsedi.* https://www.ema.europa.eu/en/medicines/human/EPAR/tegsedi (accessed August 15, 2024).
EMA. 2024d. *United States.* https://www.ema.europa.eu/en/partners-networks/international-activities/bilateral-interactions-non-eu-regulators/united-states (accessed August 15, 2024).
EMA. n.d.-a. *Accelerated assessment.* https://www.ema.europa.eu/en/human-regulatory-overview/marketing-authorisation/accelerated-assessment (accessed August 15, 2024).
EMA. n.d.-b. *Authorisation of medicines.* https://www.ema.europa.eu/en/about-us/what-we-do/authorisation-medicines (accessed March 18, 2024).
EMA. n.d.-c. *Clinical data publication.* https://www.ema.europa.eu/en/human-regulatory-overview/marketing-authorisation/clinical-data-publication (accessed July 10, 2024).
EMA. n.d.-d. *Collaborating experts.* https://careers.ema.europa.eu/content/Collaborating-Expert/?locale=en_GB (accessed August 15, 2024).
EMA. n.d.-e. *Conditional marketing authorization.* https://www.ema.europa.eu/en/human-regulatory-overview/marketing-authorisation/conditional-marketing-authorisation (accessed February 20, 2024).
EMA. n.d.-f. *European experts.* https://www.ema.europa.eu/en/about-us/how-we-work/european-medicines-regulatory-network/european-experts (accessed March 15, 2024).
EMA. n.d.-g. *European Medicines Agency (EMA).* https://european-union.europa.eu/institutions-law-budget/institutions-and-bodies/search-all-eu-institutions-and-bodies/european-medicines-agency-ema_en#:~:text=The%20European%20Medicines%20Agency%20(EMA,European%20Economic%20Area%20(EEA (accessed August 15, 2024).
EMA. n.d.-h. *Exceptional circumstances.* https://www.ema.europa.eu/en/glossary/exceptional-circumstances (accessed March 10, 2024).
EMA. n.d.-i. *How EMA evaluates medicines for human use.* https://www.ema.europa.eu/en/about-us/what-we-do/authorisation-medicines/how-ema-evaluates-medicines-human-use (accessed August 15, 2024).
EMA. n.d.-j. *How the committees work.* https://www.ema.europa.eu/en/committees/how-committees-work (accessed March 15, 2024).
EMA. n.d.-k. *Marketing authorisation.* https://www.ema.europa.eu/en/human-regulatory-overview/marketing-authorisation (accessed July 10, 2024).
EMA. n.d.-l. *Obtaining an EU marketing authorisation, step-by-step.* https://www.ema.europa.eu/en/human-regulatory-overview/marketing-authorisation/obtaining-eu-marketing-authorisation-step-step (accessed August 15, 2024).
EMA. n.d.-m. *Oprhan incentives.* https://www.ema.europa.eu/en/human-regulatory-overview/research-and-development/orphan-designation-research-and-development/orphan-incentives (accessed February 19, 2024).
EMA. n.d.-n. *Patients' and consumers' working party.* https://www.ema.europa.eu/en/committees/working-parties-other-groups/comp-working-parties-other-groups/patients-consumers-working-party (accessed August 6, 2024).
EMA. n.d.-o. *PRIME: Priority Medicines.* https://www.ema.europa.eu/en/human-regulatory-overview/research-development/prime-priority-medicines (accessed August 15, 2024).
EMA. n.d.-p. *Scientific advice and protocol assistance.* https://www.ema.europa.eu/en/human-regulatory-overview/research-development/scientific-advice-protocol-assistance (accessed March 10, 2024).
EMA. n.d.-q. *Who we are.* https://www.ema.europa.eu/en/about-us/who-we-are (accessed July 9, 2024).
EMA and FDA (U.S. Food and Drug Administration). 2021. *General principles: EMA-FDA Parallel Scientific Advice.* https://www.ema.europa.eu/en/documents/other/general-principles-european-medicines-agency-food-and-drug-administration-parallel-scientific-advice_en.pdf (accessed August 1, 2024).

European Commission. 2014. *Guideline on the format and content of applications for designation as orphan medicinal products and on the transfer of designations from one sponsor to another.* https://health.ec.europa.eu/system/files/2016-11/2014-03_guideline_rev4_final_0.pdf (accessed August 1, 2024).

European Union. 2004. *Regulation (EC) NO 726/2004 of the European Parliament and of the Council.* https://eur-lex.europa.eu/LexUriServ/LexUriServ.do?uri=OJ:L:2004:136:0001:0033:en:PDF (accessed August 1, 2024).

FDA. 2007. *Soliris: Drug approval package.* https://www.accessdata.fda.gov/drugsatfda_docs/nda/2007/125166s0000TOC.cfm (accessed August 15, 2024).

FDA. 2010. *Food and Drug Administration Transparency Task Force: Request for comments.* https://www.federalregister.gov/documents/2010/03/12/2010-5377/food-and-drug-administration-transparency-task-force-request-for-comments (accessed August 1, 2024).

FDA. 2012. *Drug approval package: Kalydeco (ivacaftor).* https://www.accessdata.fda.gov/drugsatfda_docs/nda/2012/203188s000TOC.cfm (accessed August 15, 2024).

FDA. 2014. *Expedited programs for serious conditions—Drugs and biologics: Guidance for industry.* https://www.fda.gov/media/86377/download (accessed August 1, 2024).

FDA. 2015a. *Review team responsibilities.* https://www.fda.gov/about-fda/center-drug-evaluation-and-research-cder/review-team-responsibilities (accessed August 15, 2024).

FDA. 2015b. *Transparency initiative: Phase II progress report.* https://wayback.archive-it.org/7993/20171101192954/https://www.fda.gov/AboutFDA/Transparency/TransparencyInitiative/ucm273854.htm (accessed August 15, 2024).

FDA. 2015c. *Transparency initiative: Phase III progress report.* https://wayback.archive-it.org/7993/20171101192958/https://www.fda.gov/AboutFDA/Transparency/TransparencyInitiative/ucm273856.htm (accessed August, 2024).

FDA. 2016. *Advisory committees: Critical to the FDA's product review process.* https://www.fda.gov/drugs/information-consumers-and-patients-drugs/advisory-committees-critical-fdas-product-review-process (accessed July 11, 2024).

FDA. 2017. *Best practices for communication between IND sponsors and FDA during drug development guidance for industry and review staff: Good review practice.* https://www.fda.gov/media/94850/download (accessed August 1, 2024).

FDA. 2018. *Drug approval package: Tegsedi (inotersen).* https://www.accessdata.fda.gov/drugsatfda_docs/nda/2018/211172Orig1s000TOC.cfm (accessed August 1, 2024).

FDA. 2019a. *Demonstrating substantial evidence of effectiveness for human drug and biological products: Guidance for industry.* https://www.fda.gov/media/133660/download (accessed August 1, 2024).

FDA. 2019b. *Rare diseases: Natural history studies for drug development: Guidance for industry.* https://www.fda.gov/media/122425/download (accessed August 1, 2024).

FDA. 2020. *COVID-19 update: FDA's ongoing commitment to transparency for COVID-19 EUAs.* https://www.fda.gov/news-events/press-announcements/covid-19-update-fdas-ongoing-commitment-transparency-covid-19-euas (accessed August 15, 2024).

FDA. 2022a. *New drug application (NDA).* https://www.fda.gov/drugs/types-applications/new-drug-application-nda (accessed June 25, 2024).

FDA. 2022b. *Remarks by FDA Commissioner Robert M. Califf to the 2022 NORD Breakthrough Summit.* https://www.fda.gov/news-events/speeches-fda-officials/remarks-fda-commissioner-robert-m-califf-2022-nord-breakthrough-summit-10172022 (accessed July 9, 2024).

FDA. 2023a. *Benefit-risk assessment for new drug and biological products: Guidance for industry.* https://www.fda.gov/media/152544/download (accessed August 1, 2024).

FDA. 2023b. *Demonstrating substantial evidence of effectiveness with one adequate and well-controlled clinical investigation and confirmatory evidence: Guidance for industry.* https://www.fda.gov/media/172166/download (accessed August 1, 2024).

FDA. 2023c. *Formal meetings between the FDA and sponsors or applicants of PDUFA products.* https://www.fda.gov/media/172311/download (accessed August 1, 2024).

FDA. 2023d. *Rare diseases: Considerations for the development of drugs and biological products: Guidance for industry.* https://www.fda.gov/media/119757/download (accessed August 1, 2024).

FDA. 2024a. *About the FDA patient representative program.* https://www.fda.gov/patients/learn-about-fda-patient-engagement/about-fda-patient-representative-program (accessed March 10, 2024).

FDA. 2024b. *CDER patient-focused drug development.* https://www.fda.gov/drugs/development-approval-process-drugs/cder-patient-focused-drug-development (accessed March 05, 2024).

FDA. 2024c. *International collaboration/pediatric cluster.* https://www.fda.gov/science-research/pediatrics/international-collaboration-pediatric-cluster (accessed August 15, 2024).

FDA. 2024d. *Learn about FDA advisory committees.* https://www.fda.gov/patients/learn-about-fda-advisory-committees (accessed August 15, 2024).

FDA. 2024e. *Patient Engagement Collaborative.* https://www.fda.gov/patients/learn-about-fda-patient-engagement/patient-engagement-collaborative (accessed August 15, 2024).

FDA, and EMA. 2021. *Common commentary - EMA/FDA: Common issues requested for discussion by the respective agency (EMA/PDCO and FDA) concerning paediatric oncology development plans (Paediatric Investigation Plans [PIPs] and initial Pediatric Study Plans [iPSPs]).* https://www.fda.gov/media/147197/download?attachment (accessed August 1, 2024).

Gingery, D. 2021. *FDA-EMA pilot could further push global generic harmonization, but will sponsors use it?* https://generics.citeline.com/GB151311/FDAEMA-Pilot-Could-Further-Push-Global-Generic-Harmonization-But-Will-Sponsors-Use-It (accessed August 1, 2024).

Hofer, M. P., C. Jakobsson, N. Zafiropoulos, S. Vamvakas, T. Vetter, J. Regnstrom, and R. J. Hemmings. 2015. Impact of scientific advice from the European Medicines Agency. *Nature Reviews Drug Discovery 2015* 14(5).

Ibrahim, S. 2024. *CDER's OGD and EMA's Parallel Scientific Advice pilot program for complex generics works to increase harmonization and bring generic drugs to patients.* https://www.fda.gov/drugs/our-perspective/cders-ogd-and-emas-parallel-scientific-advice-pilot-program-complex-generics-works-increase (accessed August 1, 2024).

Kweder, S. 2022. *Considering a PSA request? Summary and best practices.* https://www.fda.gov/media/164718/download (accessed August 1, 2024).

Lee, K. J., K. Tyner, and S. Thirstrup. 2023. Impact of FDA and EMA collaborative efforts: Processes to Evaluate the Safety and Efficacy of Drugs for Rare Diseases or Conditions in the United States and the European Union (Meeting 2 - Hybrid).

Lurie, P., S. H. Chahal, W. D. Sigelman, S. Stacy, J. Sclar, and B. Ddamulira. 2015. Comparison of content of FDA letters not approving applications for new drugs and associated public announcements from sponsors: Cross sectional study. *BMJ: British Medical Journal* 350:h2758.

Marks, P. 2020. *FDA and EMA collaborate to facilitate SARS-CoV-2 vaccine development.* https://www.fda.gov/news-events/fda-voices/fda-and-ema-collaborate-facilitate-sars-cov-2-vaccine-development (accessed August 1, 2024).

Nature Genetics. 2022. Rare diseases, common challenges. *Nature Genetics* 54(3):215.

Papaioannou, I., J. S. Owen, and R. J. Yáñez-Muñoz. 2023. Clinical applications of gene therapy for rare diseases: A review. *International Journal of Experimental Pathology* 104(4).

Prilla, S. 2018. *Legal basis & types of approvals.* https://www.ema.europa.eu/en/documents/presentation/presentation-legal-basis-and-types-approvals-s-prilla_en.pdf (accessed August 1, 2024).

Reaman, G., D. Karres, F. Ligas, G. Lesa, D. Casey, L. Ehrlich, K. Norga, and R. Pazdur. 2020. Accelerating the global development of pediatric cancer drugs: A call to coordinate the submissions of pediatric investigation plans and pediatric study plans to the European Medicines Agency and U.S. Food and Drug Administration. *Journal of Clinical Oncology: Official Journal of the American Society of Clinical Oncology* 38(36):4227-4230.

Regnstrom, J., F. Koenig, B. Aronsson, T. Reimer, K. Svendsen, S. Tsigkos, B. Flamion, H.-G. Eichler, S. Vamvakas, J. Regnstrom, F. Koenig, B. Aronsson, T. Reimer, K. Svendsen, S. Tsigkos, B. Flamion, H.-G. Eichler, and S. Vamvakas. 2009. Factors associated with success of market authorisation applications for pharmaceutical drugs submitted to the European Medicines Agency. *European Journal of Clinical Pharmacology* 66(1).

Richardson, E., G. Daniel, D. R. Joy, S. L. Kweder, D. M. Maloney, M. J. Raggio, and J. P. Jarow. 2018. Regional approaches to expedited drug development and review. *Therapeutic Innovation & Regulatory Science* 52(6).

Sharfstein, J. M., J. D. Miller, A. L. Davis, J. S. Ross, M. E. McCarthy, B. Smith, A. Chaudhry, G. C. Alexander, and A. S. Kesselheim. 2017. Blueprint for transparency at the US Food and Drug Administration: Recommendations to advance the development of safe and effective medical products. *The Journal of Law, Medicine & Ethics* 45(2_suppl):7-23.

Teixeira, T., S. L. Kweder, and A. Saint-Raymond. 2020. Are the European Medicines Agency, US Food and Drug Administration, and other international regulators talking to each other? *Clinical Pharmacology & Therapeutics* 107(3).

Thirstrup, S. 2023. Orphan medicines in EU: Processes to Evaluate the Safety and Efficacy of Drugs for Rare Diseases or Conditions in the United States and the European Union (Meeting 2 - Hybrid).

Thor, S., T. Vetter, A. Marcal, and S. Kweder. 2023. EMA-FDA Parallel Scientific Advice: Optimizing development of medicines in the global age. *Therapeutic Innovation & Regulatory Science* 57(4).

Tyner, K., K. J. Lee, J. Arcidiacono, and S. Zaidi. 2023. International clusters and collaboration: Processes to Evaluate the Safety and Efficacy of Drugs for Rare Diseases or Conditions in the United States and the European Union (Meeting 1 - Virtual).

Ungstrup, E., and D. Vanags. 2023. *Aligning global drug development for pediatric populations.* https://www.pharmalex.com/thought-leadership/blogs/aligning-global-drug-development-for-pediatric-populations/ (accessed August 15, 2024).

Welch, A. R. 2015. *FDA, EMA drug approval stats: Are we measuring success the wrong way?* https://www.bioprocessonline.com/doc/fda-ema-approval-stats-are-we-measuring-pharma-success-the-wrong-way-0001 (accessed August 1, 2024).

Appendix A

Biographical Sketches of Committee Members and Staff

COMMITTEE MEMBERS

Jeff (Jeffrey) Kahn, Ph.D., M.P.H. (Committee Chair), is the Andreas C. Dracopoulos Director of the Johns Hopkins Berman Institute of Bioethics, a position he assumed in July 2016. Since 2011, he has been the inaugural Robert Henry Levi and Ryda Hecht Levi Professor of Bioethics and Public Policy at the Berman Institute. He is also Professor in the Department of Health Policy and Management of the Johns Hopkins Bloomberg School of Public Health. He is an internationally recognized expert in bioethics, exploring the intersection of ethics and health/science policy, including human and animal research ethics, public health, and ethical issues in emerging biomedical technologies. Dr. Kahn has served on numerous governmental and international advisory panels, including most recently on the International Commission on the Clinical Use of Heritable Human Genome Editing. He is currently chair of the National Academies of Sciences, Engineering, and Medicine (National Academies) Committee on Aerospace Medicine and Medicine of Extreme Environments and has previously chaired the National Academies Committee on the Use of Chimpanzees in Biomedical and Behavioral Research (2011); the Committee on Ethics Principles and Guidelines for Health Standards for Long Duration and Exploration Spaceflights (2014); and the Committee on the Ethical, Social, and Policy Considerations of Mitochondrial Replacement Techniques (2016). Dr. Kahn has served as chair of the National Academy of Medicine Board on Health Sciences Policy and as a member of the National Academy of Medicine Council. He received his B.A. (microbiology) from the University of California, Los Angeles, his M.P.H. from Johns Hopkins University School of Hygiene and Public Health, and his Ph.D. (philosophy/bioethics) from Georgetown University.

Ron (Ronald) Bartek, M.Sc., is co-founder and president of Friedreich's Ataxia Research Alliance (FARA). Formerly, he was director and chair of the National Organization for Rare Disorders. He also served as past president and current member of the board of directors of the Alliance for a Stronger FDA. Mr. Bartek co-founded the NCATS Alliance, now serving as chair of its board of directors. He was formerly on the board of directors of the Alliance for Regenerative Medicine. He was a member of the NIH/NCATS National Advisory Council and the NIH Neurological Institute National Advisory Council, having previously served as chair of the NCATS Cures Acceleration Network Review Board. Mr. Bartek has been recognized by FDA Office of Orphan Drug Development as one of "30 Heroes changing lives of rare disease patients." He is a former member of the FDA/CTTI Patient Engagement Collaborative. Mr. Bartek has 20 years of federal executive and legislative experience in defense, foreign policy, and intelligence. Mr. Bartek received his B.S. from U.S. Military Academy, West Point, and his M.A. from Georgetown University.

Terry Jo Bichell, Ph.D., M.P.H., is the CEO and founder of COMBINEDBrain as well as a lecturer at Vanderbilt University. She worked primarily as a public health nurse-midwife until her youngest child, Lou, was diagnosed with Angelman syndrome in 2000. She quickly switched focus to move bench research into the first clinical trials for Angelman syndrome and to help design natural history studies. Dr. Bichell was the founding director of the A-BOM Alliance from 2016–2018. In 2019, she launched COMBINEDBrain, a pre-competitive consortium of patient advocacy organizations that works with clinicians, researchers, and pharmaceutical firms to identify outcome measures and biomarkers for rare genetic neurodevelopmental disorders. She is the vice chair of the Tennessee Rare Disease Advisory Council and teaches a course in translational neuroscience at Vanderbilt University. She previously served on the Angelman Patient Advisory Council to Hoffman La Roche, which has now been disbanded. As a parent of a child living with a rare disease, Dr. Bichell gained first-hand experience in the search for a treatment for Angelman syndrome as she accompanies her son as he participates in clinical trials. Dr. Bichell received her B.S.N. from St. Louis University, her M.P.H. from Boston University, and her Ph.D. in neuroscience from Vanderbilt University where she studied gene-environment interactions in Huntington's disease rodent models.

Edward Botchwey, Ph.D., M.E., is a professor in the Wallace H. Coulter Department of Biomedical Engineering at Georgia Tech and Emory University. His research focuses on elucidating lipid signaling mechanisms in sickle cell disease and developing novel immunomodulatory therapies to resolve inflammation and treat organ dysfunction. Dr. Botchwey has garnered over $14 million in research funding and has published extensively on bioactive lipids and resolution pharmacology for sickle cell therapies. He conducts research in affiliation with the Marcus Center for Therapeutic Cell Characterization and Manufacturing. He has also spearheaded efforts to increase diversity and inclusion in biomedical engineering, including leading the Diversity, Equity, and Inclusion Committee for the Society for Biomaterials. Dr. Botchwey received his B.S. from the University of Maryland and his MEng and Ph.D. from the University of Pennsylvania. He completed a postdoctoral fellowship in vascular biology at The Wistar Institute.

Shein-Chung Chow, Ph.D., is a professor at the Department of Biostatistics and Bioinformatics at Duke University School of Medicine. Dr. Chow is also an adjunct professor at Peking University and Beijing Capital Medical University. Previously, he was a special government employee, appointed by FDA as a voting member of the Oncologic Drug Advisory Committee and a statistical advisor to FDA. Dr. Chow previously served as associate director of the Center for Drug Evaluation and Research's Office of Biostatistics at FDA. Dr. Chow is currently serving on several Data Safety Monitoring Boards for clinical studies sponsored by Genetech and Merck via third party clinical research organizations, Syneos, Parexel, and Statistics Collaborative. Dr. Chow was the editor-in-chief of the *Journal of Biopharmaceutical Statistics* (1992–2020) and is the editor-in-chief of the Biostatistics Book Series at Chapman and Hall/CRC Press of Taylor & Francis Group. He was elected Fellow of the American Statistical Association in 1995 and elected member of the ISI (International Statistical Institute) in 1999. Dr. Chow is the author or co-author of over 200 papers and 20 books on trial design considerations and statistical methods for rare disease research. He more recently authored the book *Innovative Methods for Rare Disease Drug Development*. Dr. Chow received his B.S. from National Taiwan University and his Ph.D. from University of Wisconsin–Madison.

Hans-Georg Eichler, M.D., M.Sc., is the consulting physician at the Association of Austrian Social Insurances. Prior to this role, Dr. Eichler was the senior medical officer of the European Medicines Agency (EMA) from 2007–2021. Earlier in his career, Dr. Eichler was a professor of clinical pharmacology and head of the Department of Clinical Pharmacology, as well as vice-rector for research and international relations at the Medical

University of Vienna. During his time in academia, he gained ample experience in clinical research, including being the primary investigator of numerous academic and industry-sponsored drug trials. In his subsequent positions, he was closely involved in the development of pharmaceutical policies from the governmental, regulatory, and public payer perspectives. Dr. Eichler serve as the vice-chair of the Scientific Advisory Committee at the Centre for Innovation in Regulatory Sciences and has done pro bono work for EURORDIS-Rare Diseases Europe, a nonprofit alliance of over 1,000 rare disease patient organizations across Europe. Dr. Eichler has received several honors and awards from different European universities and learned societies. He received his M.Sc. from the University of Surrey and his M.D. from the University of Vienna.

Pat (Patricia) Furlong, R.N., is president and CEO of Parent Project Muscular Dystrophy, which focuses on Duchenne and Becker muscular dystrophy. She led the development of Draft Guidance on Duchenne, which was submitted to FDA in 2016 and updated in 2022. She serves as a member for the Duchenne Community Advisory Board in Europe. Ms. Furlong served on the National Academies of Sciences, Engineering, and Medicine Committee on Safe and Effective Medicines for Children. She is a nurse practitioner by training, spending her early career in whole organ transplantation and renal dialysis. Since 1994, Ms. Furlong has focused on rare disease research—specifically on genetic testing, standards of care, therapy development, and regulatory processes. She has led preference studies to understand the patient's perspective of benefit and risk. Ms. Furlong has worked with rare disease groups as they prepare for interactions with regulatory agencies in the United States and Europe. Ms. Furlong is a member of the World Duchenne Organization's board, data safety monitoring boards for the Rare Disease Research Network and Cooperative International Neuromuscular Research Group, and New York University's Pediatric Gene Therapy Medical Ethics Group. Ms. Furlong serves on the Clinical Trials Transformation Initiative executive committee and is a board member with the National Health Council. She received her R.N./B.S.N. degree from Mount St. Joseph University.

Steven Galson M.D., M.P.H., is a senior advisor to Boston Consulting Group and serves on the board of directors of Biocryst Pharmaceuticals and Elephas Biosciences. He is a consultant for Skyline Therapeutics. Until June 2020, Dr. Galson was a senior vice president of research and development at Amgen Inc. He spent more than 20 years in government service, including 2 years as acting surgeon general of the United States. He served as director of FDA's Center for Drug Evaluation and Research, where he provided leadership for the center's national and international programs in pharmaceutical regulation. Dr. Galson began his public health service career as an epidemiological investigator at the U.S. Centers For Disease Control and Prevention. He was also the chief medical officer at both the Environmental Protection Agency and the U.S. Department of Energy. Dr. Galson is a trustee of the Keck Graduate Institute and a member of the Executive Committee of the Clinical Trial Transformation Initiative. In 2008, he received an honorary Doctor of Public Service degree from Drexel University School of Public Health, and in 2015, he received the Jacobi Medallion Award from Icahn Mount Sinai School of Medicine. In 2018 he was named health leader of the year from the Commissioned Officers Association of the U.S. Public Health Service. Dr. Galson has been a member of the Forum on Drug Discovery Development and Translation of the National Academies of Sciences, Engineering, and Medicine for 20 years. He has also served two terms as the forum's co-chair. Dr. Galson received his B.S. from Stony Brook University, his M.P.H. from Harvard University, and his M.D. from Icahn Mount Sinai School of Medicine.

Gavin Huntley-Fenner, Ph.D., is the co-founder and principal human factors consultant at Huntley-Fenner Advisors, which provides scientific advisory services. Specializing in creative and scientifically based approaches to assessing risks and benefits, Dr. Huntley-Fenner brings more than 25 years of both academic and business experience to bear on the crafting of innovative and effective communication to consumers. Dr. Huntley-Fenner also serves as an expert legal consultant, public speaker, and facilitator of risk analysis teams, where he is noted for his ability to effectively articulate solutions to complex problems. He has served on the U.S. FDA Risk Communication Advisory Committee (2004–2009) and on the National Academies of Sciences Engineering and Medicine (National Academies) Mutual Recognition Agreements in the Regulation of Medicines Study Committee (2019–2020). He is currently a member of the National Academies Environmental Health Matters Initiative Steering Committee and is also a member of Mattel's Medical and Scientific Advisory Council. Dr. Huntley-Fenner received his Ph.D. in brain and cognitive sciences from Massachusetts Institute of Technology in 1995 and his B.A. in cognitive sciences from Vassar College in 1990.

Anaeze Offodile II, M.D., M.P.H., is an executive vice president and the chief strategy officer of Memorial Sloan Kettering Cancer Center (MSK). Dr. Offodile is a member of the Forum on Drug Discovery Development and Translation of the National Academies of Sciences, Engineering, and Medicine (National Academies). He is a double board-certified physician with clinical expertise in oncologic reconstruction, a health services researcher with a focus on alternative payment models and care redesign, and a healthcare administrator with management experience in academia. He leads strategy efforts and care transformation initiatives at MSK by continuing to develop the core infrastructure, management systems, and processes for enterprise strategy and business development. Dr. Offodile pilots new initiatives, facilitates alignment on strategic institutional priorities, leverages data sources to cultivate innovative digital analytics and products, develops collaborations with outside groups, and partners with key internal leaders to competitively position MSK for the future. He received his B.S. from Kent State University, his M.P.H. from Johns Hopkins Bloomberg School of Public Health, and his M.D. from Columbia University.

Anne Pariser, M.D., is a physician, currently working with the Indian Health Service at the Crow/Northern Cheyenne Hospital in Crow Agency, Montana. Prior to this, she was the VP, medical and regulatory affairs at Alltrna, a biotech company developing tRNAs as therapeutic agents for rare genetic diseases (through March 2024), where she continues to provide part-time consulting services. Previously, she was the director of the Office of Rare Diseases Research at the NIH National Center for Advancing Translational Sciences from 2017–2022. From 2000–2017, she worked at the FDA CDER Office of New Drugs (OND), where she led the first specialized rare diseases review team for Inborn Errors of Metabolism. In 2010, Dr. Pariser founded the Rare Diseases Program (RDP) within OND/CDER, a congressional mandate intended to accelerate and improve rare diseases drug review within FDA that focused on the development of policy, guidance, training, and coordination of regulatory science to benefit rare disease programs. Dr. Pariser's research has focused on rare diseases regulatory and translational sciences, and she is the author of approximately 50 papers on these topics. Dr. Pariser has received numerous awards from FDA, NIH, HHS and other stakeholders for her service to the rare disease community. This includes the National Organization for Rare Disorders' National Public Health Leadership Award and being named, along with the OND/CDER's Rare Diseases Program, as one of the 30 Rare Disease Heroes on the 30th anniversary of the Orphan Drug Act. She is the chair of the Regulatory Scientific Committee at the International Rare Disease Research Consortium, a collaborative initiative uniting national and international nonprofits, industry, patient advocacy organizations, and scientists to promote collaboration for rare disease research. She is also a volunteer member of the board of directors for the Undiagnosed Diseases Network Foundation—a nonprofit that fosters collaboration among patients, clinicians, and scientists to bridge diagnosis, research, and clinical care for undiagnosed patients with rare and ultra-rare diseases. Dr. Pariser received her B.S. from Bates College and her M.D. from Georgetown University School of Medicine. She is board certified in internal medicine.

Jonathan Watanabe, PharmD., Ph.D., is associate dean of assessment and quality at the UC Irvine School of Pharmacy & Pharmaceutical Sciences and director of the UCI Center for Data-Driven Drugs Research and Policy. Dr. Watanabe is a member of the Forum on Drug Discovery Development and Translation of the National Academies of Sciences, Engineering, and Medicine (National Academies). Dr. Watanabe is an appointed member of the non-partisan California Health Benefits Review Program Faculty Task Force of the University of California funded by the State of California Legislature. He has been involved in research and policy efforts salient to rare diseases, including service on the National Academies' Committee on Making Medicines Affordable and participation in the National Academies' workshop series on Examining the Impact of Real-World Evidence on Medical Product Development. The latter also entailed publication of guidance manuscripts on conducting real-world trials in special populations. Additionally, he has received grant approval for a pending industry-funded project that will use publicly available data to examine global definitions of what deems drug as a 'biosimilar.' He has published original research examining the increase in high-spend medications covered by Medicare Part D that serve small populations in the United States. He was the National Academy of Medicine (NAM) Anniversary Fellow in Pharmacy from 2016 to 2018. From 2018 to 2021, he served as a Scholar in the NAM Emerging Leaders in Health and Medicine Program. Dr. Watanabe was the inaugural recipient of the University of Washington/Allergan Global Health Economics and Outcomes Research Fellowship (2007 to 2009). He received his B.S. from the University of Washington, his Pharm.D. from the University of Southern California, and his M.S. and Ph.D. from the University of Washington Comparative Health Outcomes, Policy, and Economics Institute. He is a board-certified geriatrics pharmacist.

NATIONAL ACADEMY OF MEDICINE FELLOW

Sanket Dhruva, M.D., M.H.S., is an assistant professor of medicine at the University of California, San Francisco (UCSF) and a cardiologist at the San Francisco Veterans Affairs Medical Center. His research, clinical, and education interests focus on understanding and strengthening the evidence base for the safe and effective use of drugs and medical devices in diverse populations, with the goal of improving the quality of care and clinical outcomes for patients. He identifies solutions to improve equity in the development and dissemination of these therapies. Dr. Dhruva currently serves on the Medicare Evidence Development & Coverage Advisory Committee and Institute for Clinical and Economic Review California Technology Assessment Forum. He has authored more than 185 peer-reviewed publications and has been funded by the Greenwall Foundation, Department of Veterans

Affairs, NIH, Food and Drug Administration, National Evaluation System for Health Technology, National Institute for Health Care Management, and Arnold Ventures. Dr. Dhruva received his BA in political science and molecular and cell biology from the University of California, Berkeley. He graduated with an MD from UCSF. He completed residency in internal medicine at UCSF and fellowship in cardiovascular medicine at the University of California, Davis. He subsequently completed an MHS at Yale University

STUDY STAFF AND CONSULTANT

Carolyn K. Shore, Ph.D., is a senior program officer with the Board on Health Sciences Policy of the National Academies of Sciences, Engineering, and Medicine. She is co-director of the National Academies study on Processes to Evaluate the Safety and Efficacy of Drugs for Rare Diseases or Conditions in the United States and the European Union and staff director of the Forum on Drug Discovery, Development, and Translation. Before joining the National Academies, Dr. Shore was an officer on Pew's antibiotic resistance project, leading work on research and policies to spur the discovery and development of urgently needed antibacterial therapies. She previously served as a foreign affairs officer at the U.S. Department of State, where she led an initiative on open data and innovation-based solutions to global challenges. She also served as the State Department's representative to intergovernmental organizations focusing on food safety, plant and animal health, biosecurity, and agricultural trade policy. Previously, Dr. Shore was an American Society for Microbiology congressional fellow, working on science-based policy related to antibiotic stewardship and other public health issues. She holds a doctoral degree in microbiology and molecular genetics from Harvard University. As a graduate student, she studied antimalarial drug resistance in Senegal and worked jointly between the Medicines for Malaria Venture, Genzyme Corporation, and the Broad Institute of Harvard and MIT to discover new anti-malarial compounds. Dr. Shore was awarded a Fulbright Fellowship for work at the University of Queensland in Brisbane, Australia, and a National Institutes of Health Training Grant for postdoctoral work at the University of Iowa.

Tequam Worku, M.P.H. (Study Co-Director), is a program officer for the Board on Health Sciences Policy at the National Academies of Sciences, Engineering, and Medicine. Most recently, she worked on a study *Examining the Working Definition for Long COVID* and serves as the staff lead for an Action Collaborative on Engaging Community Practices in Clinical Trials. Her previous work with the National Academies includes directing a study on *Improving the CDC Quarantine Station Network's Response* to *Emerging Threats* with the Board on Global Health. Prior to that, she worked at the Association of State and Territorial Health Officials as a senior analyst for Clinical to Community Connections, managing federally funded projects on community health workers and ending the HIV epidemic. Her past experience also includes working on projects related to chronic diseases and the development of healthy communities, including the promotion of healthy aging and hypertension prevention and control (the Million Hearts Initiative). Ms. Worku has worked on various research projects on topics including breast cancer disparities and cultural competency in health care. Additionally, she has worked internationally supporting knowledge management and data analysis efforts at the national level. She is committed to efforts aimed at bridging disparities in health and has been actively involved in health-equity initiatives. She earned her B.A. in biology from University of Maryland Baltimore County, an M.P.H. from The George Washington University, and is currently a Dr.P.H. candidate at Morgan State University.

Carson Smith, M.S., is a research associate with the Board on Health Sciences Policy of the National Academies of Sciences, Engineering, and Medicine. Prior to joining the National Academies in August 2023, he was a research assistant for the Human Factors and Aging Laboratory at the University of Illinois at Urbana-Champaign. In this role, he supported research into usefulness, ease of use, and adoption of assistive technology among older adults. He also previously worked in research at the National Center for Human Factors in Healthcare within the MedStar Institute for Innovation. Mr. Smith received his B.S. in interdisciplinary health sciences and his M.Sc. in health technology from the University of Illinois at Urbana-Champaign.

Noah Ontjes, M.A., is an associate program officer with the Board on Health Sciences Policy of the National Academies of Sciences, Engineering, and Medicine. He currently staffs the Forum on Drug Discovery, Development, and Translation, co-leading projects on engaging community practices in clinical trials and preparing the future workforce in drug research and development. He attended Wake Forest University where he graduated with a B.S. in biology and a triple minor in bioethics, chemistry, and psychology. His interest in the multiple factors that influence one's health paired with his love of different perspectives led him to pursue an M.A. in Bioethics at Wake Forest University. During graduate school, he successfully defended his thesis on the reasonable person standard of disclosure in genetic research as well as collaborated on a published paper concerning the ethical considerations of electroconvulsive therapy on incapacitated patients. Overall, he likes to categorize himself as someone who is intellectually curious.

Kyle Cavagnini, Ph.D., is an associate program officer with the Board on Health Sciences Policy. They currently staff the Forum on Drug Discovery, Development, and Translation, where their portfolio includes pre-clinical research and clinical trial diversity. Dr. Cavagnini previously worked with the National Academies Institute for Laboratory Animal Research, where they supported the Standing Committee for the Care and Use of Animals in Research, and workshop committees engaged in the One Health field. Prior to joining the National Academies, Dr. Cavagnini completed a science policy fellowship with the Federation of American Societies for Experimental Biology and was a Fulbright Fellow in the Department of Biomedicine at the University of Bergen, Norway. They earned their Ph.D. in biological chemistry from the Johns Hopkins University School of Medicine, where their doctoral research focused on genomic contributions to metabolic sensing in the liver and other tissues. They received undergraduate degrees in biochemistry and philosophy from the University of North Carolina at Asheville.

Melvin Joppy is a senior program assistant on the Board on Health Sciences Policy of the National Academies of Sciences, Engineering, and Medicine. He previously served as a program assistant at the Department of Energy (DOE) in the Office of Basic Energy Sciences. Prior to DOE, Mr. Joppy served as the committee manager for the Presidential Advisory Council on HIV/AIDS within the U.S. Department of Health and Human Services. Mr. Joppy received his B.S. in communications from Bowie State University.

Clare Stroud, Ph.D., is senior board director for the Board on Health Sciences Policy at the National Academies of Sciences, Engineering, and Medicine. In this capacity, she oversees a program of activities aimed at fostering the basic biomedical and clinical research enterprises; addressing the ethical, legal, and social contexts of scientific and technologic advances related to health; and strengthening the preparedness, resilience, and sustainability of communities. Previously, she served as director of the National Academies' Forum on Neuroscience and Nervous System Disorders, which brings together leaders from government, academia, industry, and nonprofit organizations to discuss key challenges and emerging issues in neuroscience research, development of therapies for nervous system disorders, and related ethical and societal issues. She also led consensus studies and contributed to projects on topics such as pain management, medications for opioid use disorder, traumatic brain injury, preventing cognitive decline and dementia, supporting persons living with dementia and their caregivers, the health and well-being of young adults, and disaster preparedness and response. Dr. Stroud first joined the National Academies as a Mirzayan Science and Technology Policy Graduate Fellow. She has also been an associate at AmericaSpeaks, a nonprofit organization that engaged citizens in decision making on important public policy issues. Dr. Stroud received her PhD from the University of Maryland, College Park, with research focused on the cognitive neuroscience of language, and her bachelor's degree from Queen's University in Canada.

Erin Hammers Forstag, J.D., M.P.H., supported the study as the science writer. She has been writing for the National Academies of Sciences, Engineering, and Medicine and other organizations for over 10 years, covering topics including COVID-19, mitochondrial replacement therapy, DNA forensics, and health professionals education. She obtained her JD from Georgetown University Law Center in 2012 and her Master's in Public Health from Columbia University in 2006.

Appendix B

Disclosures of Unavoidable Conflicts of Interest

The conflict of interest policy of the National Academies of Sciences, Engineering, and Medicine (http://www.nationalacademies.org/coi) prohibits the appointment of an individual to a committee authoring a Consensus Study Report if the individual has a conflict of interest that is relevant to the task to be performed. An exception to this prohibition is permitted if the National Academies determines that the conflict is unavoidable and the conflict is publicly disclosed. A determination of a conflict of interest for an individual is not an assessment of that individual's actual behavior or character or ability to act objectively despite the conflicting interest.

Dr. Steven Galson has a conflict of interest in relation to his service on the Committee on Processes to Evaluate the Safety and Efficacy of Drugs for Rare Diseases or Conditions in the United States and the European Union based on his membership on the board of directors of BioCryst Pharmaceuticals and his ownership of stocks of BioCryst Pharmaceuticals and Amgen, Inc., both of which develop products for rare diseases.

The National Academies has concluded that in order for the committee to accomplish the tasks for which it was established, its membership must include at least one person who has relevant broad expertise and experience in FDA drug regulatory policy, knowledge of what drives FDA decision making for approval of drug products, and an understanding of how FDA and the European Medicines Agency can collaborate.

As described in his biographical summary, due to his past leadership roles at FDA and at Amgen Inc., Dr. Galson has extensive expertise and experience in FDA drug regulatory policy from a variety of perspectives.

The National Academies has determined that the experience and expertise of Dr. Galson is needed for the committee to accomplish the task for which it has been established. The National Academies could not find another available individual with the equivalent experience and expertise who does not have a conflict of interest. Therefore, the National Academies has concluded that the conflict is unavoidable.

The National Academies believes that Dr. Galson can serve effectively as a member of the committee, and the committee can produce an objective report, taking into account the composition of the committee, the work to be performed, and the procedures to be followed in completing the study.

Dr. Anaeze Offodile II has a conflict of interest in relation to service on the Committee on Processes to Evaluate the Safety and Efficacy of Drugs for Rare Diseases or Conditions in the United States and the European Union based on his role as chief strategy officer at Memorial Sloan Kettering (MSK) Cancer Center, a nonprofit oncology teaching hospital and research institute that derives a portion of its income from licensing of its pre-clinical or early-clinical stage oncology therapies, invented by its scientists to pharmaceutical or biotech companies. For example, over the past 5 years MSK has received revenues, related to rare diseases, under its licenses to Venthera Inc., Takeda Pharmaceuticals, YmAbs Therapeutics, Atara Biotherapeutics, and Theragnostics Ltd.

The National Academies has concluded that for the committee to accomplish the tasks for which it was established, its membership must include at least one person who has relevant expertise and experience in translational research with current understanding of technology transfer for drug development, particularly at the intersection of clinical care and drug development. As described in his biographical summary, due to his current role at MSK and prior role at MD Anderson Cancer Center, Dr. Offodile has extensive expertise and experience in translational research and technology transfer.

The National Academies has determined that the expertise and experience of Dr. Offodile is needed for the committee to accomplish the task for which it has been established. The National Academies could not find another available individual with the equivalent expertise and experience who does not have a conflict of interest. Therefore, the National Academies has concluded that the conflict is unavoidable.

The National Academies believes that Dr. Offodile can serve effectively as a member of the committee, and the committee can produce an objective report, taking into account the composition of the committee, the work to be performed, and the procedures to be followed in completing the study.

The National Academies believes that Dr. Offodile can serve effectively as a member of the committee, and the committee can produce an objective report, taking into account the composition of the committee, the work to be performed, and the procedures to be followed in completing the study.

Dr. Anne Pariser has a conflict of interest in relation to her service on the Committee on Processes to Evaluate the Safety and Efficacy of Drugs for Rare Diseases or Conditions in the United States and the European Union because she is vice president of medical and regulatory affairs at Alltrna, which is developing a platform technology designed to utilize tRNA as a therapeutic for a variety of genetic diseases.

The National Academies has concluded that in order for the committee to accomplish the tasks for which it was established, its membership must include at least one person who has relevant current expertise and experience in private sector product development for rare diseases

As described in her biographical summary, as vice president of medical and regulatory affairs at Alltrna, as well as through her prior roles at NIH and FDA, Dr. Pariser has expertise and experience in product development, translational research, and drug regulatory policy for rare diseases.

The National Academies has determined that the experience and expertise of Dr. Pariser is needed for the committee to accomplish the task for which it has been established. The National Academies could not find another available individual with the equivalent experience and expertise who does not have a conflict of interest. Therefore, the National Academies has concluded that the conflict is unavoidable.

The National Academies believes that Dr. Pariser can serve effectively as a member of the committee, and the committee can produce an objective report, taking into account the composition of the committee, the work to be performed, and the procedures to be followed in completing the study. In each case, the National Academies determined that the experience and expertise of the individual was needed for the committee to accomplish the task for which it was established. The National Academies could not find other available individuals who had the equivalent experience and expertise and did not have a conflict of interest. Therefore, the National Academies concluded that the conflicts were unavoidable and publicly disclosed them on its website (www.nationalacademies.org).

Appendix C

Public Meeting Agendas

COMMITTEE ON PROCESSES TO EVALUATE THE SAFETY AND EFFICACY OF DRUGS FOR RARE DISEASES IN THE UNITED STATES AND THE EUROPEAN UNION

Meeting #1: November 6 – 7, 2023: Public Agenda

MONDAY, NOVEMBER 6, 2023 2:30 – 4:30 PM: OPEN SESSION

2:30–2:35 pm	Welcome and Introductions
	JEFFREY KAHN, *Committee Chair* Andreas C. Dracopoulos Director Robert Henry Levi and Ryda Hecht Levi Professor of Bioethics and Public Policy John Hopkins Berman Institute of Bioethics
2:35–3:30 pm	Sponsor Perspective and Charge to the Committee
	KERRY JO LEE Associate Director for Rare Diseases, Division of Rare Diseases and Medicine Genetics

Office of Rare Diseases, Pediatrics, Urological, and
    Reproductive Medicines
Office of New Drugs
Center for Drug Evaluation and Research
U.S. Food and Drug Administration

SANDRA RETZKY
Director, Office of Orphan Product Development
Office of the Commissioner
U.S. Food and Drug Administration

MIRANDA RAGGIO
Expedited Programs Manager, Office of Program
    Operation
Office of New Drugs
Center for Drugs Evaluation and Research
U.S. Food and Drug Administration

JULIENNE VAILLANCOURT
Policy Advisor and Rare Disease Liaison
Office of the Director
Center for Biologics Research and Evaluation
U.S. Food and Drug Administration

KATHERINE TYNER
FDA Liaison to the European Medicines Agency,
    Europe Office
Office of Global Policy and Strategy
Office of the Commissioner
U.S. Food and Drug Administration

SARAH ZAIDI
Physician Liaison for Pediatric Cluster, Pediatric
    International Team
Office of Pediatric Therapeutics
Office of Clinical Policy and Programs
Office of the Commisssioner
U.S. Food and Drug Administration

APPENDIX C 259

Other Sponsor Stakeholders on Standby for Q&A

JUDITH ARCIDIACONO
International Regulatory Expert, Office of Therapeutic
 Products
Center for Biologics Research and Evaluation
U.S. Food and Drug Administration

ROBYN BENT
Director, Patient-Focused Drug Development Program
Center for Drug Evaluation and Research
U.S. Food and Drug Administration

KEVIN FAIN
Senior Policy Advisor, Office of New Drug Policy
Office of New Drugs
Center for Drug Research and Evaluation
U.S. Food and Drug Administration

DIONNE L. PRICE
Deputy Director, Office of Biostatistics
Office of Translational Sciences
Center for Drug Evaluation and Research
U.S. Food and Drug Administration

3:30–4:30 pm	Discussion with Committee
4:30 pm	**ADJOURN MEETING DAY 1**

TUESDAY, NOVEMBER 7, 2023

10:00 AM – 1:00 PM EST: OPEN SESSION

10:00 am	Welcome and Introductions

JEFFREY KAHN, *Committee Chair*
Andreas C. Dracopoulos Director
Robert Henry Levi and Ryda Hecht Levi Professor of
 Bioethics and Public Policy
Johns Hopkins Berman Institute of Bioethics

10:05–10:30 am	Trends in Rare Disease Drug Product Approvals and Utilization of Regulatory Pathways
	ANNA SOMUYIWA Head Centre for Innovation in Regulatory Science
	MAGDA BUJAR Senior Manager, Regulatory Programme and Strategic Partnerships Centre for Innovation in Regulatory Science
	JUAN LARA Research Analyst Centre for Innovation in Regulatory Science
10:30–11:00 am	Discussion with Committee
11:00–11:15 am	*BREAK*
11:15 am –12:30 pm	Perspectives from Rare Disease Organizations
	VIRGINIE HIVERT Therapeutic Development Director EURODIS
	SAIRA SULTAN Consultant Haystack Project
	ANNIE KENNEDY Chief of Policy, Advocacy, and Patient Engagement EveryLife Foundation
	KARIN HOELZER Director of Policy and Regulatory Affairs NORD
12:30–12:45 pm	Public Comment Public comments will provide the committee with additional insight into key issues related to the study's statement of task. These include, but are not limited to:

The use of regulatory flexibilities and supplementary data (e.g. natural history studies and patient registries) when evaluating the safety and efficacy of drugs for rare diseases and conditions; and
FDA and EMA engagement of people with lived experience when developing guidance, policies, and programs.

Public comments, alongside other materials stakeholders have shared, will be reviewed by the committee and may help inform committee deliberations on the statement of task. All comments and materials shared with the committee will be made publicly available in accordance with institutional policies. **As such, please do not send confidential or HIPAA protected information and take caution when including personally identifiable information.** Should a quote from your public comment be used word-for-word in the committee's final report, you will be contacted by study staff.

If you would like to provide a verbal comment, please limit remarks to 2-3 minutes. Requests to provide verbal public comments may submitted via the meeting registration page <u>here</u>. Public commenters will be added to the agenda based on the order in which requests are received. Please note that space is limited and not all requests may be fulfilled. **You may also submit a written public comment via email: <u>RareDiseaseregPolicyStudy@nas.edu</u>.**

Public comments made at meetings and submitted in writing are subject to the same institutional disclosure requirements.

12:45pm	*ADJOURN OPEN SESSION*

COMMITTEE ON PROCESSES TO EVALUATE THE SAFETY AND EFFICACY OF DRUGS FOR RARE DISEASES IN THE UNITED STATES AND THE EUROPEAN UNION

Meeting #2: December 4 – 5, 2023: Committee Agenda

MONDAY, DECEMBER 4, 2023

Open SESSION (10:00 AM – 1:30 PM ET)

10:00–10:10 am   Welcome and Introduction
JEFFREY KAHN, *Committee Chair*
Andreas C. Dracopoulos Director
Robert Henry Levi and Ryda Hecht Levi Professor of Bioethics and Public Policy
Johns Hopkins Berman Institute of Bioethics

10:10–11:15 am   EMA Regulatory Policies for Drugs to Treat Rare Diseases and Conditions
STEFFEN THIRSTRUP
Chief Medical Officer
European Medicines Agency

Committee Discussion (30 min)

11:15 am–12:00 pm   Panel Discussion: Similarities and Differences Between FDA and EMA

STEFFEN THIRSTRUP
Chief Medical Officer
European Medicines Agency

JACQUELINE CORRIGAN-CURAY
Principal Deputy Center Director
Center for Drug Evaluation and Research
U.S. Food and Drug Administration

CELIA WITTEN
Deputy Director
Center for Biologics Evaluation and Research
U.S. Food and Drug Administration

APPENDIX C 263

12:00–12:15 pm **BREAK**

12:15–1:15 pm **Industry Perspectives on the Application of Regulatory Flexibilities**

                              LUCY VERESHCHAGINA
                              Senior Vice President, Science and Regulatory Advocacy
                              PhRMA

                              DIEGO ARDIGÒ
                              Head of R&D, Global Rare Diseases
                              Cheisi

                              E'LISSA FLORES
                              Director, Science and Regulatory Affairs
                              BIO

                              VICTOR MAERTENS
                              Government Affairs Director
                              EUCOPE

Committee Discussion (20 min)

1:15–1:30 pm Public Comment

1:30 pm **ADJOURN OPEN SESSION**

                      TUESDAY, DECEMBER 5, 2023

                    OPEN SESSION (10 AM – 12:30 PM ET)

10:00–10:05 am Welcome and Introductions

                              JEFFREY KAHN, *Committee Chair*
                              Andreas C. Dracopoulos Director
                              Robert Henry Levi and Ryda Hecht Levi Professor of Bioethics and Public Policy
                              Johns Hopkins Berman Institute of Bioethics

10:05–11:00 am	Use of "Supplemental Data" for Regulatory Decision making

Case Study: Skyclarys approval for Friedreich's ataxia (Use of natural history data)
COLIN MEYER (*Formerly at Reata Pharmaceuticals Inc.*)
Biogen

Case Study: Elevidys approval for Duchenne's muscular dystrophy (Challenges of regulatory review without "supplemental data")
HUONG HUYNH
Director, Regulatory Science
Critical Path Institute

Case Study: Relyvrio approval for ALS (Use of natural history and open label extension [active treatment extension] data)
SABRINA PAGANONI
Physician Scientist
Healey & AMG Center for ALS

Case Study: Oxbyrta approval for Sickle Cell Disease (Use of natural history data)
LAKIEA BAILEY
Executive Director
Sickle Cell Community Consortium

Committee Discussion (20 min)

11:00–11:15 am	*BREAK*
11:15 am–12:00 pm	Trends in Designation and Approvals of Drugs for Rare Diseases and Conditions

SANDRA RETZKY
Director, Office of Orphan Product Development
Office of the Commissioner
U.S. Food and Drug Administration

LEWIS FERMAGLICH
Medical Officer, Office of Orphan Product
     Development
Office of the Commissioner
U.S. Food and Drug Administration

Committee Discussion (15 min)

12:00–12:30 pm   Impact of FDA and EMA Collaborative Efforts

KERRY JO LEE
Associate Director for Rare Diseases, Division of Rare
     Diseases and Medicine Genetics
Office of Rare Diseases, Pediatrics, Urological, and
     Reproductive Medicines
Office of New Drugs
Center for Drug Evaluation and Research
U.S. Food and Drug Administration

KATHERINE TYNER
FDA Liaison to the European Medicines Agency,
     Europe Office
Office of Global Policy and Strategy
Office of the Commissioner
U.S. Food and Drug Administration

STEFFEN THIRSTRUP
Chief Medical Officer
European Medicines Agency

Committee Discussion (15 min)

12:30 pm   *ADJOURN OPEN SESSION*

                  **CLOSED SESSION (1:30 – 4:00 PM ET) –
                  COMMITTEE MEMBERS ONLY**

4:00 pm   *ADJOURN MEETING*

COMMITTEE ON PROCESSES TO EVALUATE THE SAFETY AND EFFICACY OF DRUGS FOR RARE DISEASES IN THE UNITED STATES AND THE EUROPEAN UNION

Meeting #3: February 6 – 7, 2024: Committee Agenda

TUESDAY, FEBRUARY 6, 2024

OPEN SESSION (10:00 AM – 2:30 PM ET)

10:00–10:05 am Welcome and Introduction

JEFFREY KAHN, *Committee Chair*
Andreas C. Dracopoulos Director
Robert Henry Levi and Ryda Hecht Levi Professor of Bioethics and Public Policy
Johns Hopkins Berman Institute of Bioethics

10:05–11:00 am Trial Design for Rare Disease Drug Development
LONGITUDINAL TRIAL DESIGN
TIINA URV
Director, Rare Disease Clinical Trial Network
National Center for Advancing Translational Sciences
National Institutes of Health

MASTER PROTOCOLS
NICOLE MAYER HAMBLETT
Associate Professor of Pediatrics & Adjunct Associate Professor of Biostatistics, University of Washington
Co-Executive Director, Cystic Fibrosis Therapeutics Development Network Coordinating Center

EXTERNAL CONTROLS
WILLIAM MAIER
Vice President, Rare Diseases
ICON plc

Committee Discussion (30 min)

11:00 am – Considerations for Pediatric Trials
12:00pm

    INDUSTRY PERSPECTIVE
    THOMAS MILLER
    Global Head of the Acute, Chronic, and Pediatric
     Disease Nucleus
    Bayer, Pharmaceutical Division

    CAREGIVER PERSPECTIVE
    KARA BERASI
    CEO, Haystack Project
    Vice Chair of Board of Directors, CDG Care
     (Congenital Disorders of Glycosylation)

    REGULATORY SCIENCE PERSPECTIVE
    FLORENCE BOURGEOIS
    Associate Professor of Pediatrics, Harvard Medical
     School
    Co-Director, Harvard-MIT Center for Regulatory
     Science
    Director, Pediatric Therapeutics and Regulatory
     Science Initiative, Boston Children's Hospital

Committee Discussion (30 min)

12:00–1:00 pm LUNCH BREAK

1:00-2:00 pm Use of "Supplemental" Data

    USE OF AGGREGATE DATA
    KLAUS ROMERO
    Chief Executive Officer & Chief Science Officer
    Critical Path Institute

    Expanded Access Programs
    Alison Bateman-House
    Assistant Professor, Department of Population Health
    New York University Grossman School of Medicine

    PATIENT REGISTRIES AND NATURAL HISTORY DATA
    EDWARD NEILAN
    Chief Medical and Scientific Officer
    National Organization for Rare Disorders

Committee Discussion (30 min)

2:00 pm   ADJOURN OPEN SESSION

WEDNESDAY, FEBRUARY 7, 2024

OPEN SESSION (9:30 AM – 12:15 PM ET)

9:30–9:35 am   Welcome and Introductions

                      JEFFREY KAHN, *Committee Chair*
                      Andreas C. Dracopoulos Director
                      Robert Henry Levi and Ryda Hecht Levi Professor of Bioethics and Public Policy
                      Johns Hopkins Berman Institute of Bioethics

9:35–10:30 am   Novel Methodologies
                      ANALYSIS METHODS – BAYESIAN METHODS AND SMART DESIGN
                      KELLEY KIDWELL
                      Professor of Biostatistics
                      University of Michigan

                      Analysis Methods – Causal Inference
                      Xabier Garcia de Albinez Martinez
                      Director of Epidemiology, RTI Health Solutions
                      Visiting Scientist, Department of Epidemiology, Harvard T.H. Chan School of Public Health

                      MODEL-INFORMED DRUG DEVELOPMENT
                      Hao Zhu
                      Division Director
                      Division of Pharmacometrics, Office of Combination Products, Office of Translational Sciences
                      Center for Drug Evaluation and Research
                      U.S. Food and Drug Administration

Committee Discussion (30 min)

10:30–10:45 am   *BREAK*

10:45– 12:00 pm	Flexibilities Applied at FDA EMILY FREILICH Division Director of Division of Neurology I Center for Drug Evaluation and Research U.S. Food and Drug Administration RACHAEL ANATOL Deputy Director of Office of Therapeutic Products Center for Biologics Evaluation and Research U.S. Food and Drug Administration MARTHA DONOGHUE Associate Director of Pediatric Oncology and Rare Cancers Oncology Center of Excellence U.S. Food and Drug Administration
12:00–12:15pm	Public Comment
12:15 pm	*ADJOURN OPEN SESSION*

Appendix D

Centre for Innovation in Regulatory Science Data Analysis Methodology

INTRODUCTION

The purpose of the data analysis was to help inform the National Academies Committee on Processes to Evaluate the Safety and Efficacy of Drugs for Rare Diseases or Conditions in the United States and the European Union.[1]

The National Academies approached the Centre for Innovation in Regulatory Science (CIRS) to produce a commissioned data analysis and summary of key findings based on the marketing submissions, regulatory orphan designations, and marketing approvals of new active substances (NASs) to treat rare diseases and conditions by the U.S. Food and Drug Administration (FDA) and the European Medicines Agency (EMA). The National Academies and CIRS entered into a contract agreement and agreed on the relevant data to be collected, definitions, and the analysis to be carried out by CIRS. CIRS undertook the data collection and prepared the analysis. The analysis was presented to the committee at regular meetings. The aim of those meetings was to provide feedback on the analysis, discuss the findings, and agree on additional analysis as well as next steps. Figure D-1 shows a graphical representation of the timeline of the project.

---

[1] For more information https://www.nationalacademies.org/our-work/processes-to-evaluate-the-safety-and-efficacy-of-drugs-for-rare-diseases-or-conditions-in-the-united-states-and-the-european-union (accessed December 11, 2023).

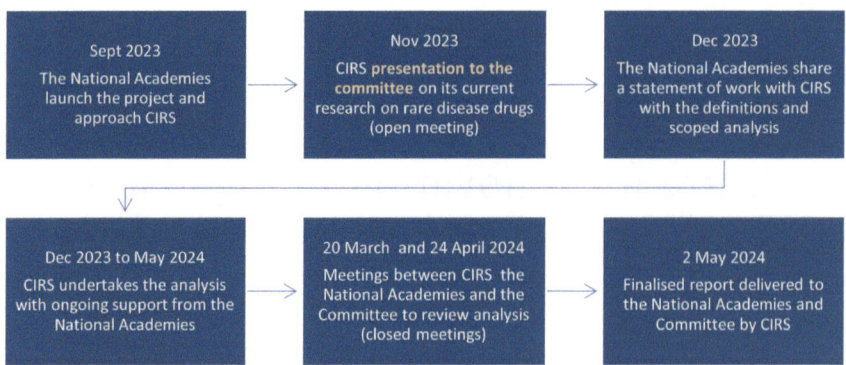

FIGURE D-1 Project timelines and steps.
SOURCE: CIRS Data Analysis, 2024.

OVERALL SCOPE

The overall analysis was limited to initial marketing authorizations by EMA and FDA and focused on new active substances (NASs).[2]

Applications that were excluded from the data analysis:

- Vaccines
- Biosimilars
- Any other application where new clinical data were submitted
- Generic applications
- Applications for which a completely new dossier was submitted from a new company for the same indications as those already approved for another company
- Applications for a new or additional name, or a change of name, for an existing compound (i.e., a "cloned" application)
- Emergency use or special authorizations derived from an emergency (e.g., COVID-19 pandemic)

The analysis was divided into two main parts as outlined in Figure D-2: part A, analysis of approval rates (applications submitted versus approved), and part B, analysis of approved products.

As a result of the lack of available data in the public domain on part A (submissions) for FDA, this information was requested and obtained directly from the agency. Similarly, information on submissions to EMA

---

[2] A new active substance (NAS) was defined as a chemical, biological, biotechnology, or radiopharmaceutical substance that has not been previously available for therapeutic use in humans and is destined to be made available as a "prescription-only medicine" to be used for the cure, alleviation, treatment, prevention, or in vivo diagnosis of diseases in humans.

was also obtained from the agency. Consequently, the data sources and products included differ when comparing parts A and B and are therefore described separately below.

For part B, data was retrieved from CIRS proprietary databases, which contains information extracted by CIRS from the public domain. Additional data points were also collected (Figure D-2).

PART A: ANALYSIS OF APPROVAL RATES

Product Scope

Products included in the analysis were NASs submitted by EMA (centralized procedure) or FDA (Center for Drug Evaluation and Research [CDER] and Center for Biologics Evaluation and Research [CBER]).

- Data obtained from FDA: New drug applications (NDAs) and biologics license applications (BLAs): Type 1 (drug product contains a new molecular entity) and Type 1,4 (combination drug product when at least one of the active ingredients is a new molecular entity).

Methods	Data sources
Part A: Analysis of approval rates	Data provided by FDA and EMA
Part B: Analysis of approved products	CIRS proprietary database
- Discordance of outcomes for orphan products approved by FDA	CIRS database + Additional data collected by CIRS
- Discordance between FDA Advisory Committees' recommendation and FDA decision	
- Use of "XYZ data"	

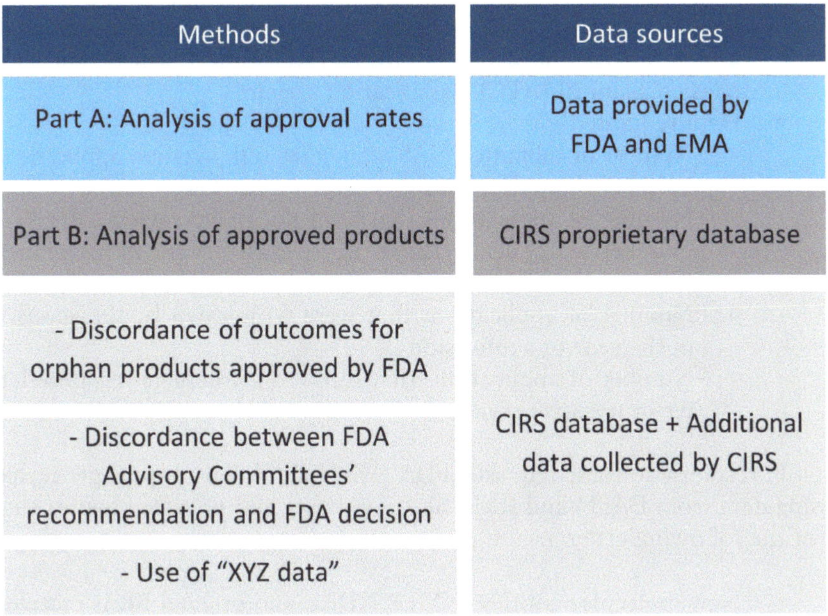

FIGURE D-2 Overall methods and data sources used based on the contract agreement with the National Academies.
SOURCE: CIRS Data Analysis, 2024.

- Data collected for EMA: Marketing authorization applications for a drug product that contains an NAS.

Caveat: These definitions differ slightly compared with the CIRS NAS definition used for Part B outlined below, resulting in a different set of products approved.

Year Ranges

Due to the fact that data provided by FDA were limited to 2015–2020, the same scope was applied to EMA in terms of the data collected from the agency.

Data Sources and Collection

FDA and EMA were approached by National Academies staff on behalf of the committee to request data relating to marketing authorization submissions and their corresponding regulatory outcomes. The following information was requested:

- Year range for analysis: 2013–2022
- Data categorization: All data broken down by year of submission cohort, orphan versus non-orphan designation, and therapeutic area following the World Health Organization Anatomical Therapeutic Chemical (ATC) classification system.
- Data requested
  - Number of submitted NAS marketing authorization applications
  - Number of applications that received marketing authorization
  - Number of applications that were not under review
  - Number of applications that were refused to file in the year of submission
  - Number of applications that were withdrawn by the sponsor in the year of submission
  - Number of applications that received a complete response letter or negative review

In response to these requests, FDA provided tabular outputs generated using data from DASH and RMS BLA databases and provided counts that met the following criteria:

- New molecular entities (NME), NDAs, and original BLAs received by CDER from January 1, 2015, to December 31, 2020.

- Original BLAs received by CBER from January 1, 2015, to December 31, 2020.
- Approval and non-approval actions (i.e., refuse to file, complete response, and withdrawals) as of December 31, 2023, stratified by the current (post-reorganization) Office of New Drugs (OND) review office and orphan designation.
- Approval and non-approval actions (i.e., refuse to file, complete response, and withdrawals as of December 31, 2023, stratified by three CBER-regulated biological product categories (i.e., cell and gene therapies; plasma-derived products; and other biological products) and orphan designation status.
- Median time to approval from FDA receipt date, regardless of filing status, is presented to account for multiple review cycles. There may be instances in which a submission received between January 1, 2015, and December 31, 2020, was reviewed more than once and did not receive an approval as of December 31, 2023. Those submissions are not included in the analysis of median time to approval from FDA receipt date.

FDA internal datasets were shared in confidence with CIRS (nonpublic data) under a contract agreement between the National Academies and CIRS. EMA provided some internal data extracts and a pivot table with links to publicly available information related to medicine that has been reviewed by the agency. Information was extracted and consolidated by CIRS.

Data Characteristics

For FDA, the following data were obtained from the agency:

- Number of applications approved by CDER and CBER between 2015 and 2020, broken down by year of submission and orphan status. CDER data was also broken down by FDA office, while CBER's data was broken down by type of product.
- Number of applications not approved (including complete response [CR] letters,[3] refusals to file and withdrawn applications) by CDER and CBER between 2015 and 2020 (lumped), broken down per orphan status. CDER data were also broken down by FDA office, while CBER's data were broken down by type of product.

---

[3] For FDA, it should be noted that certain pending applications are included (CR), whereas for EMA applications were included only where a final opinion was given (i.e., all submissions had a regulatory outcome).

For EMA, the following data were extracted by CIRS from the agency's websites:

- Databases with information on applications evaluated by EMA broken down as follows: product information (brand and generic name), orphan status, ATC code, milestone dates (validation, EMA Committee for Medicinal Products for Human Use opinion, EC decision date, etc.), type of outcome (approved, refused and withdrawn)

PART B: ANALYSIS OF APPROVED PRODUCTS

Recognizing the importance of advancing regulatory practices, CIRS has been benchmarking major regulatory agencies since 2002 using a methodology developed with the authorities (Hirako et al., 2007). The study continues today and focuses on new active substances approved by six regulatory agencies including FDA and EMA (CIRS, 2023). CIRS used its proprietary database, updated annually for the above-described study, in order to undertake the analysis of approved products. This database was supplemented with additional data points collected by CIRS as shown in Figure D-2.

Product Scope

Products included in the analysis were NASs approved by EMA (centralized procedure) or FDA (CDER and CBER).

NASs were defined by CIRS as a chemical, biological, biotechnology, or radiopharmaceutical substance that has not been previously available for therapeutic use in humans and that is destined to be made available as a "prescription only medicine" to be used for the cure, alleviation, treatment, prevention or in vivo diagnosis of diseases in humans. The term NAS also includes:

- An isomer, mixture of isomers, or a complex or derivative or salt of a chemical substance previously available as a medicinal product but differing in properties with regard to safety and efficacy from that substance previously available.
- A biological or biotech substance previously available as a medicinal product but differing in molecular structure, nature of source material, or manufacturing process and which will require clinical investigation.
- A radiopharmaceutical substance that is a radionuclide or a ligand not previously available as a medicinal product. Alternatively, the

coupling mechanism linking the molecule and the radionuclide has not been previously available.
- A combination that contains an NAS, even if it also contains another previously approved substance.

Applications that are excluded from the study:

- Any other application, where new clinical data were submitted.
- Generic applications.
- Those applications where a completely new dossier was submitted from a new company for the same indications as already approved for another company.
- Applications for a new or additional name, or a change of name, for an existing compound (i.e., a "cloned" application).

Data Sources

Data were collected from public assessment reports from the agency websites.

For EMA
- https://www.ema.europa.eu/sites/default/files/Medicines_output_european_public_assessment_reports.xlsx

For FDA

- https://www.accessdata.fda.gov/scripts/cder/daf/index.cfm
- https://www.fda.gov/vaccines-blood-biologics/licensed-biological-products-supporting-documents. For EMA and FDA—specific to discordance of outcomes for orphan NAS approved by FDA and EMA:

The rationale for non-approval of certain NASs in one agency but not the other was extracted from the public domain, such as from agency websites, pharmaceutical company websites, and news articles.

Data Collection Process

For CIRS proprietary databases, a review of the product inclusion against the NAS definition as well as data collection was performed by three CIRS researchers. One researcher extracted the data, and a second researcher validated the data through an independent review. Discrepancies were discussed until consensus was reached, and the third researcher facilitated adjudication of any differences.

For additional information collected by CIRS for the purpose of this project:

- Alternative and confirmatory data: Based on a working definition and list of keywords provided by National Academies staff,[4] two CIRS researchers worked on developing a method that was reviewed and adjudicated by a third CIRS researcher. Following, agreement on the method, which was also reviewed by the National Academies staff, one researcher collected the information, and the second researcher validated a subset of applications to ensure consistency of the method applied. Disagreements were adjudicated by a third CIRS researcher to reach agreement.
- Discordance: The method was developed by three CIRS researchers and reviewed with National Academies. Data collection was undertaken by one researcher and reviewed by the second. Disagreements were adjudicated by a third CIRS researcher to reach agreement.

Collected Characteristics

In addition to the brand name, generic name, and sponsor (applicant), the collected variables are outlined in Table D-1.

Year Ranges

The focus of the analysis was on NASs approved between January 1, 2013, and December 31, 2022.

---

[4] For purposes of this data analysis, "alternative and confirmatory data" refers to marketing authorization data submitted to FDA or EMA that falls outside of an adequate and well controlled trial and may have been used by a given regulatory agency to evaluate safety or effectiveness of a drug product. Sources of supplemental data may include:
- Natural history studies (e.g., patient registries)
- Expanded-access programs
- Open-label extension studies
- External control groups (concurrent and historical)
- Case reports
- Extrapolation based on data from related drug products or indications
- Mechanistic correlation (pharmacokinetic and pharmacodynamic data)
- Nonclinical studies (e.g., stability and quality control data)
- Passive data collection (e.g., digital phenotyping)
- Patient and caregiver reported outcomes (including preference data)
- Real world evidence
- Literature reviews

TABLE D-1 Variables and Data Points Collected for Each New Active Substance

Variable	Data point	Note on definition
Therapy area	Anatomical therapeutic chemical (ATC) code	As defined by the World Health Organization.
Regulatory pathway	Expedited	FDA: fast track, breakthrough therapy, priority review, accelerated approval, real-time oncology review and rolling review.
		EMA: PRIME, conditional approval, accelerated assessment, exceptional circumstances, and rolling review.
		Caveat: Multiple pathways may be applied to one product.
	Traditional	Products which do not fall under the above criteria.
Orphan status	Orphan designation	
Approval milestone dates	Sponsor submission date	Date of receipt of dossier by the agency.
	Regulatory approval date	Date of marketing authorisation.
		Caveat: For EMA this refers to European Commission decision date.
Review cycles (FDA only)	1st cycle, 1st cycle with major amendment approval, more than one cycle, more than one cycle with major amendments approved	As defined by FDA.

continued

TABLE D-1 Continued

Variable	Data point	Note on definition
Discordance between FDA advisory committee's recommendation and FDA decision	FDA advisory committee meeting held	
	Nature of the advisory committee vote	Votes in favor, votes against, abstentions.
		Caveat: Split votes were excluded. In meetings with multiple votes, overall approval questions were prioritized if available over specific questions asking about safety or efficacy separately. This analysis was limited to approved products only; therefore, the study only includes cases where the advisory committee did not recommend a product which was approved by FDA. Products that were recommended by the committee and not approved by FDA were not included.
Discordance of outcomes for orphan NAS approved by FDA and EMA	NAS not submitted	This combines a number of scenarios, such as development is in progress (based on FDA investigational new drug or EMA pediatric investigation plan or orphan designation received); or (in the case of EMA) that the product was not submitted to EMA but to EU member states. Lack of submission could not always be verified from the public domain and was assumed where no information was found.
	NAS still in review	
	NAS not approved	EMA: refused. FDA: complete response letter.
	NAS withdrawn by the sponsor	

TABLE D-1 Continued

Variable	Data point	Note on definition
Acceptance of alternative and confirmatory data to support regulatory decision-making	Natural history studies (e.g., patient registries) Expanded access programs Open-label extension studies External control groups (concurrent and historical) Case reports Extrapolation based on data from related drug products or indications Mechanistic correlation (pharmacokinetic and pharmacodynamic data) Nonclinical studies (e.g., stability and quality control data) Passive data collection (e.g., digital phenotyping) Patient- and caregiver-reported outcomes (including preference data) Real-world evidence Literature EMA, FDA, and NAS reviews	Alternative and confirmatory data accepted by the agency (i.e., information supported the approval and articulated in the public assessment report). *Caveat: The concept and definition for alternative and confirmatory data were developed by the committee. This variable was only collected for orphan products.*

NOTES: EMA = European Medicines Agency; FDA = U.S. Food and Drug Administration; NAS = National Academy of Sciences.

Caveat:

- The collection of alternative and confirmatory data was limited to the following year ranges: 2013–2014, 2017–2018, 2021–2022. The sample was selected to manage the volume of data collection required, while still providing an overview of the decade.
- Discordance on the approval of orphan NAS between agencies: this analysis investigated regulatory review outcomes for orphan NASs approved by either FDA or EMA from 2018 through 2022; however, regulatory outcomes were tracked (at the other agency) into 2024 (public domain last accessed in April 2024).

Analysis of Time

For timelines, medians and percentiles (25th and 75th percentiles) were analyzed to facilitate the understanding of the variation around the median (50th percentile). The following time periods were calculated:

- Approval time: Time calculated from sponsor submission date to regulatory approval date. This time includes agency and company time. EMA time includes European Commission time.
- Submission gap: Date of submission at the first regulatory agency to the date of regulatory submission to the subsequent regulatory agency.
- Rollout time: Time between the date of submission at the first regulatory agency to the date of approval by the target agency.

Caveat: All timelines were calculated in calendar days (hereafter "days").

REFERENCES

Hirako, M., N. McAuslane, S. Salek, C. Anderson, and S. Walker. 2007. A comparison of the drug review process at five international regulatory agencies. *Therapeutic Innovation & Regulatory Science* 41:291-308.

CIRS (Centre for Innovation in Regulatory Science). 2023. R&D Briefing 88: New drug approvals in six major authorities 2013–2022: Focus on orphan designation and facilitated regulatory pathways. London: Centre for Innovation in Regulatory Science. https://cirsci.org/publications/cirs-rd-briefing-88-new-drug-approvals-in-six-major-authorities-2013-2022-focus-on-orphan-designation-and-facilitated-regulatory-pathways/ (accessed July 12, 2024).

Appendix E

Qualitative Interview Summary and Methodology

PURPOSE

The National Academies Committee on Processes to Evaluate the Safety and Efficacy of Drugs for Rare Diseases or Conditions in the United States and the European Union sought qualitative information from biopharmaceutical and biotechnology companies to better understand:

- How regulatory flexibilities have been applied by the U.S. Food and Drug Administration (FDA) and the European Medicines Agency (EMA) towards drugs to treat rare diseases or conditions.
- The use of alternative and confirmatory data (e.g., open label extension studies, expanded access programs, natural history studies, and patient registries) for informing regulatory decision-making.
- The impact of collaboration between FDA and EMA on review/approval of drugs for rare diseases or conditions.

TYPE OF RESEARCH

A series of semi-structured qualitative interviews were conducted by National Academies staff to supplement information gathered from the published literature and public statements made by industry representatives and other stakeholders. All interviewees were asked the same set of starting questions (see methodology), which covered the following topics:

- Regulatory flexibilities, authorities, and mechanisms
- Use of alternative and confirmatory data during the review process
- Collaborative efforts between FDA and EMA
- Inclusion of pediatric populations in rare disease trials
- Use of patient and caregiver input

Coverage of these topics varied depending on time available and breadth of interviewee expertise. Information shared by interviewees was collected and summarized in this document by National Academies staff. Interviewee responses to questions were anonymized and statements were not attributed to specific interviewees or companies to protect the identification of individuals who agreed to participate and enable more open sharing of information. A more in-depth description of the methodology is located at the end of this document.

Aggregated, de-identified results of the semi-structured interviews may help inform deliberations of the committee on the study statement of task and may be included in the final published report of the committee.

Exemption from Institutional Review Board (IRB) approval for this work was obtained February 19, 2024, from the Committee to Review Human Subjects, acting as the National Academies of Sciences, Engineering, and Medicine's IRB (#IRB00000281; expires February 17, 2026).

INFORMATION ON INTERVIEWEES

Companies represented: AMO Pharma; AbbVie; Affinia Therapuetics; Agios; Bayer; BioMarin Pharmaceuticals; Biogen; BridgeBio; Dyne Therapeutics; GlaxoSmithKline; Glycomine; Janssen Pharmaceutical Companies of Johnson & Johnson; Mahzi Therapeutics; Prilenia Therapeutics; Reata; Recordati; Roche; Sanofi; Stealth BioTherapeutics; Takeda; Ultragenyx Pharmaceutical Inc.

Roles: Clinical Development and Operations; Medical; Regulatory Policy; Patient Advocacy; Product Development; Research and Development

Invitation Summary

Invitations Sent	Responses Received	Interviews Held	Interview Success Rate
95	28	21	22.1%

Company Type

Pharma	9
Biotech	6
Pre-revenue	6

FDA/EMA Experience

Both	17
FDA Only	4
EMA Only	0

Therapeutic Area

Neurology	13
Metabolic Disorders	9
Hematology	4
Nephrology	3
Oncology	2
Endocrinology	2
Cardiology	1
Pulmonology	1
Infectious Diseases	1
General Pediatrics	1

INTERVIEWEE RESPONSES RE: REGULATORY FLEXIBILITIES, AUTHORITIES, AND MECHANISMS

Interview Questions

- What has been your experience engaging with FDA and/or EMA on drugs to treat rare diseases or conditions? What worked well? What could be improved upon and how?
- Based on your experience, how have regulatory flexibilities been applied by FDA and/or EMA for marketing applications for drugs to treat rare diseases or conditions?
- If you could wave a magic regulatory wand, what would you like to see change as it relates to the review and approval of drugs to treat rare diseases and conditions?

Summary of Responses Organized by Theme

Agency Structure

FDA

- Interviewees said that FDA engagement with drug sponsors seems inconsistent across divisions. They pointed to differences at the division-level when it comes to whether or not FDA grants a meeting requested by a sponsor.
- There seem to be differences in the level of engagement between individual FDA employees and a given sponsor.
- Interviewees appreciate the overall structure of the agency, which enables the same FDA staff to support sponsor engagement throughout a program's lifespan.
- Interviewees indicated that FDA provides predictable timelines for sponsors, but the advice provided by the agency can be unpredictable.

EMA

- Interviewees said that EMA's organizational structure and procedures for sponsor engagement can be difficult for companies to navigate.
- The decentralized structure of EMA was described by one interviewee as a "daunting and difficult process."
- Interviewees pointed to the requirement of first engaging national regulatory bodies within the European Union before EMA as a barrier to regulatory submission.
- Interviewees suggested that smaller, pre-revenue companies may be particularly vulnerable to these types of organizational/structural barriers.
- The rapporteur process employed by EMA Committee for Medicinal Products for Human Use (CHMP) may add another layer of difficulty for sponsors.

Alignment between FDA and EMA

- Interviewees said that FDA and EMA both understand unmet medical need for rare indications and appreciate the difficulties that accompany rare disease drug development.
- At the same time, interviewees said that approaches for facilitating rare disease drug development varies between the agencies. For

example, FDA seems to provide clearer guidance documents on rare disease drug development while EMA seems to provide more feedback to an individual sponsor.
- Interviewees who have worked with FDA and EMA described inconsistencies that may be the result of differences between the organization/structure of the agencies.
- There are cases in which the two agencies have diverging guidance – specifically statistical methodology.
- Interviewees noted that the two agencies often arrive at the same regulatory decision.

Sponsor Support

- Interviewees said that current mechanisms for interacting with FDA are generally favored by sponsors. In part, this may be due to well-defined and shorter timelines for advice from FDA compared to EMA, which may be seen as more formal and rigid in their approach.
  - Interviewees noted that both FDA and EMA employ helpful sponsor support strategies. They also suggested that both agencies provide an appropriate level of guidance to help bring treatments to market.
  - Interviewees said that EMA provides more detail and clarity in their advice than FDA.
  - Interviewees said that meetings with regulators are helpful and can make the drug development process easier. It was specifically stated that the best alignment between sponsors and regulators come out of formal meetings. However, interviewees also pointed out that FDA seems to have made a shift away from granting meetings in recent years.
  - Interviewees expressed frustration at being 'stuck' with a written response from FDA. A written response feedback from FDA can make it difficult for sponsors to understand the nuance of the response, which can lead to delays in bringing treatments to market.

Wish List

- Interviewees called for greater transparency in decision making and consistency in reasoning for FDA and EMA decision making, both internally and between the agencies. This type of information could cut out some of the ambiguities that slow drug development, help guide future product development, better inform the research and patient community on strategies sponsors plan to take, reduce

duplicative efforts, and document examples of drug products that received marketing authorization approval.
- It was stated that, "readily accepting the qualification of biomarkers for accelerated approval using scientific and pharmacologic criteria would transform rare disease drug development."
- Interviewees expressed a desire for the pediatric voucher to not sunset.
- Interviewees indicated a need for more in-person or teleconference meetings with FDA throughout the development process, timely explanations for why flexibilities were or were not applied, and increased expertise in rare diseases among reviewers.
- Interviewees noted the following changes to regulatory flexibility and the acceptance of alternative and confirmatory data:
  ○ Increased consistency within FDA;
  ○ Increased use of data from other development programs;
  ○ Increased use of the patient's voice; and
  ○ New ways to get promising products to market.
- Consistency in the application of regulatory flexibilities within FDA was the most common request for change. Interviewees suggested that better resources for FDA reviewers and other staff would help increase consistency across the agency and acceptance of these data.
- Interviewees called for greater acceptance of real-world data (RWD) and less dependence on p-values.
- Interviewees suggested the following data resources would also be helpful:
  ○ Use of data from other drug development programs and repurposing of data;
  ○ Curated natural history data, registry data, and control data to inform the development and use of external controls; and
  ○ Patient experience data.
- Interviewees said increased regulatory flexibility around the use of endpoints (e.g., decreasing rigor; validating/accepting endpoints) would help to bring promising products to market.
- Interviewees said the substantial evidence needed for drugs to treat rare diseases and conditions could be altered to allow more flexibility.

INTERVIEWEE RESPONSES RE: USE OF ALTERNATIVE AND CONFIRMATORY DATA DURING THE REVIEW PROCESS

Interview Questions

- Have you incorporated "supplemental data" (e.g., data from open label extension studies, expanded access programs, natural history studies, or use of real-world data (RWD)) in submission materials to FDA or EMA? Why or why not?
- If you could wave a magic regulatory wand, what would you like to see change as it relates to the review and approval of drugs to treat rare diseases and conditions?

Summary of Responses Organized by Theme

Variability Between FDA and EMA

- Interviewees suggested that FDA and EMA are both flexible in accepting alternative and confirmatory data (ACD).
- Interviewees provided conflicting examples and perspectives that highlighted variability between the agencies on their application of flexibility and acceptance of ACD for specific drug development programs.
- Interviewees said that FDA has been less likely to use RWD, specifically for labeling decisions, than EMA.
- FDA tends to rely on placebo controls more heavily than EMA.
- Interviewees recounted instances of FDA leadership impacting agency decisions. In contrast, there seems to be limited opportunity for sponsors to engage EMA leadership.

Intra-FDA Variability

- Within FDA, there are inter-center and inter-divisional differences in the application of flexibility and acceptance of ACD.
- Interviewees expressed that FDA's Center for Biologics Evaluation and Research (CBER) tends to be more flexible in its acceptance of ACD than the FDA's Center for Drug Evaluation and Research (CDER). Interviewees identified neurology and oncology as areas within FDA with the greatest application of regulatory flexibilities.
- Differences in regulatory flexibility were attributed to a lack of experience with regulating rare disease products. The endocrinology

division was specifically called out for a lack of experience in the rare disease space and lack of flexibility.
- Several interviewees noted that increased application of regulatory flexibility and acceptance of ACD seems to be spreading throughout FDA. However, there are still issues with FDA decisions and data being siloed by divisions, which may limit the ability of divisions to learn from one another.
- The lack of consistency and reliance on precedence can lead to issues for drug development given that sponsors design programs based on regulatory certainty.
- Interviewees raised the issue of inconsistency between individual reviewers. Interviewees suggested that less experienced reviewers seemed less flexible. Some sponsors have been able to circumvent this issue by engaging FDA leadership, particularly within FDA/CBER.
- Interviewees suggested that the thoughts and beliefs of FDA leadership do not seem to trickle down to the reviewer level.

INTERVIEWEE RESPONSES RE: COLLABORATIVE EFFORTS

Interview Questions

- Have you used or considered the FDA–EMA Parallel Scientific Advice (PSA) Program? Why or why not?
- If you could wave a magic regulatory wand, what would you like to see change as it relates to the review and approval of drugs to treat rare diseases and conditions?

Summary of Responses Organized by Theme

Collaborative Efforts – Parallel Scientific Advice (PSA)

- Interviewees expressed that the usefulness of PSA seems dependent on timing and need for advice. For example, PSA may not be useful for sponsors if accessed too early in development and the product is too far from the market.
- Sponsors are trying to "ask the right question at the right time to the right agency," meaning that sponsors may need to ask a specific question to only one agency and PSA could hinder that ability.
- Interviewees said that the opportunity to harmonize feedback would be beneficial, but this would need to result in a more efficient development plan.

- One interviewee provided a favorable perspective of PSA, noting that PSA can be used to streamline the regulatory process and the company used that PSA given the significant investment in the drug development process.
- Interviewees listed issues with PSA that stem from the timing of the program, non-binding nature of PSA, misalignment of advice, and the influence of one agency on the other:
    ○ PSA utilizes EMA timelines for scientific advice, which are less favored than FDA timelines. Thus, sponsors view PSA as adding steps to the development process that slows the time to getting approval;
    ○ PSA is also non-binding which does not decrease sponsors' uncertainty in the development process, a key aspect to PSA usefulness;
    ○ The distinction was made that PSA is not joint, only parallel. Thus, the agencies often provide their own advice; and
    ○ The misalignment of advice further exacerbates issues with timing and speed.
- Sponsors are able to leverage the differences in flexibilities employed by agencies to their advantage. They can strategically plan development in the more flexible region to improve the issues with rigidity in the other region.
- Interviewees suggested there is fear on the part of sponsors that the agencies may influence each other in a negative way:
    ○ There is the perception that through PSA, the more rigid (less flexible) opinion tends to prevail, resulting in a less flexible development in both regions; and
    ○ There is a general perception that the 'worst common denominator' will dominate the advice.
- Interviewee quote: "PSA meetings can be protracted, discordant, and non-binding. Sponsors need them to be rapid, concordant, and binding."

Wish List

- Interviewees said that concordance between the two agencies is important and divergent feedback leads to fear/uncertainty on the part of sponsors.
- Interviewees specifically called for alignment on approvable endpoints and harmonization for validated biomarkers and standards for rare disease drug development. For example, a joint EMA/FDA group that validates biomarkers could be helpful, but there is concern that the "worst common denominator" may dominate

decision making and limit flexibility on the part of the regulatory agencies. Interviewees noted that it can cost almost a million dollars to go through the steps to validate measures and noted that companies have gone out of business pursing this to "please the FDA with validation."

INTERVIEWEE RESPONSES RE: INCLUSION OF PEDIATRIC POPULATIONS IN RARE DISEASE TRIALS

Interview Question

- Have you included or considered the inclusion of pediatric populations as part of your submission to FDA or EMA? Why or why not?

Summary of Responses Organized by Theme

Pediatric Inclusion

- Interviewees indicated that the type of disease and age of onset is the largest driver for pediatric inclusion. They said they have no issues following the regulatory pathways for pediatric studies for submission to either agency.
- Interviewees indicated that the process of starting in adults to collect data and ensure safety before moving into pediatrics works well for sponsors, but this may not always be practical in practice.
- For indications primarily among adults, it is seen as helpful to determine if the drug works before being required to conduct a study in a pediatric population by EMA.
    - Both agencies have adequate scrutiny of safety data before entering into pediatric populations.
- FDA often prefers to see RCTs in pediatrics and do not question whether children can burden a placebo control
- early on in the drug development process, sponsors submitting for approval in EMA for adult or pediatric populations are required to submit a Pediatric Investigation Plan (PIP). PIPs are a binding agreement between the sponsor and EMA which outline a development plan and identify the particular studies needed to gather the necessary data to support the authorization of a drug for children.
- One interviewee suggested that EMA uses PIPs to avoid massive off-label use of drugs and ensure sponsors complete post-approval studies to protect children from more unregulated use.

- Interviewees noted the involvement of EMA's Paediatric Committee (PDCO), and the Committee for Medicinal Products for Human Use (CHMP) can be burdensome as they are not always aligned.
- PIP requirements are often viewed as inefficient and procedural, with interviewees stressing the requirements often cause delays in authorization by EMA which is not always advantageous for sponsors. Interviewees suggested that some issues surrounding PIPs may be a result of EMA binding PIPs to incentives (rewards linked with obligations).
- For pediatric inclusion, interviewees noted FDA has a more pragmatic approach for pediatric study development while EMA has a more conversative approach. This is in part due to the exemption from needing a pediatric plan within FDA for orphan products
- One interviewee drew upon a specific experience in which, based on recommendations from FDA, they included an additional study for pediatric safety concerns that EMA flagged as unnecessary. The interviewee noted that EMA and FDA have a mechanism to discuss and work out these types of issues.

INTERVIEWEE RESPONSES RE: USE OF PATIENT & CAREGIVER INPUT

Interview Question

- Have you invited patients and/or caregiver representatives to participate in meetings with FDA? Why or why not?

Summary of Responses Organized by Theme

Patient Inclusion

- In seeking input on how the agencies tend to approach the use of patient and caregiver input, interviewees said that their inclusion in some manner is important as it allows discussions to become more personal and the patient voice to be considered by reviewers.
- Patient input may be better utilized when it is preplanned (e.g., prospective rather than post-hoc).
- Patient involvement with FDA is sometimes seen as complicated because FDA does not require sponsors to incorporate the patient voice.

- EMA seems more formal with patient inclusion as the agency selects patient groups to be present for certain meetings and requires that sponsors verify that they have included the patient voice.

FDA

- Interviewees shared mixed opinions on the value of including patient input during program specific meetings.
- Some interviewees stated it was clear how FDA incorporated patient input into their decision making account, others noted that it is not clear, especially for written responses.
- Interviewees commented on their success with patient inclusion and noted that FDA is amenable, acknowledges the importance of inclusion, and that it helped enlighten the agencies' thinking on topics such as unmet need and the impact of available treatment on risk-benefit ratios.
- Interviewees highlighted the potential benefit of public Patient Focused Drug Development (PFDD) meetings. Interviewees also said benefit comes from product-specific meetings, which include FDA, the sponsor, as well as patients who can provide valuable input and added context for a particular treatment.
- Interviewees expressed that they do not include patients in meetings with FDA, holding the belief that meetings with FDA and sponsors should be data driven and objective and patients may not have the expertise needed for these conversations. Instead, these interviewees opt to include key opinion leaders or clinicians and suggested that the PFDD and listening sessions are adequate mechanisms for FDA to gather patient input.
- Interviewees also suggested that meetings between patients and FDA, without sponsors present, work better than PFDD and listening sessions, given potential concerns that FDA may view sponsor-invited patients as biased.
- PFDD meetings and listening sessions are becoming the more common form of patient inclusion for FDA.
- Interviewees shared that there seems to be an overall lack of clarity on how these meetings are considered during the review process, noting that FDA could do a better job of applying the knowledge gained form these meetings.
- PFDD meetings may not be as effective as intended.
- Interviewees suggested that PFDD meetings listening sessions can be a waste of advocacy group resources as a great number of patients are needed to provide a comprehensive perspective and it may cost up to $100,000 for a PFDD meeting and $25,000 for a listening session.

METHODOLOGY

Interview Question and Guide Development

Semi-structured interview questions were developed by the committee to better understand (1) how regulatory flexibilities have been applied by FDA and EMA towards drugs to treat rare diseases or conditions, (2) the use of "supplemental data" (e.g., open label extension studies, expanded access programs, natural history studies, and patient registries), and (3) the impact of collaboration between FDA and EMA on drug review/approval for rare diseases or conditions.

The use of pre-determined questions included flexibility for follow-up questions to allow for further clarification of interviewee experiences as needed. Information gathered on the interviewees (e.g., organization type, products approved, and circumstances surrounding product approval) also helped inform follow-up questions.

During the interview, National Academies staff asked interviewees the following questions:

- Of the rare disease drug products that you have worked on:
    a. Which disease/condition or therapeutic area(s) were these products intended to treat?
    b. Do you have experience submitting a marketing authorization application for a rare disease drug product to FDA or EMA?
- What has been your experience engaging with FDA and/or EMA on drugs to treat rare diseases or conditions?
- Based on your experience, how have regulatory flexibilities been applied by FDA and/or EMA for marketing applications for drugs to treat rare diseases or conditions?
- Have you incorporated "supplemental data" (e.g., data from open label extension studies, expanded access programs, natural history studies, or use of real-world data) in submission materials to FDA or EMA? Why or why not?
- Have you used or considered FDA-EMA Parallel Scientific Advice (PSA) Program? Why or why not?
- Have you included or considered the inclusion of pediatric populations as part of your submission to FDA or EMA?
- Have you invited patients and/or caregiver representatives to participate in meetings with FDA? Why or why not?
- If you could wave a magic regulatory wand, what would you like to see change as it relates to the review and approval of drugs to treat rare diseases and conditions?

These interview questions were included in a note-taking template to standardize response recording to and simplify the analysis.

Selection of Interviewees

Recruitment of interviewees was purposive, based on their expertise in leading clinical development and regulatory submission of rare disease drug products. The following criteria were used to identify and select interviewees:

- Individuals with expertise in FDA and/or EMA regulatory policy and who have direct experience working with one or both regulatory agencies (e.g., through submitting marketing approval packets for drug products that treat rare diseases and conditions).
- Individuals who serve in a clinical development, R&D strategy, and/or regulatory affairs leadership/decision making role within a company.
- Individuals who work at companies that have applied for FDA or EMA marketing authorization for a drug to treat a rare disease or condition within the past 5 years.
- Individuals who led the clinical development and marketing authorization submission of rare disease drug products that used "supplementary data" (e.g., open label extension studies, expanded access programs, natural history studies, and patient registries) to demonstrate evidence for effectiveness.

After identifying the final list of interviewees, National Academies staff will contact selected individuals by email to inform them of the study and qualitative interview process and gauge interest in participation. The invitation email will include a subject line which clearly states that it is an interview invitation to provide input for the study. National Academies staff will attach an interview process overview and FAQ document to ensure all interviewees understand the purpose and process for participation. Interviewees will be made aware that their participation is voluntary and that they have the opportunity to retract responses up to when the committee holds its last meeting on May 23, 2024. They will also be made aware upfront that should they choose to retract their responses, all materials related to their interview will be deleted immediately.

National Academies staff assembled an initial list of 89 individuals who represent companies based in the United States and European Union and cover a range of rare disease therapeutic areas. These individuals were contacted by email to inform them of the study, the qualitative interview process, and gauge interest in participation. National Academies staff provided documentation on the interview process and FAQs to ensure all interviewees understood the purpose and process for interview participation. An additional 6 individuals were identified from a snowballing process – individuals who received an invitation to participate in the interview process were asked for suggestions of other people who might be added to the list.

A total of 95 individuals received an email invitation to participate in the interview process. 28 of the individuals responded to the invitation and 21 individuals were interviewed by National Academies staff.

Interview Process

Once interviewees agreed to participate, 45-minute Zoom interviews were scheduled via a Calendly account with each interviewee. Prior to invitation emails being sent, all interviewees were assigned a unique identification (ID) number using the RAND function in Microsoft Excel. This enabled all internal references to individual interviewees to be anonymized after they agreed to participate.

Interviews were conducted via videoconference between February 23, 2024, and March 22, 2024, by at least two National Academies staff—one to facilitate the interview and one to capture notes in the note-taking template. When conducting each interview, National Academies staff followed an interview guide, which included an overview of the interview process and efforts taken to anonymize responses. National Academies staff obtained verbal consent to proceed with the interview and saved an audio recording for note-taking purposes if interviewees explicitly agreed to this request. If an interviewee did not agree to recording, staff would verify statements with the interviewee to ensure the notes taken during the interview were accurate. Prior to each interview, note-taking templates were labeled by interviewee unique IDs to help protect interviewee identification and anonymization of their responses.

Qualitative Analysis

Following each interview, National Academies staff reviewed notes taken during the interview and confirmed the content based on available audio recordings. After reviewing three randomly selected interview notes, National Academies staff developed a set of common themes and subthemes for each set of questions (see *Interview Themes and Sub-Themes* for list and description of themes). Once themes and subthemes were developed, National Academies staff reviewed and organized all interviewee responses into a filterable Excel file based on these themes and subthemes. To add context for each interviewee, the following additional information was included in the Excel file: type of company (clinical stage/pre-revenue/

biotech/pharma), FDA experience, EMA experience, and therapeutic area. To aggregate responses, National Academies staff used the Excel file to filter responses to a particular theme and subtheme. All responses for a particular theme and subtheme were then aggregated.

Data Anonymization

All interviewees were assigned a unique identification (ID) number using the RAND function in Microsoft Excel. The key for anonymization of interviewees will be stored on the private drive of a National Academies study staff member whose laptop is password protected and requires a personal identification number and VPN application to access.

Interviews were conducted by two individuals and, as such, data could not be blinded. However, all interview materials (audio, transcript, notes, and rubric analysis) were tagged with a unique ID to anonymize responses. The following steps were used to help protect interviewee identification:

1. Once interviewees use Calendly to schedule an interview, all zoom meetings will be updated such that their name is tagged with the interviewee's unique ID. This will help ensure that audio transcripts will be saved with the appropriate file name. Passcodes and waiting rooms will be used for each meeting to prevent unwanted third parties from joining.
2. Note taking templates will be pre-saved with interviewee's assigned unique IDs. Within the document, only the unique ID will be used to refer to the interviewee.
3. At the beginning of each Zoom meeting, National Academies staff will change the interviewees name in Zoom to their unique ID.
4. After notes are taken, staff will delete all references to the name of an interviewee's employer. Names of specific products discussed (both generic and trade names) will be also deleted from notes. Product names will not be mentioned in aggregate analysis to prevent external audiences from tracing responses back to the interviewee.
5. Note-taking templates will be pre-saved with interviewee's assigned unique ID.

Data Storage and Destruction

Interview audio recordings, transcripts and notes will be stored on a private folder on SharePoint, accessible only to the National Academies study team.

Zoom audio recordings will be stored on a local drive before being moved to SharePoint. All local drive recordings will be promptly deleted after being moved to SharePoint. Following the development of interview analysis (using an inductive approach), audio recordings will be deleted permanently.

After the release of the pre-publication version of the report in August 2024, all materials containing identifiable information (e.g., the anonymization key) and de-identified meeting transcripts will be deleted permanently. The original notes and analysis will be deleted after the final electronic version of the report, prepared by the National Academies Press, is submitted to the sponsor in October 2024.

Any identifying information on interviewees will be anonymized. Only aggregated, de-identified information will be made available to the full committee. Only a summary of key themes will be included in the study's public access file.

Interview Themes and Subthemes

Themes: The themes below were identified by using three randomly selected interview notes to identify common topics raised by interviewees in response to each question.

Subthemes: The subthemes below were identified by using the same process as above, but serve to further categorize responses within a theme. The subthemes were used to review and organize interviewee responses to each question.

Themes and subthemes identified based on interviewee responses to questions on regulatory flexibilities, authorities, and mechanisms:

Theme	Subtheme
Sponsor Support by FDA and EMA	Speed
	Type of Engagement (e.g., oral, in-person, written, etc.)
	Generic vs. Tailored Feedback
Agency Structure	FDA: Consistency/Inconsistency Between Divisions
	EMA: Committee Engagement, Decentralization, and National-Level Engagement
Alignment/Misalignment Between FDA and EMA	Guidance
	Submissions Requirements

Themes and subthemes identified based on interviewee responses to questions on FDA and EMA use of regulatory flexibilities and acceptance alternative and confirmatory data

Theme	Subtheme
Openness	FDA
	EMA
Rigidity	FDA
	EMA
FDA and EMA Variability	Use of Biomarkers/Surrogate Endpoints
	Acceptance of Trial Design/ACD
	Guidance Documents
Intra-FDA Variability	Center/Division Differences
	Application of Lessons across Centers/Divisions
	Leadership Influence

Themes and subthemes identified based on interviewee responses to questions on FDA and EMA collaboration

Theme	Subtheme
General	Considerations of when to use PSA
Favorable	*No subtheme here*
Unfavorable	Misalignment Between FDA and EMA advice
	Influence of one agency over the other
	Non-binding nature of advice
	Timing of PSA

Themes and subthemes identified based on interviewee responses to questions on inclusion of pediatric populations in trials

Theme	Subtheme
Practicality of policies	Timeline for inclusion (e.g., initiation in adults vs. children)
	Data requirements
Pediatric Plans (iPSP & PIP)	Timeline for plan development/submission
	Difficulties with PIP/PSP approval
	Orphan exemption

Themes and subthemes identified based on interviewee responses to questions on use of patient and caregiver input

Theme	Subtheme
Program Specific Inclusion	FDA
	EMA
General Patient Engagement/Inclusion	PFDD
	Listening Sessions

Themes and subthemes identified based on interviewee responses to questions on changes to the rare disease regulatory processes

Theme	Subtheme
Regulatory Authorities & Mechanisms	Sponsor Engagement
	Internal Expertise
Regulatory Flexibilities & Acceptance of ACD	Inclusion of Patient Voice/Input
	Intra-FDA Consistency
	Use of data from other clinical dev. programs
FDA-EMA Collaboration	Harmonized advice
	Aligned acceptance of trial design, endpoints, and ACD
	Joint validation of/consensus on endpoints
	Collaboration Programs

Appendix F

Non-Exhaustive List of Patient Focused Drug Development Meetings and Patient Listening Sessions for Rare Diseases Between 2013 and 2023[1]

Disease/Condition Name	Meeting Type	Meeting Date
Narcolepsy	FDA-led PFDD meeting	9/24/2013
Sickle cell disease	FDA-led PFDD meeting	2/7/2014
Pulmonary arterial hypertension (PAH)	FDA-led PFDD meeting	5/13/2014
Hemophilia A, hemophilia B, von Willebrand disease (VWB), and other heritable bleeding disorders	FDA-led PFDD meeting	9/22/2014
Idiopathic pulmonary fibrosis (IPF)	FDA-led PFDD meeting	9/26/2014
Huntington's disease (HD)	FDA-led PFDD meeting	9/22/2015
Alpha-1 antitrypsin deficiency	FDA-led PFDD meeting	9/29/2015
Non-tuberculous mycobacterial (NTM) lung infections	FDA-led PFDD meeting	10/15/2015
Amyloidosis	EL-PFDD meeting Host: The Amyloidosis Research Consortium	11/16/2015
Myotonic dystrophy (DM)	EL-PFDD meeting Host: Myotonic Dystrophy Foundation	9/15/2016

---

[1] For more information on these meetings such as summaries and agendas, see FDA (2024k): https://www.fda.gov/industry/prescription-drug-user-fee-amendments/condition-specific-meeting-reports-and-other-information-related-patients-experience (accessed July 1, 2024).

Disease/Condition Name	Meeting Type	Meeting Date
Spinal muscular atrophy (SMA)	EL-PFDD meeting Host: Cure SMA	4/18/2017
Friedreich's ataxia (FA)	EL-PFDD meeting Host: Friedreich's Ataxia Research Alliance	6/2/2017
Tuberous sclerosis complex (TSC)	EL-PFDD meeting Host: Tuberous Sclerosis Alliance	6/21/2017
Alopecia areata	FDA-led PFDD meeting	9/11/2017
Hereditary angioedema (HAE)	FDA-led PFDD meeting	9/25/2017
Pachyonychia congenita (PC)	EL-PFDD meeting Host: Pachyonychia Congenita Project	4/6/2018
Barth syndrome (BTHS)	EL-PFDD meeting Host: The Barth Syndrome Foundation	7/18/2018
Alport syndrome	EL-PFDD meeting Host: National Kidney Foundation and the Alport Syndrome Foundation	8/3/2018
Charcot-Marie-Tooth and inherited neuropathies (CMT/IN)	EL-PFDD meeting Host: Hereditary Neuropathy Foundation	9/28/2018
Fabry disease	Patient listening session	12/4/2018
Niemann-Pick type C (NPC)	EL-PFDD meeting Host: Ara Parseghian Medical Research Fund at Notre Dame, Hide & Seek Foundation, Dana's Angels Research Trust, Hope for Marian, National Niemann-Pick Disease Foundation, Niemann-Pick Canada, Firefly Fund, and Johnathon's Dreams	3/18/2019
Fibrodysplasia ossificans progressiva (FOP)	Patient Listening session	5/29/2019
Neurofibromatosis (NF)	Patient Listening session	6/13/2019
Immune thrombocytopenia (ITP)	EL-PFDD meeting Host: Platelet Disorder Support Association	7/26/2019
IgA nephropathy (IgAN)	EL-PFDD meeting Host: National Kidney Foundation and the IgA Nephropathy Foundation of America	8/19/2019
Osteogenesis imperfecta (OI)	Patient listening session	9/17/2019

APPENDIX F

Disease/Condition Name	Meeting Type	Meeting Date
Pyruvate kinase deficiency	EL-PFDD meeting Host: National Organization for Rare Disorders (NORD)	9/20/2019
Cerebral cavernous malformation (CCM)	Patient listening session	11/6/2019
Gastroparesis	Patient listening session	12/2/2019
Ocular melanoma (OM)	Patient listening session	1/27/2020
Von Hippel Lindau (VHL)	Patient listening session	6/11/2020
Homocystinuria (HCU)	Patient listening session	6/26/2020
Pulmonary alveola proteinosis (PAP)	Patient listening session	7/8/2020
Pompe disease	EL-PFDD meeting Host: Muscular Dystrophy Association	7/13/2020
Progressive multifocal leukoencephalopathy (PML)	Patient listening session	7/22/2020
Smith-Magenis syndrome (SMS)	Patient listening session	8/12/2020
Focal segmental glomerulosclerosis (FSGS)	EL-PFDD meeting Host: National Kidney Foundation and NephCure Kidney International	8/28/2020
Guillain-Barre' syndrome (GBS)	Patient listening session	9/29/2020
Primary hyperoxaluria (PH)	EL-PFDD meeting Host: The Oxalosis and Hyperoxaluria Foundation	10/5/2020
Systemic sclerosis	FDA-led PFDD meeting	10/13/2020
Limb-girdle muscular dystrophies (LGMD)	Patient listening session	10/20/2020
Primary sclerosing cholangitis (PSC)	EL-PFDD meeting Host: PSC Partners Seeking a Cure	10/23/2020
Gorlin syndrome (GS)	Patient listening session	11/9/2020
SYNGAP1	EL-PFDD meeting Host: SYNGAP1 Foundation	11/19/2020
Acromegaly	EL-PFDD meeting Host: Acromegaly Community, Inc	1/21/2021
Pemphigus and pemphigoid	Patient listening session	2/8/2021
Fragile X syndrome (FXS)	EL-PFDD meeting Host: National Fragile X Foundation	3/3/2021

Disease/Condition Name	Meeting Type	Meeting Date
Frontotemporal degeneration (FTD)	EL-PFDD meeting Host: Association for Frontotemporal Degeneration (AFTD)	3/5/2021
Glycogen storage disease (GSD) type 1 – adult patients	Patient listening session	3/18/2021
Glycogen storage disease (GSD) type 1 – caregivers to pediatric patients	Patient listening session	3/25/2021
Cystic fibrosis (PM – nonsense mutations	Patient listening session	7/15/2021
Cerebrotendinous xanthomatosis (CTX)	EL-PFDD meeting Host: United Leukodystrophy Foundation of America	9/14/2021
Ichthyosis	Patient listening session	9/17/2021
Mastocytosis	Patient listening session	9/28/2021
Gorlin syndrome (GS)	EL-PFDD meeting Host: Gorlin Syndrome Alliance	10/8/2021
Hypothalamic obesity (HO)	Patient listening session	10/22/2021
Adult polyglucosan body disease	Patient listening session	10/28/2021
Thymidine kinase 2 deficiency (TK2)	Patient listening session	1/31/2022
Dravet syndrome (DS)	EL-PFDD meeting Host: The Dravet Syndrome Foundation	2/3/2022
Primary biliary cholangitis (PBC)	EL-PFDD meeting Host: Global Liver Institute	2/4/2022
Glycogen storage disease (GSD) type 1B	Patient listening session	3/3/2022
Rett syndrome	EL-PFDD meeting Host: Rett Syndrome Research Trust (RSRT)	3/11/2022
Chronic inflammatory demyelinating polyneuropathy (CIDP)	EL-PFDD meeting Host: GBS|CIDP Foundation International	3/25/2022
Congenital muscular dystrophy (CMD)	EL-PFDD meeting Host: Cure CMD	7/1/2022
Succinic semialdehyde dehydrogenase deficiency (SSADHD)	EL-PFDD meeting Host: SSADH Association	7/8/2022
Short bowel syndrome (SBS)	Patient listening session	7/19/2022

Disease/Condition Name	Meeting Type	Meeting Date
X-linked adrenoleukodystrophy (ALD)	EL-PFDD meeting Host: ALD Connect	7/22/2022
Huntington's disease (HD) pre-symptomatic population	Patient listening session	7/25/2022
Spinal muscular atrophy (SMA)	Patient listening session	8/4/2022
Narcolepsy and idiopathic hypersomnia (IH)	Patient listening session	8/8/2022
Galactosemia	EL-PFDD meeting Host: National Organization for Rare Disorders (NORD)	9/1/2022
Fabry disease	EL-PFDD meeting Host: National Kidney Foundation and Fabry Support & Information Group	9/19/2022
Alström syndrome	EL-PFDD meeting Host: Alstrom International	9/22/2022
Limb–girdle muscular dystrophies (LGMD)	EL-PFDD meeting Host: Coalition to Cure Calpain 3, CureLGMD2i, the Kurt+Peter Foundation, the LGMD2D Foundation, the McColl-Lockwood Laboratory for Muscular Dystrophy Research, and the Speak Foundation	9/23/2022
Metachromatic leukodystrophy (MLD)	EL-PFDD meeting Host: Cure MLD, The Calliope Joy Foundation, MLD Foundation, The United Leukodystrophy Foundation, and the Global Leukodystrophy Initiative	10/21/2022
Phelan-McDermid syndrome (PMS)	EL-PFDD meeting Host: CureSHANK	11/8/2022
Kennedy's disease (KD)/spinal and bulbar muscular atrophy (SBMA)	EL-PFDD meeting Host: Kennedy's Disease Association	11/9/2022
Hypophosphatasia (HPP)	EL-PFDD meeting Host: Soft Bones, Inc., The US Hypophosphatasia Foundation	11/15/2022
Proteus syndrome	Patient listening session	12/1/2022
Cerebral creatine deficiency syndromes (CCDS)	EL-PFDD meeting Host: Association for Creatine Deficiencies	1/24/2023

Disease/Condition Name	Meeting Type	Meeting Date
Pemphigus and pemphigoid	EL-PFDD meeting Host: International Pemphigus and Pemphigoid Foundation	1/25/2023
Autoimmune hepatitis (AIH)	EL-PFDD meeting Host: Autoimmune Hepatitis Association	1/27/2023
Wiskott-Aldrich syndrome (WAS)	EL-PFDD meeting Host: Wiskott-Aldrich Foundation	2/3/2023
Bronchopulmonary dysplasia (BPD)	Patient listening session	3/20/2023
Sickle cell disease	Patient listening session	5/5/2023
Prader-Willi syndrome (PWS)	EL-PFDD meeting Host: PWSA|USA	6/22/2023
Pyruvate dehydrogenase complex deficiency (PDCD)	Patient listening session	9/8/2023
Atypical hemolytic uremic syndrome (aHUS)	Patient listening session	9/21/2023
Spinocerebellar ataxia type 3 (SCA3)	Patient listening session	9/22/2023
Amyotrophic lateral sclerosis (ALS)	N/A	N/A

SOURCE: U.S. Food and Drug Administration. 2024. *Condition-specific meeting reports and other information related to patients' experience.* https://www.fda.gov/industry/prescription-drug-user-fee-amendments/condition-specific-meeting-reports-and-other-information-related-patients-experience (accessed August 15, 2024).

Appendix G

List of Orphan Approvals by FDA or EMA Between 2018 and 2022

Brand name	Generic Name	Approved by EMA	EMA Approved as Orphan	EMA Approval Year	Approved by FDA	FDA Approved as Orphan	FDA Approval Year	Divergent Decision	Therapeutic Area	Reason for non-approval in EMA	Reason for non-approval in FDA
Abecma	idecabtagene vicleucel	Y	Y	2021	Y	Y	2021	N	L01		
Adakveo	crizanlizumab	Y	Y	2020	Y	Y	2019	N	B06		
Alofisel	darvadstrocel	Y	Y	2018	N	N	#N/A	Y	L04		Not submitted
Amondys 45	casimersen	N	N	#N/A	Y	Y	2021	Y	M09	Not submitted	
Amvuttra	vutrisiran sodium	Y	Y	2022	Y	Y	2022	N	N07		
Andexxa	coagulation factor Xa [recombinant], inactivated-zhzo	Y	N	2019	Y	Y	2018	N	B02		
ANTHIM	obiltoxaximab	Y	Y	2020	Y	Y[a]	2016	N	J01		
Artesunate Amivas	Artesunate	Y	Y	2021	Y	Y	2020	N	P01		
Asparlas	calaspargase pegol-mknl	N	N	#N/A	Y	Y	2018	Y	L01	Not submitted	
Ayvakit	Avapritinib	Y	Y	2020	Y	Y	2020	N	L01		
Besremi	ropeginterferon alfa-2b	Y	N	2019	Y	Y	2021	N	L03		
Blenrep	belantamab mafodotin	Y	Y	2020	Y	Y	2020	N	L01		
Braftovi	encorafenib	Y	N	2018	Y	Y	2018	N	L01		

311

Breyanzi	lisocabtagene maraleucel	Y	N	2022	Y	Y	2021	N	L01
Brukinsa	zanubrutinib	Y	N	2021	Y	Y	2019	N	L01
Bylvay	odevixibat	Y	Y	2021	Y	Y	2021	N	A05
Cablivi	caplacizumab	Y	Y	2018	Y	Y	2019	N	B01
Camzyos	mavacamten	Y	N	2023	Y	Y	2022	N	C01
Carvykti	ciltacabtagene autoleucel	Y	Y	2022	Y	Y	2022	N	L01
Copiktra	duvelisib	Y	N	2021	Y	Y	2018	N	L01
Crysvita	burosumab	Y	Y	2018	Y	Y	2018	N	M05
Cytalux	pafolacianine sodium	N	N	#N/A	Y	Y	2021	Y	V04	Not submitted
Danyelza	naxitamab-gqgk	N	N	#N/A	Y	Y	2020	Y	L01	Not submitted
Daurismo	glasdegib	Y	Y	2020	Y	Y	2018	N	L01
Detectnet	copper Cu 64 dotatate injection	N	N	#N/A	Y	Y	2020	Y	V09	Not submitted
Diacomit	stiripentol	Y	Y[a]	2007	Y	Y	2018	N	N03
Dojolvi	triheptanoin	N	N	#N/A	Y	Y	2020	Y	A16	Not submitted
Ebanga	ansuvimab-zykl	N	N	#N/A	Y	Y	2020	Y	J05	Not submitted
Ebvallo	Tabelecleucel	Y	Y	2022	N	N	#N/A	Y	L01	Not submitted

continued

Brand name	Generic Name	Approved by EMA	EMA Approved as Orphan	EMA Approval Year	Approved by FDA	FDA Approved as Orphan	FDA Approval Year	Divergent Decision	Therapeutic Area	Reason for non-approval in EMA	Reason for non-approval in FDA
EGATEN	triclabendazole	N	N	#N/A	Y	Y	2019	Y	P02	Not submitted	
Elahere	mirvetuximab soravtansine-gynx	N	N	#N/A	Y	Y	2022	Y	L01	Still in review	
Elzonris	tagraxofusp	Y	Y	2021	Y	Y	2018	N	L01		
Empaveli	pegcetacoplan	Y	Y	2021	Y	Y	2021	N	L04		
Enjaymo	sutimlimab	Y	Y	2022	Y	Y	2022	N	L04		
Enspryng	satralizumab	Y	Y	2021	Y	Y	2020	N	L04		
Epidiolex	cannabidiol	Y	Y[a]	2019	Y	Y	2018	N	N03		
Evkeeza	evinacumab	Y	N	2021	Y	Y	2021	N	C10		
Evrysdi	risdiplam	Y	Y	2021	Y	Y	2020	N	M09		
Exkivity	mobocertinib succinate	N	N	#N/A	Y	Y	2021	Y	L01	Withdrawn by the sponsor	
Fexinidazole	fexinidazole	N	N	#N/A	Y	Y	2021	Y[a]	P01	Not submitted	
Firdapse	amifampridine	Y	Y[a]	2009	Y	Y	2018	N	N07		
Galafold	migalastat hydrochloride	Y	Y[a]	2016	Y	Y	2018	N	A16		
Gamifant	emapalumab-lzsg	N	N	#N/A	Y	Y	2018	Y	L04	Refused	
Gavreto	pralsetinib	Y	N	2021	Y	Y	2020	N	L01		

Givlaari	givosiran	Y	Y	2020	Y	2019	N	A16	
Hemgenix	etranacogene dezaparvovec-drlb	Y	Yᵃ	2023	Y	2022	N	B02	
Hepcludex	bulevirtide	Y	Y	2020	N	#N/A	Y	J05	Still in review
Idefirix	imlifidase	Y	Y	2020	N	#N/A	Y	L04	Not submitted
Imcivree	setmelanotide	Y	Y	2021	Y	2020	N	A08	
Imjudo	tremelimumab-actl	Y	N	2023	Y	2022	N	L01	
Inmazeb	atoltivimab, maftivimab, and odesivimab-ebgn	N	N	#N/A	Y	2020	Y	J05	Not submitted
Inqovi	decitabine and cedazuridine	Y	N	2023	Y	2020	N	L01	
Inrebic	fedratinib	Y	Y	2021	Y	2019	N	L01	
Isturisa	osilodrostat	Y	Y	2020	Y	2020	N	H02	
Kimmtrak	tebentafusp	Y	Y	2022	Y	2022	N	L01	
Koselugo	selumetinib	Y	Y	2021	Y	2020	N	L01	
Krazati	adagrasib	Y	N	2024	Y	2022	N	L01	
Krintafel	tafenoquine	N	N	#N/A	Y	2018	Y	P01	
Kymriah	tisagenlecleucel	Y	Y	2018	Yᵃ	2017	N	L01	Not submitted
Lampit	nifurtimox	N	N	#N/A	Y	2020	Y	P01	Not submitted
Lamzede	velmanase alfa	Y	Y	2018	Yᵃ	2023	N	A16	

continued

Brand name	Generic Name	Approved by EMA	EMA Approved as Orphan	EMA Approval Year	Approved by FDA	FDA Approved as Orphan	FDA Approval Year	Divergent Decision	Therapeutic Area	Reason for non-approval in EMA	Reason for non-approval in FDA
Libmeldy	Autologous CD34+ cells encoding ARSA gene	Y	Y	2020	Y	Y	2024	N	N07		
Livmarli	maralixibat chloride	Y	Y	2022	Y	Y	2021	N	A05		
Livtencity	maribavir	Y	Y	2022	Y	Y	2021	N	J05		
Lorbrena	lorlatinib	Y	N	2019	Y	Y	2018	N	L01		
Lumakras	sotorasib	Y	N	2022	Y	Y	2021	N	L01		
Lumoxiti	moxetumomab pasudotox-tdfk	N	N	#N/A	Y	Y	2018	Y	L01	Withdrawn by the sponsor	
Lunsumio	Mosunetuzumab	Y	Y	2022	Y	Y	2022	N	L01		
Lutathera	lutetium (177Lu) oxodotreotide	Y	Y[a]	2017	Y	Y	2018	N	V10		
Luxturna	voretigene neparvovec	Y	Y	2018	Y	Y[a]	2017	N	S01		
Lytgobi	futibatinib	Y	N	2023	Y	Y	2022	N	L01		
Mektovi	binimetinib	Y	N	2018	Y	Y	2018	N	L01		
Mepsevii	vestronidase alfa	Y	Y	2018	Y	Y[a]	2017	N	A16		
Monjuvi	tafasitamab-cxix	Y	Y	2021	Y	Y	2020	N	L01		
Moxidectin	moxidectin	N	N	#N/A	Y	Y	2018	Y	P02	Not submitted	

MYALEPT (BLA #125390)	METRELEPTIN	Y	Y	2018	Y	Y[a]	2014	N	A16
Mylotarg	gemtuzumab ozogamicin	Y	Y	2018	Y	Y[a]	2000	N	L01
Nexviazyme	avalglucosidase alfa-ngpt	Y	N	2022	Y	Y	2021	N	A16
Ngenla	somatrogon	Y	Y	2022	Y	Y[a]	2023	N	H01
Nulibry	fosdenopterin hydrobromide dihydrate	Y	Y	2022	Y	Y	2021	N	A16
Omegaven	fish oil triglycerides	N	N	#N/A	Y	Y	2018	Y	B05
Onpattro	patisiran sodium	Y	Y	2018	Y	Y	2018	N	N07
Opdualag	nivolumab, relatlimab	Y	N	2022	Y	Y	2022	N	L01
Orladeyo	berotralstat	Y	N	2021	Y	Y	2020	N	B06
Oxbryta	voxelotor	Y	Y	2022	Y	Y	2019	N	B06
Oxervate	recombinant human nerve growth factor (rhNGF)	Y	Y[a]	2017	Y	Y	2018	N	S01
Oxlumo	lumasiran	Y	Y	2020	Y	Y	2020	N	A16
Palynziq	pegvaliase	Y	Y	2019	Y	Y	2018	N	A16
Pemazyre	pemigatinib	Y	Y	2021	Y	Y	2020	N	L01

Not submitted

continued

315

Brand name	Generic Name	Approved by EMA	EMA Approved as Orphan	EMA Approval Year	Approved by FDA	FDA Approved as Orphan	FDA Approval Year	Divergent Decision	Therapeutic Area	Reason for non-approval in EMA	Reason for non-approval in FDA
Pepaxto	melphalan flufenamide hydrochloride	Y	Y[a]	2022	Y	Y	2021	N	L01		
Polivy	polatuzumab vedotin	Y	Y	2020	Y	Y	2019	N	L01		
Poteligeo	mogamulizumab	Y	Y	2018	Y	Y	2018	N	L01		
Dovprela	pretomanid	Y	Y	2020	Y	Y	2019	N	J04		
Prevymis	letermovir	Y	Y	2018	Y	Y[a]	2017	N	J05		
Pyrukynd	mitapivat sulfate	Y	Y	2022	Y	Y	2022	N	B06		
Qinlock	ripretinib	Y	Y	2021	Y	Y	2020	N	L01		
Reblozyl	luspatercept	Y	Y	2020	Y	Y	2019	N	B03		
Relyvrio	sodium phenylbutyrate and taurursodiol	N	N	#N/A	Y	Y	2022	Y	N07	Refused	
Retevmo	selpercatinib	Y	N	2021	Y	Y	2020	N	L01		
Revcovi	elapegademase-lvlr	N	N	#N/A	Y	Y	2018	Y	L03	Not submitted	
Rezlidhia	olutasidenib	N	N	#N/A	Y	Y	2022	Y	L01	Not submitted	
Rezurock	belumosudil mesylate	N	N	#N/A	Y	Y	2021	Y	L04	Not submitted	
Roctavian	valoctocogene roxaparvovec	Y	Y	2022	Y	Y[a]	2023	N	B02		

Rozlytrek	entrectinib	Y	N	2020	Y	2019	N	L01
Rubraca	rucaparib	Y	Y	2018	Y	2016	N	L01
Rylaze	asparaginase erwinia chrysanthemi (recombinant)-rywn	Y	N	2023	Y	2021	N	L01
Sarclisa	isatuximab	Y	N	2020	Y	2020	N	L01
Scemblix	asciminib hydrochloride	Y	Y	2022	Y	2021	N	L01
Scenesse	afamelanotide	Y	Y[a]	2014	Y	2019	N	D02
Skysona	elivaldogene autotemcel	Y	Y	2021	Y	2022	N	A16
Skytrofa	lonapegsomatropin	Y	Y	2022	Y	2021	N	H01
Sogroya	somapacitan	Y	Y	2021	N	2020	N	H01
Spevigo	spesolimab	Y	N	2022	Y	2022	N	L04
Sunosi	solriamfetol	Y	N	2020	Y	2019	N	N06
Symdeko	tezacaftor; ivacaftor	Y	Y	2018	Y	2018	N	R07
Tabrecta	capmatinib dihydrochloride monohydrate	Y	N	2022	Y	2020	N	L01
Takhzyro	lanadelumab	Y	Y	2018	Y	2018	N	B06
Tavalisse	fostamatinib	Y	N	2020	Y	2018	N	B02
Tavneos	avacopan	Y	Y	2022	Y	2021	N	L04

continued

Brand name	Generic Name	Approved by EMA	EMA Approved as Orphan	EMA Approval Year	Approved by FDA	FDA Approved as Orphan	FDA Approval Year	Divergent Decision	Therapeutic Area	Reason for non-approval in EMA	Reason for non-approval in FDA
Tazverik	tazemetostat	N	N	#N/A	Y	Y	2020	Y	L01	Not submitted	
Tecartus	brexucabtagene autoleucel	Y	Y	2020	Y	Y	2020	N	L01		
Tecvayli	teclistamab	Y	N	2022	Y	Y	2022	N	L01		
Tegsedi	inotersen sodium	Y	Y	2018	Y	Y	2018	N	N07		
Tepezza	teprotumumab-trbw	N	N	#N/A	Y	Y	2020	Y	L04	Not submitted	
Tepmetko	tepotinib hydrochloride monohydrate	Y	N	2022	Y	Y	2021	N	L01		
Terlivaz	terlipressin	N	N	#N/A	Y	Y	2022	Y	H01	Not submitted	
Tibsovo	ivosidenib	Y	Y[a]	2023	Y	Y	2018	N	L01		
TPOXX	tecovirimat	Y	N	2022	Y	Y	2018	N	J05		
TRIKAFTA (copackaged)	elexacaftor, ivacaftor, tezacaftor	Y	Y	2020	Y	Y	2019	N	R07		
Trogarzo	ibalizumab	Y	N	2019	Y	Y	2018	N	J05		
Truseltiq	infigratinib phosphate	N	N	#N/A	Y	Y	2021	Y	L01	Withdrawn by the sponsor	
Tukysa	tucatinib	Y	N	2021	Y	Y	2020	N	L01		
TURALIO	pexidartinib hydrochloride	N	N	#N/A	Y	Y	2019	Y	L01	Refused	

319

Brand	Generic	C3	C4	C5	C6	Year	C8	ATC	Notes
Ukoniq	umbralisib tosylate	N	N	Y	Y	#N/A	2021	Y	L01	Not submitted
Ultomiris	ravulizumab	Y	N	Y	Y	2019	2018	N	L04	
Uplizna	Inebilizumab	Y	N	Y	Y	2022	2020	N	L04	
Upstaza	eladocagene exuparvovec	Y	Y	N	N	2022	#N/A	Y	N07	Still in review
Viltepso	viltolarsen	N	N	Y	Y	#N/A	2020	Y	M09	Not submitted
Vitrakvi	larotrectinib sulfate	Y	N	Y	Y	2019	2018	N	L01	
Vizimpro	dacomitinib monohydrate	Y	N	Y	Y	2019	2018	N	L01	
Vonjo	pacritinib	N	N	Y	Y	#N/A	2022	Y	L01	Withdrawn by the sponsor
Voraxaze	glucarpidase	Y	Y	Y	Y^a	2022	2012	N	V03	
Voxzogo	vosoritide	Y	Y^a	Y	Y	2021	2021	N	M05	
VYNDAQEL	tafamidis meglumine	Y	Y^a	Y	Y	2011	2019	N	N07	
VYONDYS 53	golodirsen	N	N	Y	Y	#N/A	2019	Y	M09	Not submitted
Vyvgart	efgartigimod alfa	Y	Y	Y	Y	2022	2021	N	L04	
Wakix	pitolisant	Y	Y^a	Y	Y	2016	2019	N	N07	
Waylivra	volanesorsen sodium	Y	Y	N	N	2019	#N/A	Y	C10	Complete Response

continued

Brand name	Generic Name	Approved by EMA	EMA Approved as Orphan	EMA Approval Year	Approved by FDA	FDA Approved as Orphan	FDA Approval Year	Divergent Decision	Therapeutic Area	Reason for non-approval in EMA	Reason for non-approval in FDA
Welireg	belzutifan	N	N	#N/A	Y	Y	2021	Y	L01	Not submitted	
Xenpozyme	olipudase alfa	Y	Y	2022	Y	Y	2022	N	A16		
Xospata	gilteritinib fumarate	Y	Y	2019	Y	Y	2018	N	L01		
XPOVIO	selinexor	Y	N	2021	Y	Y	2019	N	L01		
Yescarta	axicabtagene ciloleucel	Y	Y	2018	Y	Y[a]	2017	N	L01		
Zepzelca	lurbinectedin	N	N	#N/A	Y	Y	2020	Y	L01	Not submitted	
Zokinvy	lonafarnib	Y	Y	2022	Y	Y	2020	N	A16		
Zolgensma	onasemnogene abeparvovec	Y	Y	2020	Y	Y	2019	N	M09		
Ztalmy	ganaxolone	Y	Y[a]	2023	Y	Y	2022	N	N03		
Zynlonta	loncastuximab tesirine	Y	Y	2022	Y	Y	2021	N	L01		
Zynteglo	betibeglogene autotemcel	Y	Y	2019	Y	Y	2022	N	B06		

[a] These data points were corrected after release of the prepublication version of the report to accurately reflect the orphan status of the drugs and decisions made by FDA and EMA.

NOTES: Ga-68-DOTATOC (gallium [68Ga] edotreotide, known as Somakit TOC in Europe) was approved as an Orphan drug by FDA in 2019 and recommended for authorization as an Orphan drug by EMA in 2016. However, FDA's orphan designation was withdrawn or revoked on December 9, 2020. Thus, the drug did not fall into the criteria for this analysis; includes approvals outside of year range, 2018–2022, if approved by the other agency within the date range.

SOURCE: Centre for Innovation in Regulatory Science, 2024 (unpublished). Data analysis and summary to help inform the National Academies committee on Processes to Evaluate the Safety and Efficacy of Drugs for Rare Diseases or Conditions in the United States and the European Union. Data analysis commissioned by the committee on Processes to Evaluate the Safety and Efficacy of Drugs for Rare Diseases or Conditions in the United States and the European Union, National Academies of Sciences, Engineering, and Medicine, Washington, DC.

Appendix H

Select Examples of Rare Disease Drug Products

ELEVIDYS (*DELANDISTROGENE MOXEPARVOVEC-ROKL*)

Condition (Therapeutic Area):
Duchenne muscular dystrophy (DMD)

Year of Approval (by Agency):
Approved by FDA in June 2023 (FDA, 2023a);
Not yet submitted to EMA.

Context of Approval (e.g., Standard of Care):
Elevidys was approved for the treatment of ambulatory patients, aged 4 through 6 years of age with DMD with a confirmed mutation in the DMD gene (FDA, 2023a). It was the first approval of a gene therapy for DMD (FDA, 2023c).

Regulatory Pathway Used:
Elevidys was approved under FDA's accelerated pathway (FDA, 2023a).

Designations/Expedited Programs Used:
FDA granted the drug Orphan Product designation and Fast Track (FDA, 2023a).

Novel Trial Design Elements:
Approval relied on three separate studies submitted: two were open-label studies and one was a randomized, placebo-controlled cross-over trial

(cross-over trial formed the primary base of the decision). The studies used of a surrogate endpoint of expression of ELEVIDYS micro-dystrophin; correlated to North Star Ambulatory Assessment score (FDA, 2023a).

"Supplemental Data" Used:
Open Label Extension Study and use of natural history data used as the external control (FDA, 2023a).

Advisory Committee and Patient Community Engagement:
A virtual Advisory Committee was held on May 12, 2023. FDA expanded the public hearing to 90 minutes, allowing for public testimony as well as videos of individuals who had participated in studies. Parents, clinicians, and others presented what they referenced as real world data to demonstrate benefit of Elevidys. Individuals who had received Elevidys demonstrated the increased ability to jump, climb and ride bikes, activities that were impossible prior to receiving the therapy. The advisory committee voted 8 to 6 in favor of Elevidys (FDA, 2023a).

Regulatory Flexibilities Deployed:
FDA:
FDA approval demonstrated flexibility expressed in FDA guidance allowing for submissions based on "one adequate and well controlled study with confirmatory evidence." That "confirmatory evidence" included the use of natural history data used as an "external control" in comparison to subjects in the open label extension of the single study. Despite the Review Committee's determination, that there was insufficient evidence to use micro-dystrophin as a surrogate endpoint, the Center Director overrode the decision leading to approval of Elevidys (FDA, 2023a).

MEPSEVII (*VESTRONIDASE ALFA*)

Condition (Therapeutic Area):
Mucopolysaccharidosis (MPS) VII, Sly Syndrome

Year of Approval (by Agency):
Approved by FDA November 2017 (FDA, 2017);
Recommended for authorization by EMA in April 2018 (EMA, 2018b);
Authorized by European Commission in August 2018 (EMA, 2018b).

Context of Approval (e.g., Standard of Care):
First treatment approved for MPS VII. Prior to approval of Mepsevii, there were no disease-modifying treatments available; treatment consisted of supportive care and management of disease complications (FDA, 2017).

APPENDIX H

Regulatory Pathway Used:
FDA granted Mepsevii standard approval (FDA, 2017).
EMA used Exceptional Circumstances approval to approve Mepsevii (EMA, 2018b).

Designations/Expedited Programs Used:
FDA granted Mepsevii Orphan and Fast Track designation as well as Priority Review (FDA, 2017).
EMA had designated the drug an orphan product (EMA, 2018b).

Novel Trial Design Elements:
FDA: Approval based on totality of evidence approach on a per subject basis. There was no pre-specified primary endpoint for the study (FDA, 2017)
EMA: Approval based on a surrogate biomarker uGAG (EMA, 2018b)

"Supplemental Data" Used:
FDA: Natural history (informal)—no organized natural history data collection, but consideration of the known chronic progressive nature of the disease, disease complications/manifestations, and extrapolation of findings from other related MPS's and ERT approvals for these conditions. FDA also considered pharmacologic effect of the drug from nonclinical studies (FDA, 2017).
EMA: relied upon knowledge of the disease, severity and life-threatening nature of the illness, lack of available treatments, and reliance upon a biomarker for clinical outcome (EMA, 2018b).

Advisory Committee and Patient Community Engagement:
There are no advisory committees or patient engagement documented for this drug

Regulatory Flexibilities Deployed:
Both FDA and EMA relied upon efficacy and safety data from 17 patients exposed to Mepsevii.

FDA:
Although limitations in the clinical program were noted relating to the quantity of the evidence, FDA considered that given the rarity of the disease and the limited patient availability, it was not feasible to conduct a traditional parallel group, placebo-controlled trial (FDA, 2017).

EMA:
EMA considered the limited amount of data from clinical studies, the life-threatening and debilitating nature of MPS7, and lack of authorized medicines available to treat the disease, all of which supported an MA under "exceptional circumstances" (EMA, 2018b).

NEXVIAZYME® (*AVALGLUCOSIDASE ALFA*)

Condition (Therapeutic Area):
Late-onset Pompe disease

Year of Approval (by Agency):
Approved by FDA August 2021 (FDA, 2021b);
Recommended for authorization by EMA in November 2021 (EMA, 2024b);
Authorized by European Commission in June 2022 (EMA, 2024b).

Context of Approval (e.g., Standard of Care):
First treatment.

Regulatory Pathway Used:
FDA granted Nexviazyme approval using priority review (FDA, 2021b);
EMA used standard approval to approve Nexviazyme (EMA, 2024b).

Designations/Expedited Programs Used:
FDA granted Nexviazyme Breakthrough Therapy, Fast Track, and Orphan designations (FDA, 2021b).
EMA had originally granted Nexviazyme an orphan designation. However, at the time of authorization, the dug was not found to provide a significant benefit over an existing treatment. Thus, the orphan designation was removed (EMA, 2022a)

Novel Trial Design Elements:
FDA: Approval based on totality of evidence approach which included open label data and g an analysis of covariance (ANCOVA) model (FDA, 2021b)
EMA: Approval based on a benefit risk analysis (EMA, 2024b)

"Supplemental Data" Used:
Open label data was used to support approval in both FDA and EMA (EMA, 2024b; FDA, 2021b).

APPENDIX H

Advisory Committee and Patient Community Engagement:
There are no advisory committees or patient engagement documented for this drug

Regulatory Flexibilities Deployed:
Both FDA and EMA relied on open label data

FDA:
Despite a non-statistically significant analysis, FDA reviewed the totality of evidence

OGSIVEO (*NIROGACESTAT*)

Condition (Therapeutic Area):
Progressing, unresectable, recurrent or refractory desmoid tumors

Year of Approval (by Agency):
Approved by FDA in November 2023 (FDA, 2023e);
Submitted to EMA – no opinion yet. EMA validated the Marketing Authorization Application in February 2024 (SpringWorks Therapeutics, 2024).

Context of Approval (e.g., Standard of Care):
First product approved for desmoid tumors (FDA, 2023e)

Regulatory Pathway Used:
FDA granted Ogsiveo standard approval (FDA, 2023e)

Designations/Expedited Programs Used:
FDA granted Orphan designation, Breakthrough Therapy, Fast Track, and Priority Review (FDA, 2023e).
EMA granted Orphan designation (EMA, 2019a)

Novel Trial Design Elements:
Phase 3 randomized (1:1), double-blind, placebo-controlled trial with 142 patients in an international multicenter setting (FDA, 2023e).

"Supplemental Data" Used:
Patient-reported outcomes such as pain, physical functioning, health-related quality of life, and desmoid tumor specific symptoms (FDA, 2023e)

Advisory Committee and Patient Community Engagement:
There are no advisory committees or patient engagement documented for this drug

Regulatory Flexibilities Deployed:
FDA:
The program utilized the real-time oncology review (RTOR) pilot program; it entails a rapid-cycle and streamlined data submission process prior to the application filing. The approval also included a post-marketing requirement for the presence of ovarian toxicity risk increase. Risk-benefit profile was in favor of an approval, and this is why a REMS or risk management plan was not indicated (FDA, 2023e).

QALSODY (*TOFERSEN*)

Condition (Therapeutic Area):
Amyotrophic lateral sclerosis (ALS)

Year of Approval (by Agency):
Approved by FDA April 2023 (FDA, 2023g);
Recommended for authorization by EMA in February 2024 (EMA, 2024c);
Not yet authorized by European Commission (EMA, 2024c).

Context of Approval (e.g., Standard of Care):
Qalsody is the first drug specific to SOD1 mutation; progressive disease with rapid morbidity and mortality with standard of care (FDA, 2023f).

Regulatory Pathway Used:
FDA used Accelerated Approval (based on surrogate endpoint) to approve Qalsody (FDA, 2023g).
EMA recommended marketing authorization under exceptional circumstances (EMA, 2024d).

Designations/Expedited Programs Used:
FDA granted Qalsody orphan designation and Priority Review (FDA, 2023g).
EMA granted orphan designation (EMA, 2024d).

Novel Trial Design Elements:
One randomized, double-blinded, placebo-controlled trial; post-hoc analyses; open-label extension study (post-hoc exploratory analyses); use of novel surrogate endpoint (NfL)

APPENDIX H

"Supplemental Data" Used:
Open-label extension study (FDA, 2023g)

Advisory Committee and Patient Community Engagement:
FDA advisory committee which unanimously voted in favor of Qalsody (FDA, 2023g).

Regulatory Flexibilities Deployed:
FDA:
Qalsody failed its primary endpoint in the one pivotal trial. FDA accepted the significant reduction of NfL, a marker of neuronal degeneration and a secondary endpoint in the study as a reasonably likely surrogate endpoint to predict clinical benefit and thus support accelerated approval (FDA, 2023g).

EMA:
The CHMP positive opinion was "based on a reduction in the levels of SOD1 in the cerebrospinal fluid, a reduction in the levels of plasma neurofilament light chain (a marker of neuronal damage), and a numerically favorable effect on the ALSFRS-R physical ability scale" (EMA, 2024d)

RELYVIO (*SODIUM PHENYLBUTYRATE AND TAURURSODIOL*) KNOWN AS ALBRIOZA IN EU

Condition (Therapeutic Area):
Amyotrophic lateral sclerosis (ALS)

Year of Approval (by Agency):
Approved by FDA September 29, 2022 (FDA, 2022b);
Negative opinion for authorization by EMA in December 2023 (EMA, 2024a);
Refusal of marketing authorization by European Commission in May 2024 (EMA, 2024a).

Context of Approval (e.g., Standard of Care):
Two other drugs approved in United States (FDA, 2022b);
One other drug approved in EU (EMA, 2023).
Alternative products offer only modest clinical benefits. Patients have rapid morbidity and mortality on existing therapy (EMA, 2023; FDA, 2022b).

Regulatory Pathway Used:
FDA granted Relyvrio standard approval (FDA, 2022b).

Designations/Expedited Programs Used:
FDA granted Relyvrio orphan designation and Priority Review (FDA, 2022b). EMA granted orphan designation (EMA, 2023).

Novel Trial Design Elements:
Phase 3, double-blind, placebo-controlled trial—post-hoc long-term analysis (FDA, 2022b).

"Supplemental Data" Used:
Open-label extension study and Natural History Database (FDA, 2022b).

Advisory Committee and Patient Community Engagement:
United States: Two Advisory Committees. First AC voted down approval. Reconvened AC to discuss a major amendment to application, and committee voted in favor of the drug (FDA, 2022b).
EU: Scientific Advisory Group Review (EMA, 2023)

Regulatory Flexibilities Deployed:
FDA and EMA analyzed the same data from a Phase II study with open label extension; both sought input from outside scientific advisors and both received extensive input from patient groups. FDA and EMA both assessed that there were limitations in the clinical dataset.

FDA:
FDA noted that although these limitations were greater than usually were seen in drugs that meet the approval standard, they considered that the serious nature of the disease and the un-met need warranted use of regulatory flexibility. Applying this flexibility, they found that the benefits outweighed the risk and approved the drug (FDA, 2022b). In 2024, Relyvrio failed a Phase 3 trial. The company has withdrawn the drug from U.S. market (Amylyx Pharmaceuticals, 2024).

EMA:
EMA rejected the application based on its assessment that the efficacy data was neither robust nor statistically compelling (EMA, 2023)

SKYCLARYS (*OMAVELOXOLONE*)

Condition (Therapeutic Area):
Friedreich's ataxia

APPENDIX H   *329*

Year of Approval (by Agency):
Approved by FDA February 28, 2023 (FDA, 2023h);
Recommended for authorization by EMA in December 2023 (EMA, 2024e);
Authorized by European Commission in February 2024.

Context of Approval (e.g., Standard of Care):
SkyClarys is the first approved treatment for Friedreich's ataxia in the United States (FDA, 2023d) and in Europe (Biogen Inc., 2024).

Regulatory Pathway Used:
Both agencies granted SkyClarys a standard approval (EMA, 2024e; FDA, 2023h).

Designations/Expedited Programs Used:
FDA granted the drug Orphan Product designation, Rare Pediatric Disease Priority Review Voucher program, Expedited Review, and Fast Track (FDA, 2023h).
EMA had designated it an Orphan Product (EMA, 2024e).

Novel Trial Design Elements:
External control in comparison to subjects in the open-label extension (OLE) (FDA, 2023h)

"Supplemental Data" Used:
Open-label extension study and use of natural history data used as the external control (Biogen Inc., 2024; FDA, 2023h)

Advisory Committee and Patient Community Engagement:
A patient advocacy organization, the Friedreich's Ataxia Research Alliance (FARA), engaged with both FDA and EMA during the drug development process.

Regulatory Flexibilities Deployed:
FDA:
FDA approval demonstrated flexibility expressed in FDA guidance allowing for submissions based on "one adequate and well controlled study with confirmatory evidence." That "confirmatory evidence" included the use of natural history data used as an "external control" in comparison to subjects in the Open Label Extension (OLE) of the single study (FDA, 2023h).

EMA:
EMA received the same clinical study data and supplemental data/confirmatory evidence as FDA, assessed them very similarly, and reached the same

conclusion—recommending market approval 10 months after submission (EMA, 2024e).

TAFLINAR (*DABRAFENIB*) & MEKINIST (*TRAMETINIB*)

Condition (Therapeutic Area):
Unresectable or metastatic melanoma with a BRAF V600 mutation

Year of Approval (by Agency):
Approved by FDA in June 2022 (FDA, 2022a);
FDA indication update to include pediatric patients with low-grade glioma in March 2023 (FDA, 2023b);
EMA adopted a positive opinion to a change in the marketing indication for the combination therapy for resected Stage III melanoma (adjuvant treatment) in July 2018 (EMA, 2018a).

Context of Approval (e.g., Standard of Care):
This combination therapy was also approved as first-line therapy for pediatric patients with low-grade glioma driven by BRAF V600E mutation (FDA, 2023b).

Regulatory Pathway Used:
FDA used Accelerated Approval to approve the combination treatment (FDA, 2022a).

Designations/Expedited Programs Used:
FDA granted the drugs Priority Review (FDA, 2022a).

Novel Trial Design Elements:
Notable for the use of a basket trial design (NCI-MATCH and ROAR trials) inclusive or rare and non-rare cancer across 24 indications. Three trials and supporting evidence from 2 studies (FDA, 2022a).

"Supplemental Data" Used:
Patient reported outcomes specifically PROMIS Parent Proxy Global Health 7+2 were also used in the FDA approval process (FDA, 2022a).

Advisory Committee and Patient Community Engagement:
There are no advisory committees or patient engagement documented for this drug

APPENDIX H

Regulatory Flexibilities Deployed:
FDA:
This FDA approval is a first-in-class tumor agnostic indication for BRAF V600E mutation in solid tumors and expands the pool of biomarker targeted therapies in the marketplace. Additionally, this approval was facilitated by leveraging "Project Orbis," an initiative designed by FDA Oncology Center of Excellence that entails a pathway for simultaneous review of oncology-focused therapies with international partners (FDA, 2023b)

EMA:
EMA approval is limited to a single-disease (melanoma) as opposed to the tumor agnostic framework of FDA and based on the results of a single Phase 3 RCT (EMA, 2018a)

WAKIX® (*PITOLISANT*)

Condition (Therapeutic Area):
Excessive daytime sleepiness (EDS) or cataplexy in adults with narcolepsy.

Year of Approval (by Agency):
Approved by FDA in October 2020 (FDA, 2021a);
Recommended for authorization by EMA on November 19, 2015 (EMA, n.d.);
Authorized by European Commission on March 31, 2016 (EMA, n.d.).]

Context of Approval (e.g., Standard of Care):
Wakix, which was approved in the United States and Europe to treat narcolepsy, is now being trialed in United States for a rare disease, Prader-Willi syndrome. Ten families in the United States obtained the medication at FDA's discretion via personal importation and documented their experiences of improved sleep profiles and cognitive indicators (Pullen et al., 2019). The drug is now in clinical trials as a treatment for Prader Willi syndrome.

Regulatory Pathway Used:
FDA used priority review to approve Wakix (FDA, 2021a)

Designations/Expedited Programs Used:
FDA granted the drug orphan status for treatment of narcolepsy and Prader-Willi syndrome (FDA, n.d.). FDA also granted the drug Fast Track and Breakthrough Therapy designations for the cataplexy indication, but only Fast Track designations for the EDS indication (FDA, 2021a).
EMA granted the drug Orphan Product designation (EMA, n.d.)

Novel Trial Design Elements:
A study of Pitolsant in patients with Prader-Willi Syndrome began in April, 2024. The study is a "Phase 3, randomized, double-blind, placebo-controlled, multicenter, global clinical study" (NIH, 2024). The study will include an open-label extension period (NIH, 2024).

"Supplemental Data" Used:
None

Advisory Committee and Patient Community Engagement:
There are no advisory committees or patient engagement documented for this drug (FDA, 2021a).

Regulatory Flexibilities Deployed:
FDA allowed for personal importation of the treatment for off-label use before the drug was approved in the United States.

WAYLIVRA (*VOLANESORSEN*)

Condition (Therapeutic Area):
Familial Chylomicronemia Syndrome (FCS)

Year of Approval (by Agency):
Not approved – complete response letter from FDA in August 2018 (Ionis Pharmaceuticals, 2018);
Recommended for authorization by EMA on February 28, 2019 (EMA, 2022b);
Authorized by European Commission on May 3, 2019 (EMA, 2022b).

Context of Approval (e.g., Standard of Care):
Waylivra was approved for patients in whom other medicines to reduce triglycerides have not worked (EMA, 2022b).

Regulatory Pathway Used:
EMA used conditional approval to approve Waylivra (EMA, 2022b).

Designations/Expedited Programs Used:
EMA granted the drug Orphan Product designation (EMA, 2022b).

Novel Trial Design Elements:
One pivotal controlled study in conjunction with open label extension and additional control from a previous study (EMA, 2022b).

"Supplemental Data" Used:
Open-label extension study (EMA, 2019b).

Advisory Committee and Patient Community Engagement:
An ad hoc expert group was convened to address questions raised by the CHMP on June 19, 2018. The CHMP considered the views of the ad hoc expert group as presented in the minutes of that meeting and, between June 28, 2018, and November 15, 2018, sent three additional lists of outstanding issues to the applicant (EMA, 2019b).

Regulatory Flexibilities Deployed:
EMA:
EMA stated "The overall safety database is therefore relatively limited but acceptable in the context of a rare and orphan disease like FCS" when discussing the limited data available (EMA, 2019b).

ZOLGENSMA (ONASEMNOGENE ABEPARVOVEC-XIOI)

Condition (Therapeutic Area):
Spinal muscular atrophy (SMA)

Year of Approval (by Agency):
Approved by FDA May 24, 2019 (FDA, 2019b);
Recommended for authorization by EMA in March 2020 (EMA, 2022c);
Authorized by European Commission in May 2020 (EMA, 2022c).

Context of Approval (e.g., Standard of Care):
Zolgensma was the first approved gene therapy to treat SMA in children younger than 2 years old (FDA, 2019a).

Regulatory Pathway Used:
FDA used priority review to approve Zolgensma (FDA, 2019b).
EMA used Conditional approval to approve Zolgensma (EMA, 2022c).

Designations/Expedited Programs Used:
FDA designated the drug an Orphan Product, a Rare Pediatric Disease, and Fast Track (FDA, 2019b).
EMA had designated it an Orphan Product and an Advanced therapy medicinal product (EMA, 2022c).

Novel Trial Design Elements:
External control in comparison to subjects in the open-label extension (FDA, 2019b).

"Supplemental Data" Used:
Open-label extension study and use of natural history data used as the external control (FDA, 2019b).

Advisory Committee and Patient Community Engagement:
There are no advisory committees or patient engagement documented for this drug

Regulatory Flexibilities Deployed:
FDA:
FDA granted approval based on a Phase 1 trial evaluating safety and preliminary efficacy and an ongoing Phase 3 trial evaluating the efficacy and safety. Both studies were open-label extension studies with 15 patients in the first study and 21 in the second. FDA demonstrated flexibility by approving Zolgensma based on increase in survival when compared with a natural history control (FDA, 2019b).

EMA:
EMA used the same data to approve Zolgensma but provided a conditional approval pending the final outcome of the Phase 3 trial (EMA, 2022c).

REFERENCES

Amylyx Pharmaceuticals. 2024. *Amylyx Pharmaceuticals announces formal intention to remove Relyvrio®/Albrioza™ from the market; provides updates on access to therapy, pipeline, corporate restructuring, and strategy.* https://www.amylyx.com/news/amylyx-pharmaceuticals-announces-formal-intention-to-remove-relyvrior/albriozatm-from-the-market-provides-updates-on-access-to-therapy-pipeline-corporate-restructuring-and-strategy (accessed August 15, 2024).

Biogen Inc. 2024. *Biogen received European Commission approval for SkyClarys® (omaveloxolone), the first therapy to treat Friedreich's ataxia.* https://investors.biogen.com/news-releases/news-release-details/biogen-received-european-commission-approval-skyclarysr (accessed August 15, 2024).

EMA (European Medicines Agency). 2018a. *Mekinist: Summary of opinion (post authorisation).* https://www.ema.europa.eu/system/files/documents/smop/wc500252515_en.pdf (accessed August 1, 2024).

EMA. 2018b. *Mepsevii: EPAR.* https://www.ema.europa.eu/en/medicines/human/EPAR/mepsevii (accessed August 15, 2024).

EMA. 2019a. EU/3/19/2214 - orphan designation for treatment of soft tissue sarcoma. https://www.ema.europa.eu/en/medicines/human/orphan-designations/eu-3-19-2214 (accessed August 1, 2024)

EMA. 2019b. *Waylivra: Assessment report.* https://www.ema.europa.eu/en/documents/assessment-report/waylivra-epar-public-assessment-report_en.pdf (accessed August 1, 2024).

EMA. 2022a. *Nexviadyme: Orphan maintenance assessment report.* https://www.ema.europa.eu/en/documents/orphan-maintenance-report/nexviadyme-epar-orphan-maintenance-assessment-report-initial-authorisation_en.pdf (accessed August 1, 2024).

APPENDIX H

EMA. 2022b. *Waylivra: EPAR.* https://www.ema.europa.eu/en/medicines/human/EPAR/waylivra (accessed August 15, 2024).
EMA. 2022c. *Zolgensma: An overview of Zolgensma and why it is authorised in the EU.* https://www.ema.europa.eu/en/medicines/human/EPAR/zolgensma (accessed August 1, 2024).
EMA. 2023. *Albrioza: Assessment report.* https://www.ema.europa.eu/en/documents/assessment-report/albrioza-epar-refusal-public-assessment-report_en.pdf (accessed August 1, 2024).
EMA. 2024a. *Albrioza: EPAR.* https://www.ema.europa.eu/en/medicines/human/EPAR/albrioza (accessed August 15, 2024).
EMA. 2024b. *Nexviadyme.* https://www.ema.europa.eu/en/medicines/human/EPAR/nexviadyme (accessed August 15, 2024).
EMA. 2024c. *Qalsody: EPAR.* https://www.ema.europa.eu/en/medicines/human/EPAR/qalsody (accessed August 15, 2024).
EMA. 2024d. *Qalsody: Summary of opinion.* https://www.ema.europa.eu/en/documents/smop-initial/chmp-summary-positive-opinion-qalsody_en.pdf (accessed August 1, 2024).
EMA. 2024e. *SkyClarys: EPAR.* https://www.ema.europa.eu/en/medicines/human/EPAR/skyclarys (accessed August 15, 2024).
EMA. n.d. *Wakix.* https://www.ema.europa.eu/en/medicines/human/EPAR/wakix (accessed August 15, 2024).
FDA (U.S. Food and Drug Administration). 2017. *Mepsevii (vestronidase alfa-vjbk) injection: Review.* https://www.accessdata.fda.gov/drugsatfda_docs/nda/2017/761047Orig1s000TOC.cfm (accessed August 15, 2024).
FDA. 2019a. *FDA approves innovative gene therapy to treat pediatric patients with spinal muscular atrophy, a rare disease and leading genetic cause of infant mortality.* https://www.fda.gov/news-events/press-announcements/fda-approves-innovative-gene-therapy-treat-pediatric-patients-spinal-muscular-atrophy-rare-disease (accessed August 15, 2024).
FDA. 2019b. *Zolgensma: Summary basis for regulatory action.* https://www.fda.gov/media/127961/download?attachment (accessed August 1, 2024).
FDA. 2021a. *Drug approval package: Wakix.* https://www.accessdata.fda.gov/drugsatfda_docs/nda/2021/211150Orig2s000TOC.cfm (accessed August 15, 2024).
FDA. 2021b. *Nexviazyme: Integrated assessment.* https://www.accessdata.fda.gov/drugsatfda_docs/nda/2021/761194Orig1s000IntegratedR.pdf (accessed August 1, 2024).
FDA. 2022a. *FDA grants accelerated approval to dabrafenib in combination with trametinib for unresectable or metastatic solid tumors with BRAF V600E mutation.* https://www.fda.gov/drugs/resources-information-approved-drugs/fda-grants-accelerated-approval-dabrafenib-combination-trametinib-unresectable-or-metastatic-solid (accessed August 15, 2024).
FDA. 2022b. *Relyvrio: Summary review.* https://www.accessdata.fda.gov/drugsatfda_docs/nda/2022/216660Orig1s000SumR.pdf (accessed August 1, 2024).
FDA. 2023a. *Elevidys: Summary basis for regulatory action.* https://www.fda.gov/media/169746/download?attachment (accessed August 1, 2024).
FDA. 2023b. *FDA approves dabrafenib with trametinib for pediatric patients with low-grade glioma with a BRAF V600E mutation.* https://www.fda.gov/drugs/resources-information-approved-drugs/fda-approves-dabrafenib-trametinib-pediatric-patients-low-grade-glioma-braf-v600e-mutation (accessed August 1, 2024).
FDA. 2023c. *FDA approves first gene therapy for treatment of certain patients with Duchenne muscular dystrophy.* https://www.fda.gov/news-events/press-announcements/fda-approves-first-gene-therapy-treatment-certain-patients-duchenne-muscular-dystrophy (accessed August 15, 2024).

FDA. 2023d. *FDA approves first treatment for Friedreich's ataxia.* https://www.fda.gov/drugs/news-events-human-drugs/fda-approves-first-treatment-friedreichs-ataxia (accessed August 15, 2024).

FDA. 2023e. *FDA approves nirogacestat for desmoid tumors.* https://www.fda.gov/drugs/resources-information-approved-drugs/fda-approves-nirogacestat-desmoid-tumors (accessed August 15, 2024).

FDA. 2023f. *FDA approves treatment of amyotrophic lateral sclerosis associated with a mutation in the SOD1 gene.* https://www.fda.gov/drugs/news-events-human-drugs/fda-approves-treatment-amyotrophic-lateral-sclerosis-associated-mutation-sod1-gene#:~:text=Qalsody%20is%20an%20antisense%20oligonucleotide%20that%20targets%20SOD1,blood-based%20biomarker%20of%20axonal%20%28nerve%29%20injury%20and%20neurodegeneration (accessed August 15, 2024).

FDA. 2023g. *Qalsody: Integrated review.* https://www.accessdata.fda.gov/drugsatfda_docs/nda/2023/215887Orig1s000IntegratedR.pdf (accessed August 1, 2024).

FDA. 2023h. *SkyClarys: Summary review.* https://www.accessdata.fda.gov/drugsatfda_docs/nda/2023/216718Orig1s000SumR.pdf (accessed August 1, 2024).

FDA. n.d. *Orphan Drug Database.* https://www.accessdata.fda.gov/scripts/opdlisting/oopd/index.cfm (accessed August 15, 2024).

Ionis Pharmaceuticals. 2018. *Akcea and Ionis receive complete response letter for Waylivra from FDA.* https://ir.ionispharma.com/news-releases/news-release-details/akcea-and-ionis-receive-complete-response-letter-waylivra-fda (accessed August 15, 2024).

NIH (National Institutes of Health). 2024. A study of pitolisant in patients with Prader-Willi Syndrome: ClinicalTrials.gov.

Pullen, L., M. Picone, L. Tan, C. Johnston, and H. Stark. 2019. Pitolisant treatment improves multiple clinical symptoms of Prader-Willi Syndrome (PWS) in children (P3.6-024). *Neurology* 92(15_supplement):P3.6-024.

SpringWorks Therapeutics. 2024. *SpringWorks therapeutics announces European Medicines Agency validation for marketing authorization application of Nirogacestat for the treatment of adults with desmoid tumors.* https://ir.springworkstx.com/news-releases/news-release-details/springworks-therapeutics-announces-european-medicines-agency (accessed August 15, 2024).

Appendix I

FDA and EMA Resources, Policies, and Programs Relevant for Drug Development for Rare Diseases and Conditions

This appendix summarizes a non-exclusive list of resources, polices, and programs that the U.S. Food and Drug Administration (FDA) and European Medicines Agency (EMA) have in place to support drug development for rare disease and conditions. Each section provides a brief summary on the topic and lists relevant FDA and EMA resources (e.g., guidance, program websites, and other publications).

While FDA and EMA are considered regulatory counterparts, there are a few key differences in their jurisdiction and authority as well as how the organizations operate. FDA is a centralized regulatory body that oversees the evaluation of safety and efficacy of drugs approved in the United States and has a dedicated workforce and authority to issue guidance and make regulatory decisions on medications and medical devices. EMA is a decentralized agency of the European Union (EU) that is responsible for evaluating the safety and efficacy of drugs in Europe. However, it does not have the authority to approve medications. Instead, EMA can issue guidance and make authorization recommendations on medical products that the European Commission ultimately approves for marketing in the European Union (EMA, n.d.-j). Day-to-day operations at EMA are carried out by dedicated staff that rely on a network of experts from across Europe and collaboration with member states to pool resources and coordinate work to regulate medicines for use in humans (EMA, n.d.-v).

FDA and EMA each have regulatory policies in place to support and incentivize drug development for rare diseases and conditions, including mechanisms for facilitating expedited regulatory review, and opportunities for engagement with sponsors and people with lived rare disease experience.

ORPHAN DRUG DESIGNATION

Both FDA and EMA offer an orphan designation for drugs that are targeted at rare diseases. The criteria are similar but not identical. FDA offers orphan designation to products that treat conditions affecting fewer than 200,000 individuals in the United States, or that affect more than 200,000 individuals but there is no reasonable expectation that the cost of developing a drug for the condition would be recovered by sales of the drug. EMA offers orphan designation to products that treat conditions affecting not more than 5 in 10,000 individuals in the European Union, or that affect more than 5 in 10,000 individuals but the market is unlikely to generate sufficient return on the investment. EMA further requires that the product targets a condition for which there is either no treatment available, or the product provides a "significant benefit" over available treatments. This significant benefit may be related to either improvements in clinical outcomes or patient care (e.g., ease of use). FDA also has a program for Rare Pediatric Disease Designation (FDA, 2024t), while EMA does not have a designation specifically for rare pediatric conditions.

For the purposes of orphan designation, FDA and EMA define "condition" slightly differently. FDA requires that a product be targeted at a distinct condition, as determined by a variety of factors. A product targeted at a subset of a more common condition may be eligible if the drug itself has properties that make it inappropriate for patients with the more common version of the condition; for example, a drug that is only effective in patients with a specific biomarker may be eligible, whereas those without the biomarker or drug-target would not be expected to respond (for example, mutationally-defined cancers).[1] EMA also specifies that the targeted condition must be clearly distinct from other conditions, and notes that differences in severity or stages do not make a condition distinct (European Commission, 2014). A treatment targeted at a subtype of the condition may be eligible if the characteristics of the subtype make the treatment ineffective for patients with the more common version of the condition; biomarkers of a subtype are not currently accepted as evidence of a distinct condition (Thirstrup, 2023). For these reasons, it can be more difficult for a drug product to be granted and keep an orphan designation by EMA.

---

[1] 78 FR 35117.

As stated in Chapter 1, orphan designation in the United States qualifies sponsors for incentives (see Box 1-1). Similarly, in the European Union, sponsors may also receive incentives including (EMA, n.d.-m):

- Reduced fees for regulatory activities, which may include reduced fees for protocol assistance, marketing-authorisation applications, inspections before authorisation, applications for changes to marketing authorisations made after approval, and reduced annual fees; and
- Potential 10 years market exclusivity after approval.

EMA has not issued guidance on drug development for rare diseases and conditions. However, EMA has issued several disease-specific guidelines, many of which concern rare diseases, and held a workshop in 2015 on the demonstration of significant benefit of orphan medicines (EMA, 2016). In addition, there are EMA guidelines and reflection papers on a number of topics that are relevant to the collection of data on rare disease drug development. The details of these guidelines are discussed further in Chapter 4.

FDA Resources	EMA Resources

• Orphan Designation Resource Repository (FDA, 2024i)
   ○ Frequently Asked Questions (FDA, 2023k)
• Guidance Documents for Rare Disease Drug Development (FDA, 2024n)
• Rare Diseases: Considerations for the Development of Drugs and Biological Products—FINAL Guidance (FDA, 2023o)
	• Orphan Designation (EMA, n.d.-n)
	   ○ How to Apply (EMA, n.d.-c)
	   ○ Post Designation Procedural Advice (EMA, 2023c)
	   ○ Orphan Designation Fact Sheet (EMA, 2018)
	• Workshop Report: Demonstrating Significant Benefit of Orphan Medicines—Concepts, Methodology and Impact on Access (EMA, 2015)

INCENTIVES FOR ORPHAN DRUG DEVELOPMENT

Once designated as an orphan drug by FDA, sponsors receive the following incentives (Michaeli et al., 2023):

- Tax credits worth 25 percent of costs for qualified clinical trials;
- Waiver of the Prescription Drug User Fee ($4 million for FY 2024); and
- Potential 7 years of market exclusivity after approval.

In addition, the Orphan Drug Act established the Orphan Product Grants Program to provide funding for developing products for rare diseases or conditions. Products that receive EMA orphan designation can access a number of incentives (EMA, n.d.-m). First, sponsors can request protocol assistance from EMA at a reduced fee; this allows sponsors to get answers to questions about what types of studies are necessary to demonstrate the quality, benefits, risks, and significant benefit of the drug. Second, a product with orphan designation is mandated to use the centralized marketing approval process conducted by EMA. Third, products maintaining orphan designation at the time of approval receive 10 years of market exclusivity; this is extended to 12 years for products with an approved pediatric investigation plan. Fourth, sponsors applying for orphan designation pay reduced fees for regulatory activities, including marketing authorization application fees, inspections before authorization, and applications for post-approval changes. In addition, sponsors may be eligible for incentives available through individual EU member states. For companies classified as small and medium-sized enterprises (SMEs) that are developing a product with orphan designation, there may also be administrative and procedural assistance from EMA's SME office and fee reduction.

FDA Resources	EMA Resources
• Orphan Drug Designation Program (FDA, 2024i) • Orphan Products Grant Program (FDA, 2023m)	• Orphan Incentives (EMA, n.d.-m)

EVIDENTIARY STANDARDS

As discussed in Chapters 2 and 3, FDA and EMA each define standards of evidence in different ways. By statute, FDA approval of a drug product requires a demonstration of "substantial evidence of effectiveness," which has generally been interpreted as requiring at least two adequate and well-controlled studies (FDA, 2019b). However, amendments have clarified that substantial effectiveness may be demonstrated with one adequate and well-controlled study along with confirmatory evidence (FDA, 2023h). FDA and EMA approval processes require a risk-benefit assessment that requires consideration of many complex factors (e.g., therapeutic context, seriousness of condition). FDA has published a number of guidance documents that are relevant to rare disease drug development, including *Demonstrating Substantial Evidence of Effectiveness for Human Drug and Biological Products* (FDA, 2019b), *Rare Diseases: Considerations for the Development of Drugs and Biological Products* (FDA, 2023o), *Benefit–Risk Assessment for New Drug and Biological Products* (FDA, 2023a), *Demonstrating Substantial Evidence of Effectiveness with One Adequate and Well-Controlled Clinical Investigation and Confirmatory Evidence* (FDA, 2023h), and *Rare*

Diseases: Natural History Studies for Drug Development (FDA, 2019c). EMA has not issued general guidance on drug development for rare diseases and conditions, but there are a number of publications that apply to issues involved in rare disease drug development, including clinical trials in small populations, real-world evidence, registry-based studies, single arm trials, and use of one pivotal study in drug application.

FDA Resources	EMA Resources
• Providing Clinical Evidence of Effectiveness for Human Drug and Biological Products—FINAL Guidance (FDA, 1998) • Benefit–Risk Assessment for New Drug and Biological Products—FINAL Guidance (FDA, 2023a) • Demonstrating Substantial Evidence of Effectiveness for Human Drug and Biological Products—DRAFT Guidance (FDA, 2019b) • Rare Diseases: Considerations for the Development of Drugs and Biological Products—FINAL Guidance (FDA, 2023o) • Demonstrating Substantial Evidence of Effectiveness with One Adequate and Well-Controlled Clinical Investigation and Confirmatory Evidence—DRAFT Guidance (FDA, 2023h) • Rare Diseases: Natural History Studies for Drug Development—DRAFT Guidance (FDA, 2019c)	• ICH-E9 Statistical Principles for Clinical Trials—FINAL Guidance (ICH, 1998) • ICH-E8(R1) General Considerations for Clinical Studies—FINAL Guidance (ICH, 2021) • General Overview of Clinical Efficacy and Safety (EMA, n.d.-f) • Benefit-Risk Methodology Project (EMA, 2009) • Guideline on the Investigation of Subgroups in Confirmatory Clinical Trials—FINAL Guidance (EMA, 2019) • Data Quality Framework for EU Medicines Regulation—DRAFT Guidance (EMA, 2023a) • Single-arm Trials as Pivotal Evidence for the Authorisation of Medicines in the EU—Reflection Paper (EMA, 2023d) • Guideline on Clinical Trials in Small Populations (EMA, 2006) • Real-World Evidence Provided by EMA (EMA, 2024b) • Guideline on Registry-Based Studies (EMA, 2021a) • Application with 1. Meta-Analyses; 2. One Pivotal Study—Scientific Guideline (EMA, 2001)

EXPEDITED REGULATORY PATHWAYS

FDA and EMA both offer a number of expedited pathways that allow products to be approved on a shorter timeline and/or with preliminary or limited data.

Approval on a Shortened Review Timeline

FDA's breakthrough therapy designation and EMA's Priority Medicines (PRIME) scheme are similar programs; they are both designed to assist sponsors of products developed for conditions with an unmet need and offer the potential for shortened review. Breakthrough therapy designation is for products that are intended to treat a serious or life-threatening condition, and where preliminary clinical evidence indicates a substantial improvement on a clinically significant endpoint over available therapies (FDA, 2018c). For PRIME designation, an applicant must provide data that demonstrate a meaningful improvement of clinical outcomes (EMA, n.d.-q). Breakthrough therapy designation offers intensive guidance on drug development, meetings and communication with FDA staff, and the potential for accelerated approval or priority review. PRIME offers similar benefits including meetings with EMA experts, iterative and expedited scientific advice, and the potential for accelerated assessment.

FDA has one program that shortens review time, called Priority Review (FDA, 2018h). EMA also has one program, called Accelerated Assessment (EMA, n.d.-a). Priority Review is for products aimed at a serious condition that demonstrate a significant improvement in safety or effectiveness and offers review of the application in 6 months. EMA's Accelerated Assessment is for products that are of "major public health interest," particularly ones that involve innovations or improvements for unmet needs. The program reduces the timeframe for application assessment from 210 days to 150 days.

Approval Based on Preliminary Data

Both agencies have a mechanism that allows a product to be approved with preliminary data which is to be followed by confirmatory data after approval. FDA's Accelerated Approval pathway can be used when a product has a meaningful advantage over available therapies, and evidence demonstrates an effect on a surrogate or intermediate endpoint that is reasonably likely to predict clinical benefit (FDA, 2024b). This pathway allows for a shorter development timeline and requires sponsors to collect data after approval to confirm the clinical benefit. EMA's Conditional Marketing Authorization is used when there is an unmet need and the benefits of making the product available to the public outweigh the risks; sponsors are required to collect additional data after approval to confirm the benefit-risk analysis (EMA, n.d.-g).

Approval Based on Limited Data

Only EMA has a mechanism for approving a product for which comprehensive data on safety and efficacy are not available. Under the Exceptional Circumstances pathway, EMA may grant approval to a product if it is not possible to collect comprehensive data because of the current state of scientific knowledge, the condition is too rare, or it would be unethical (EMA, n.d.-k).

Both agencies have the legal authority to exercise a great degree of flexibility in the amount and type of data necessary for rare disease product approval.

FDA Programs	EMA Programs
Shorten Review Timelines • Breakthrough Therapy Designation (FDA, 2018c) • Fast Track (FDA, 2018f) • Priority Review (FDA, 2018h)	Shorten Review Timelines • Accelerated Assessment (EMA, n.d.-a) • Priority Medicines (PRIME) (EMA, n.d.-q)
Preliminary Approval Pending Additional Data • Accelerated Approval (FDA, 2024b)	Preliminary Approval Pending Additional Data • Conditional Marketing Authorization (EMA, n.d.-g)
Approval Based on Limited Data—N/A	**Approval Based on Limited Data** • Exceptional Circumstances (EMA, n.d.-k)

Other Programs
• Rare Pediatric Disease Priority Review Vouchers (FDA, 2019d)
• Project Orbis (FDA, 2024r)
	Other Programs
	• Innovation in medicines (EMA, n.d.-u)
	   ○ Innovation Task Force (EMA, 2014)
	   ○ EU Innovation Network (EMA, n.d.-i)
	• Rolling Review (EMA, 2020)

RARE DISEASE PROGRAMS

FDA has several programs dedicated to rare diseases, several of which are in pilot form:

- Accelerating Rare disease Cures (ARC) program: CDER launched the ARC Program in 2022; its mission is "to drive scientific and regulatory innovation and engagement to accelerate the availability of treatments for patients with rare diseases" (FDA, 2024c)
- Learning and Education to Advance and Empower Rare Disease Drug Developers (LEADER 3D): ARC launched the LEADER 3D initiative in 2023. Through LEADER 3D, FDA seeks input from stakeholders who design and conduct rare disease drug development programs in order to identify gaps in knowledge about the regulatory process (FDA, 2024o).

- Rare Disease Endpoint Advancement (RDEA) pilot program: The RDEA pilot program is a joint CDER and CBER program that seeks to advance rare disease drug development by providing a mechanism for sponsors to collaborate with FDA throughout the efficacy endpoint development process (FDA, 2024s).
- Support for clinical Trials Advancing Rare disease Therapeutics (START) pilot program: START is a joint CBER and CDER pilot program that was launched in late 2023. It augments currently available formal meetings by addressing issues through more rapid, ad hoc communication mechanisms (FDA, 2023q; Lee et al., 2023).
- The Rare Disease Cures Accelerator-Data and Analytics Platform (RDCA-DAP®): RDCA-DAP®, funded by FDA and operated by the Critical Path Institute in collaboration with the National Organization for Rare Disorders, is a centralized database and analytics hub that contains standardized data on a growing number of rare diseases and allows secure sharing of data collected across multiple sources, including natural history studies/patient registries, control arms of clinical trials, longitudinal observational studies, and real-world data. Since RDCA-DAP® was launched in 2021, the platform has enabled access to data from over 30 rare disease areas with more data being added over time (Critical Path Institute, n.d.-b).

EMA does not currently have programs specific to rare disease drug development. However, one of EMA's stated goals is to encourage and facilitate the use of innovative methods in the development of medicines (EMA, n.d.-m). To this end, EMA has several initiatives that support the development of innovative methods by fostering collaboration with academia and across the regulatory network. In addition to PRIME (described above), two of these initiatives are particularly relevant to rare diseases: the Innovation Task Force (ITF) and the EU Innovation Network (EU-IN).

There are two rare disease programs funded by the European Commission:

- **The European Partnership on Rare Diseases** is an implementation tool of Horizon Europe, a broad research and innovation funding scheme by the European Commission. The Rare Disease Partnership seeks to advance innovation for rare diseases by coordinating local, national, and regional research activities. It will succeed the European Joint Programme on Rare Diseases (European Comission, 2022).
- **The European Joint Programme on Rare Diseases (EJP RD)** facilitates rare disease research collaboration across the EU member

states as well as associated states and the UK & Canada (European Joint Programme on Rare Diseases, n.d.).

U.S. Programs	EU Programs
• Learning and Education to Advance and Empower Rare Disease Drug Developers (LEADER 3D) (FDA, 2024o) **Critical Path Institute Programs** • Rare Disease Cures Accelerator-Data and Analytics Platform (RDCA-DAP) (Critical Path Institute, n.d.-b) • Rare Disease Clinical Outcome Assessment Consortium (RD-COA) (Critical Path Institute, n.d.-a)	• European Partnership on Rare Diseases (European Comission, 2022) • European Joint Programme on Rare Diseases (EJP RD) (European Joint Programme on Rare Diseases, n.d.) • Support to SMEs (EMA, n.d.-t)

SPONSOR ENGAGEMENT

Sponsors developing new drugs must navigate a range of complex challenges when designing and conducting a study for regulatory submission. Clinical trials for regulatory submission require a combination of clinical, safety, biostatistical, and regulatory expertise, as well an understanding of the patient populations a drug is intended to treat to maximize the likelihood that study results meet regulatory requirements to gain market approval. These challenges are heightened when it comes to rare diseases and conditions. Additionally, many companies developing rare disease drugs are small and medium-sized enterprises, which may have fewer resources and less in-house expertise than large pharmaceutical companies. For these reasons, it is critically important for sponsors developing rare disease drug products to engage with the agency early and often.

Both agencies offer sponsors the opportunity to engage throughout the development and approval process. Sponsors may request a meeting with FDA at any time during drug development. In general, communication with the agency is through the regulatory project manager and sponsors are discouraged from contacting reviewers directly (FDA, 2017). Sponsors may solicit advice on a variety of topics and may also request a formal meeting at critical junctures of development. EMA offers preparatory meetings for sponsors early in the development process in order to avoid major issues, and sponsors are encouraged to reach out at any time for feedback. Scientific advice is available from EMA for a fee; the fee can be waived for orphan medicines, smaller sponsors, and in the case of public emergencies (EMA, n.d.-s).

FDA Resources	EMA Resources
• Formal Meetings Between FDA and Sponsors or Applicants—FINAL Guidance (FDA, 2009) • Early Drug Development and the Role of Pre-IND Meetings—DRAFT Guidance (FDA, 2018i) • Formal Meetings Between FDA and Sponsors or Applicants of PDUFA Products—DRAFT Guidance (FDA, 2023j) • CDER's Small Business and Industry Assistance (SBIA)—FDA's SBIA office guides small pharmaceutical businesses navigate FDA's resources and assists them in understanding human drug product regulation (FDA, 2022a)	• Scientific Advice and Protocol Assistance (EMA, n.d.-s) ○ Frequently Asked Questions (EMA, 2022d) • Framework of Collaboration with Academia (EMA, 2017a) • Support to SMEs (EMA, n.d.-t)

PATIENT ENGAGEMENT

FDA and EMA both have several mechanisms for engaging with patients, caregivers, and patient groups. FDA uses the Patient-Focused Drug Development (PFDD) program as a systematic approach for incorporating patient perspectives into drug development (FDA, 2024f), while EMA utilizes the Patients' and Consumers' Working Party (PCWP) to provide a platform for the exchange of information between the agency and patients (EMA, n.d.-p). Individual patients can serve on FDA advisory committees and provide advice to FDA through the Patient Representative Program (FDA, 2024a), while at EMA patients and organizations can apply to be part of a database of patients that can be called on by EMA during the drug evaluation process (EMA, 2022c). Although there are differences in how each agency engages with patients there is no evidence that one agency's methods are superior.

    • **Methodological Guidance Series**: A series of guidance that is intended to promote the use of systematic approaches for incorporating patient and caregiver input in medical product development and regulatory decision-making (FDA, 2024k).

    • **Clinical Outcome Assessments (COA) and their Related Endpoints Pilot Grant Program**: A pilot grant program to support the development of publicly available COAs and their related endpoints. In 2021, a grant was awarded for a project developing an observer measure of communications abilities of individuals with rare, neurodevelopmental disorders (FDA, 2024g).

FDA's PFDD initiative, which was established under the fifth authorization of the Prescription Drug User Fee Act (PDUFA), is a systematic approach to help ensure that patients' experiences, perspectives, needs, and priorities are meaningfully incorporated into drug development and evaluation" (FDA, 2024f). Patient listening sessions, similar to PFDD meetings, serve to inform FDA on the concerns of the patient community. However, patient listening sessions are nonpublic and only FDA, patients, caregivers, advocates, and community representatives can participate in the session, and they are non-interactive, in that the agency participants are listening but not conversing with other participants (FDA, 2024l).

Organizations, patients, and caregivers interact with EMA in a variety of ways all along the regulatory pathway (EMA, n.d.-l), a practice that is underpinned by EMA's broader engagement framework to engage patients and consumers throughout a medical product's lifecycle (EMA, 2022c). Depending on the activity, patients may interact as representatives of their community, representing an organization, or as individual experts. Specific opportunities for engagement include serving on EMA's Management Board and scientific committees, attending consultations and workshops, assisting with providing advice on science and protocols, and involvement in the PCWP (EMA, n.d.-l).

EMA also has several avenues to promote patient engagement, including public hearings, participation on review, scientific advice, and other consultative committees, and involvement in preparing guidelines.

FDA Resources	EMA Resources
• Collecting Comprehensive and Representative Input—FINAL Guidance (FDA, 2020c) • Methods to Identify What Is Important to Patients—FINAL Guidance (FDA, 2022f) • Selecting, Developing, or Modifying Fit-for-Purpose Clinical Outcome Assessments—DRAFT Guidance (FDA, 2022g) • Incorporating Clinical Outcome Assessments Into Endpoints for Regulatory Decision-Making—DRAFT Guidance (FDA, 2023n)	• Engagement Framework: EMA and Patients, Consumers and their Organisations (EMA, 2022c) • Presentation: Patient engagement at EMA (Bere and Garcia, 2020) ◦ Getting Involved (EMA, n.d.-l)

FDA Programs	EMA Programs

• Patient-Focused Drug Development
  ○ FDA-led PFDD Meetings (FDA, 2024j)
  ○ Externally-led PFDD Meetings (FDA, 2022b)
• Patient Listening Sessions
  ○ FDA-led Listening Sessions (FDA, 2024m)
  ○ Patient-led Listening Sessions (FDA, 2024q)
	• Patients' and Consumers' Working Party (PCWP) (EMA, n.d.-p)

INCLUSION OF PEDIATRIC POPULATIONS

In 2012, the Food and Drug Administration Safety and Innovation Act added a provision to section 505B of the FD&C Act,[2] often referred to by the acronym of the legislation that created section 505B, the Pediatric Research Equity Act (PREA), that requires sponsors to submit an initial pediatric study plan (iPSP) "before the date on which the sponsor submits the required assessments or investigation and no later than either 60 days after the date of the end-of-Phase 2 meeting or such other time as agreed upon between FDA and the sponsor" (FDA, 2020d). The iPSP must include the following: (1) "an outline of the pediatric study or studies that the sponsor plans to conduct (including, to the extent practicable, study objectives and design, age groups, relevant endpoints, and statistical approach); (2) "any request for a deferral or waiver . . . if applicable, along with any supporting information; and (3) "other information specified in the regulations promulgated under paragraph (7)."[3]

A sponsor should not submit a marketing application or supplement until FDA confirms agreement on the iPSP, and the total review period for iPSPs should not exceed 210 days. PREA provides an exemption from iPSP requirements for applications for drugs that have orphan designation.[4] In 2017, PREA was amended by the FDA Reauthorization Act of 2017,[5] by including the RACE for Children Act[6] to lift the orphan exemption for rare pediatric cancers, requiring sponsors to submit iPSPs for these indications. This amendment has required that sponsors submit a planned approach for studying drugs in pediatric populations if they intend to apply for approval of adult cancer drugs (GAO, 2023).

---

[2] Public Law 112-144, 126 Stat. 993 (July 9, 2012).
[3] 21 U.S.C. § 355c(e)(2)(B).
[4] 21 U.S.C. § 355c(k)(1).
[5] P. L. 115-52, § 504. FDA Reauthorization Act of 2017 (August 18, 2017).
[6] H.R.1231—RACE for Children Act—115th Congress (2017–2018).

In EMA, the paediatric investigation plan (PIP) serves to ensure all needed data to support a marketing authorization for children are collected. PIPs are required to be submitted when the Phase 2 dose is selected at the end of Phase 1 (Ungstrup and Vanags, 2023). All medicines seeking marketing authorization have to include a PIP unless the treatment is exempt due to referral or waiver (EMA, n.d.-e). Typically, waivers are provided to treatments that are likely to be ineffective or unsafe in children, intended for adult-only conditions, or unlikely to provide significant benefit over current treatment available to children (EMA, n.d.-e). The PIP is reviewed and agreed upon by the drug sponsor and EMA's Paediatric Committee (EMA, n.d.-o). In early 2023, EMA launched a stepwise PIP pilot program which is designed to allow greater flexibility for sponsors that are developing innovative treatments (EMA, 2023b). The stepwise PIP will allow sponsors to continue with development with a partial PIP in place rather than waiting for more data to support a full PIP (Al-Faruque, 2023). Sponsors indicated that the PIP can be restrictive to drug development and expect the stepwise program to ease some of the issues.

FDA has a program for Rare Pediatric Disease Designation, while EMA does not have a designation specifically for rare pediatric conditions.

FDA Resources	EMA Resources
• Pediatric Study Plans: Content of and Process for Submitting Initial Pediatric Study Plans and Amended Initial Pediatric Study Plans—FINAL Guidance (FDA, 2020d) • General Clinical Pharmacology Considerations for Pediatric Studies of Drugs, Including Biological Products—DRAFT Guidance (FDA, 2022c)	• Guideline on Pharmaceutical Development of Medicines for Paediatric Use—FINAL Guidance (EMA, 2013) • Paediatric Investigation Plans (EMA, n.d.-o) ◦ Class Waivers (EMA, n.d.-d) • Guidance for Stepwise PIP Pilot—FINAL Guidance (EMA, 2023b)

INNOVATIVE CLINICAL TRIAL DESIGN

Due to the complex biology underpinning rare diseases and conditions, low disease prevalence, and patient heterogeneity, it is often challenging to design traditional randomized controlled trials (RCTs) for studying drugs that treat rare diseases or conditions. As such, clinical trials for rare diseases and conditions are often smaller than for other more prevalent conditions and may require the use of novel design elements to meet evidentiary standards.

In general, both agencies have demonstrated an openness to the use of alternative and confirmatory data (e.g., natural history studies), as well as novel approaches for data analysis (e.g., Bayesian statistical methods).

To assist sponsors, FDA's Complex Innovative Trial Design Meeting program (also referred to as the Complex Innovative Trial Paired Meeting Program) offers sponsors up to two meetings with FDA to discuss their proposed complex innovative design elements during late-stage clinical development (FDA, 2023c). In guidance, FDA explains that there is no fixed definition of a complex innovative design because what is considered innovative may change over time, and that the determination of whether a specific novel design is appropriate for regulatory use is made on a case-by-case basis (FDA, 2020b). The guidance provides examples of innovative design approaches (e.g., adaptive designs, Bayesian inference), and gives sponsors suggestions on common elements that should be included in a proposal for this program (FDA, 2020b). EMA, in collaboration with the European Commission and member state heads of medicines agencies, launched the Accelerating Clinical Trials in the EU (ACT EU) program to improve regional clinical trials infrastructure in the European Union through several action areas (EMA, n.d.-b). Those most relevant to rare diseases are: (1) Implementation of the Clinical Trial Regulation, (2) Clinical Trial Methodologies, (3) Scientific Advice, and (4) Clinical Trials Training Curriculum.

FDA Resources	EMA Resources
Trial Design	**Trial Design**
• Adaptive Designs for Clinical Trials of Drugs and Biologics—FINAL Guidance (FDA, 2019a) • Master Protocols: Efficient Clinical Trial Design Strategies to Expedite Development of Oncology Drugs and Biologics—FINAL Guidance (FDA, 2022d) • Clinical Pharmacology Considerations for the Development of Oligonucleotide Therapeutics—FINAL Guidance (FDA, 2024h)	• Complex Clinical Trials—Questions and Answers (EMA, 2022a) • IHC-E20 Adaptive Clinical Trials—FINAL Guidance (ICH, 2019) • Concept Paper on Platform Trials (EMA, 2022b)
Decentralized Trials	**Decentralized Trials**
• E17 General Principles for Planning and Design of Multiregional Clinical Trials—FINAL Guidance (FDA, 2018e) • Decentralized Clinical Trials for Drugs, Biological Products, and Devices—DRAFT Guidance (FDA, 2023g)	• IHC-E17 General Principles for Planning and Design of Multi-regional Clinical Trials—FINAL Guidance (EMA, 2017b)

FDA Programs	EMA Programs
• Complex Innovative Trial Design Paired Meeting Program (FDA, 2023c) ○ Interacting with FDA on Complex Innovative Trial Designs for Drugs and Biological Products—FINAL Guidance (FDA, 2020b) • Model-Informed Drug Development Paired Meeting Program (FDA, 2024p) • Support for clinical Trials Advancing Rare disease Therapeutics (START) Pilot Program (FDA, 2024u)	• Accelerating Clinical Trials in the EU (ACT EU) (EMA, n.d.-b) • The EU Decentralised Clinical Trials (EU DCT) Project (European Union, 2022)

ENDPOINT SELECTION AND BIOMARKER DEVELOPMENT

Attributable to the small number of patients with rare diseases, an inherent challenge is accruing study sample sizes large enough to adequately power all endpoints. This commonly translates to disproportionate focus on the primary endpoint and concomitant emphasis on the population most relevant for that endpoint. Criteria that focus on power to detect a difference for the study primary endpoint may obfuscate statistical efficacy measurement on important secondary endpoints. Conversely, study eligibility criteria attempting to enroll patients for all endpoints often slows accrual. For these reasons, endpoint selection and utilization of biomarkers are particularly crucial in rare disease treatment development where small sample sizes impact statistical power for efficacy and safety determinations.

FDA guidance acknowledges that, given limited sample size, flexibility may be needed in qualifying biomarkers (FDA, 2018a) and that such strategies as exit interviews or surveys may be needed for COAs (FDA, 2023n) to add greater depth to data for rare diseases (FDA, 2022f). EMA's 2006 *Guideline on Clinical Trials in Small Populations* has several pertinent statements related to the choice of endpoints that indicate regulatory flexibility (EMA, 2006):

- Recognition that there may be too few patients to validate endpoints and test treatments.
- Adequate follow-up in time to progression or time to remission can be obtained in open-label extension studies.
- Given that the mode of action of the treatment may not be sufficiently well known, EMA states that "the usual approach of pre-specifying the primary endpoint may be too conservative, and more knowledge may be gained from collecting all sensible/possible endpoints and then presenting all the data in the final study report. Still, every effort should be made to identify an appropriate

hierarchy in the endpoints. If, collectively, the data look compelling, then a Marketing Authorisation may be grantable" (EMA, 2006).

FDA Resources	EMA Resources
Endpoint Selection	**Endpoint Selection**
• Clinical Trial Endpoints for the Approval of Cancer Drugs and Biologics—FINAL Guidance (FDA, 2018d) • Multiple Endpoints in Clinical Trials—FINAL Guidance (FDA, 2022e)	• ICH-E9 Statistical Principles for Clinical Trials—FINAL Guidance (ICH, 1998)
Biomarker Development and Qualification	**Biomarker Development and Qualification**
• Biomarker Qualification: Evidentiary Framework—DRAFT Guidance (FDA, 2018b) • E16 Biomarkers Related to Drug or Biotechnology Product Development: Context, Structure, and Format of Qualification Submissions—FINAL Guidance (FDA, 2011)	• ICH-M10 Bioanalytical Method Validation and Study Sample Analysis—FINAL Guidance (EMA, 2022f) • ICH-E16 Genomic Biomarkers Related to Drug Response: Context, Structure and Format of Qualification Submissions—FINAL Guidance (EMA, 2010)
Other	
• Qualification Process for Drug Development Tools—FINAL Guidance (FDA, 2020e)	
FDA Programs	**EMA Programs**
• Biomarker Qualification Program (FDA, 2024e) • Clinical Outcome Assessment (COA) Qualification Program (FDA, 2023b) • Rare Disease Endpoint Advancement (RDEA) Pilot Program (FDA, 2024s)	• Qualification of Novel Methodologies for Medicine Development—This provides the Committee for Medicinal Products for Human Use (CHMP) a procedure to issue an opinion on acceptable use of a method, including novel biomarkers (EMA, n.d.-r)

STATISTICAL ANALYSIS AND USE OF REAL-WORLD DATA

Beyond the choice in study design, researchers must consider the analytical challenges that arise when sample sizes are small and data are limited. It is often more difficult to achieve the statistical power necessary to demonstrate substantial evidence of effectiveness for a drug to treat a rare vs a common disease or condition. Innovative statistical methods (e.g. Bayesian analysis, extrapolation of adult data for pediatric uses, and network meta-analysis) and the use of real-world sources of data (e.g. expanded access programs, open label extension studies, natural history data, and patient registries) are additional tools that can be applied for studying rare disease drug products.

Bayesian statistics enable the incorporation of prior and external information, which may be a useful approach for the study of drugs to treat rare diseases or conditions. For example, a Bayesian approach could apply information from a study of a drug in adult populations towards understanding the effect of the same drug in children. Though FDA does not have guidance solely focused on the use of Bayesian methods in drug trials, it does cover this topic in guidance for adaptive trial designs and dedicates it as a focal point in the Complex Innovative Trial Design Paired Meeting Program (FDA, 2023r). Furthermore, it is documenting instances in which Bayesian methods have been used within CBER and CDER, with the aim of issuing draft guidance on applying them in drug trials by the end of the fiscal year 2025 (Ionan et al., 2023). EMA briefly covers Bayesian methods in guidance on clinical trials in small populations (EMA, 2006) and more thoroughly in a 2022 Q&A on complex clinical trials (EMA, 2022a).

External sources of data can help supplement RCT data for rare disease drug development and strengthen the evidence base for regulatory decision-making. FDA has issued several guidance, such as draft guidance on the design and conduct of externally controlled trials (FDA, 2023d), as well as draft guidance on the utilization of natural history studies (FDA, 2019c) and patient registries (FDA, 2023p). EMA has issued guidance on choice of control groups (ICH, 2001), including external control groups, and registry-based studies (EMA, 2021a). Additionally, EMA has outlined the role of real-world evidence in regulatory decision-making (Flynn et al., 2022).

FDA Resources	EMA Resources
Innovative Statistical Techniques • Meta-Analyses of Randomized Controlled Clinical Trials to Evaluate the Safety of Human Drugs or Biological Products—DRAFT Guidance (FDA, 2018g) • Use of Bayesian Statistics in Medical Device Clinical Trials—DRAFT Guidance (FDA, 2010) • Documentation on the use of Bayesian methods for drugs and biologics (Ionan et al., 2023) **External Sources of Data** • Rare Diseases: Natural History Studies for Drug Development—DRAFT Guidance (FDA, 2019c) • Real World Data: Assessing Registries to Support Regulatory Decision-Making for Drug and Biological Products—FINAL Guidance (FDA, 2023p) • Considerations for the Use of Real-World Data and Real-World Evidence to Support Regulatory Decision-Making for Drug and Biological Products—FINAL Guidance (FDA, 2023e) • Data Standards for Drug and Biological Product Submissions Containing Real-World Data—FINAL Guidance (FDA, 2023f) • Considerations for the Design and Conduct of Externally Controlled Trials for Drug and Biological Products—DRAFT Guidance (FDA, 2023d)	**Innovative Statistical Techniques** • Points to Consider on Applications with 1. Meta-Analyses; 2. One Pivotal Study—FINAL Guidance (EMA, 2001) • Bayesian methods o Guideline on Clinical Trials in Small Populations—FINAL Guidance (EMA, 2006) • Complex Clinical Trials—Questions and Answers (EMA, 2022a) **External Sources of Data** • ICH-E10 Choice of Control Group in Clinical Trials—FINAL Guidance (ICH, 2001) • Guideline on Registry-Based Studies—FINAL Guidance (EMA, 2021a) • A Vision for Use of Real-World Evidence in EU Medicines Regulation (EMA, 2021b) • Good Practice Guide for the Use of Metadata Catalogue of Real-World Data Sources (EMA, 2022e) • Contribution of RWE to Marketing Authorization (Flynn et al., 2022)
FDA Programs	**EMA Programs**
• CURE ID—A program designed to use clinician-reported data to support drug repurposing (FDA, 2020a) • Advancing Real-World Evidence Program (FDA, 2024d)	• Data Analysis and Real World Interrogation Network (DARWIN EU)—A coordination center that provides "timely and reliable evidence on the use, safety, and effectiveness" of drugs from health care databases across the EU. Data supports regulatory decision-making by expanding sources of observational data, providing a source of validated real world data, and addressing specific questions via non-interventional studies (EMA, n.d.-h)

FDA AND EMA COLLABORATIVE EFFORTS

Despite some key differences, FDA and EMA have similar approaches to the evaluation and approval of drugs for rare diseases. Given this overlap, there are many existing mechanisms for close collaboration between the two agencies, as well as opportunities for enhanced collaboration in the future. Since the signing of a confidentiality agreement in 2003, which permits the agencies to share nonpublic information, including confidential commercial information, FDA and EMA have created multiple formalized mechanisms to facilitate communication and collaboration. These collaborations cover a wide range of topics and activities, including scientific advice, orphan designations, marketing authorizations, post-authorization requirements, inspections, pharmacovigilance, guidance documents, and other topics (EMA, 2024c) (see Figure 5-7).

One of the primary formal mechanisms for collaboration between EMA and FDA are so-called "clusters"—regular virtual meetings between EMA and FDA staff, which are focused on specific topics and therapeutic areas that would benefit from an "intensified exchange of information and collaboration" (EMA, 2024a). Documents exchanged within clusters may include draft guidances/guidelines; assessment reports; review memos; and meeting minutes. The agencies typically set the agenda for what is discussed at a cluster meeting. However, sponsors also have the option of asking that a drug program or topic be discussed. Topics discussed within clusters range from emerging scientific and ethical issues to challenges in product development to issues with the review of marketing authorization applications.

Established in 2005, the Parallel Scientific Advice (PSA) program is a voluntary mechanism through which FDA and EMA can concurrently provide scientific advice to sponsors during the development of new drugs, biological products, vaccines, or advanced therapies (EMA and FDA, 2021). The goals of the PSA program are to: (1) increase dialogue early on in the product lifecycle, (2) deepen understanding of regulatory decisions, (3) optimize product development, and (4) avoid unnecessary or duplicative testing (Thor et al., 2023). The program does not guarantee EMA and FDA alignment, but can offer a number of potential benefits for sponsors, including agency convergence on approaches to development, a better understanding of each agency's concerns and requirements, and opportunity for sponsors and agencies to ask and answer questions (Thor et al., 2023).

FDA Programs	EMA Programs
• International Agreements and Information Sharing (FDA, 2023l) • FDA–EMA Parallel Scientific Advice (PSA) Program (FDA, 2023i)	• International Agreements: United States Cluster Activities (EMA, 2024a)

REFERENCES

Al-Faruque, F. 2023. *EMA launches stepwise 'PIP' pilot*. https://www.raps.org/news-and-articles/news-articles/2023/2/ema-launches-stepwise-pip-pilot (accessed March 12, 2024).

Bere, N., and J. Garcia. 2020. *Patient engagement at EMA*. https://www.ema.europa.eu/en/documents/presentation/presentation-patient-engagement-ema-progressing-concept-patient-centered-development-practice-nbere-jgarcia-ema_en.pdf (accessed August 1, 2024).

Critical Path Institute. n.d.-a. *Rare Disease Clinical Outcome Assessment consortium*. https://c-path.org/program/rare-disease-clinical-outcome-assessment-consortium/ (accessed August 6, 2024).

Critical Path Institute. n.d.-b. *Rare Disease Cures Accelerator-Data and Analytics Platform*. https://c-path.org/program/rare-disease-cures-accelerators-data-and-analytics-platform/ (accessed March 7, 2024).

EMA (European Medicines Agency). 2001. *Points to consider on application with 1. Meta-analyses; 2. One pivotal study*. https://www.ema.europa.eu/en/documents/scientific-guideline/points-consider-application-1meta-analyses-2one-pivotal-study_en.pdf (accessed August 1, 2024).

EMA. 2006. *Guideline on clinical trials in small populations*. https://www.ema.europa.eu/en/documents/scientific-guideline/guideline-clinical-trials-small-populations_en.pdf (accessed August 1, 2024).

EMA. 2009. *Benefit-risk methodology project*. https://www.ema.europa.eu/en/documents/report/benefit-risk-methodology-project_en.pdf (accessed August 1, 2024).

EMA. 2010. *ICH guideline E16 on genomic biomarkers related to drug response: Context, structure and format of qualification submissions*. https://www.ema.europa.eu/en/documents/scientific-guideline/ich-guideline-e16-genomic-biomarkers-related-drug-response-context-structure-and-format-qualification-submissions-step-5_en.pdf (accessed August 1, 2024).

EMA. 2013. *Guideline on pharmaceutical development of medicines for paediatric use*. https://www.ema.europa.eu/en/documents/scientific-guideline/guideline-pharmaceutical-development-medicines-paediatric-use_en.pdf (accessed August 1, 2024).

EMA. 2014. *Mandate of the EMA Innovation Task Force (ITF)*. https://www.ema.europa.eu/en/documents/other/mandate-european-medicines-agency-innovation-task-force-itf_en.pdf (accessed August 1, 2024).

EMA. 2015. *Workshop on demonstrating significant benefit of orphan medicines: Concepts, methodology, and impact on access*. https://www.ema.europa.eu/en/events/workshop-demonstrating-significant-benefit-orphan-medicines-concepts-methodology-impact-access (accessed August 6, 2024).

EMA. 2016. *Demonstrating significant benefit of orphan medicines: Concepts, methodology and impact on access: Workshop report*. https://www.ema.europa.eu/en/documents/report/workshop-report-demonstrating-significant-benefit-orphan-medicines-concepts-methodology-and-impact-access_en.pdf (accessed August 1, 2024).

EMA. 2017a. *Framework of collaboration between the European Medicines Agency and academia*. https://www.ema.europa.eu/en/documents/regulatory-procedural-guideline/framework-collaboration-between-european-medicines-agency-and-academia_en.pdf (accessed August 1, 2024).

EMA. 2017b. *ICH guideline E17 on general principles for planning and design of multi-regional clinical trials*. https://www.ema.europa.eu/en/documents/scientific-guideline/ich-guideline-e17-general-principles-planning-and-design-multi-regional-clinical-trials-step-5-first-version_en.pdf (accessed August 1, 2024).

EMA. 2018. *Rare diseases, orphan medicines: Getting the facts straight*. https://www.ema.europa.eu/en/documents/other/rare-diseases-orphan-medicines-getting-facts-straight_en.pdf (accessed August 1, 2024).

EMA. 2019. *Guideline on the investigation of subgroups in confirmatory clinical trials.* https://www.ema.europa.eu/en/documents/scientific-guideline/guideline-investigation-subgroups-confirmatory-clinical-trials_en.pdf (accessed August 1, 2024).

EMA. 2020. *EMA starts first rolling review of a COVID-19 vaccine in the EU.* https://www.ema.europa.eu/en/news/ema-starts-first-rolling-review-covid-19-vaccine-eu (accessed August 15, 2024).

EMA. 2021a. *Guideline on registry-based studies.* https://www.ema.europa.eu/en/documents/scientific-guideline/guideline-registry-based-studies_en.pdf-0 (accessed August 1, 2024).

EMA. 2021b. *A vision for use of real-world evidence in EU medicines regulation.* https://www.ema.europa.eu/en/news/vision-use-real-world-evidence-eu-medicines-regulation (accessed August 15, 2024).

EMA. 2022a. *Complex clinical trials—Questions and answers.* https://health.ec.europa.eu/system/files/2022-06/medicinal_qa_complex_clinical-trials_en.pdf (accessed August 1, 2024).

EMA. 2022b. *Concept paper on platform trials.* https://www.ema.europa.eu/en/documents/scientific-guideline/concept-paper-platform-trials_en.pdf (accessed August 1, 2024).

EMA. 2022c. *Engagement framework: EMA and patients, consumers and their organizations.* https://www.ema.europa.eu/system/files/documents/other/updated_engagement_framework_-_ema_and_patients_consumers_and_their_organisations_2022-en.pdf (accessed August 1, 2024).

EMA. 2022d. *European Medicines Agency guidance for applicants seeking scientific advice and protocol assistance.* https://www.ema.europa.eu/en/documents/regulatory-procedural-guideline/european-medicines-agency-guidance-applicants-seeking-scientific-advice-and-protocol-assistance_en.pdf

EMA. 2022e. *Good practice guide for the use of the metadata catalogue of real-world data sources.* https://www.ema.europa.eu/en/documents/regulatory-procedural-guideline/good-practice-guide-use-metadata-catalogue-real-world-data-sources_en.pdf (accessed August 1, 2024).

EMA. 2022f. *ICH guideline M10 on bioanalytical method validation and study sample analysis.* https://www.ema.europa.eu/en/documents/scientific-guideline/ich-guideline-m10-bioanalytical-method-validation-step-5_en.pdf (accessed August 1, 2024).

EMA. 2023a. *Data quality framework for EU medicines regulation.* https://www.ema.europa.eu/en/documents/regulatory-procedural-guideline/data-quality-framework-eu-medicines-regulation_en.pdf (accessed August 1, 2024).

EMA. 2023b. *Guidance for stepwise PIP pilot.* https://www.ema.europa.eu/en/documents/regulatory-procedural-guideline/guidance-stepwise-pip-pilot_en.pdf (accessed August 1, 2024).

EMA. 2023c. *Procedural advice for post-orphan medicinal product designation activities.* https://www.ema.europa.eu/en/documents/other/procedural-advice-post-orphan-medicinal-product-designation-activities-guidance-sponsors_en.pdf (accessed August 1, 2024).

EMA. 2023d. *Reflection paper on establishing efficacy based on single arm trials submitted as pivotal evidence in a marketing authorisation.* https://www.ema.europa.eu/en/documents/scientific-guideline/reflection-paper-establishing-efficacy-based-single-arm-trials-submitted-pivotal-evidence-marketing-authorisation_en.pdf (accessed August 1, 2024).

EMA. 2024a. *Cluster activities.* https://www.ema.europa.eu/en/partners-networks/international-activities/cluster-activities (accessed August 15, 2024).

EMA. 2024b. *Real-world evidence provided by EMA.* https://www.ema.europa.eu/en/documents/other/guidance-real-world-evidence-provided-ema-support-regulatory-decision-making_en.pdf (accessed August 1, 2024).

EMA. 2024c. *United States.* https://www.ema.europa.eu/en/partners-networks/international-activities/bilateral-interactions-non-eu-regulators/united-states (accessed August 15, 2024).

EMA. n.d.-a. *Accelerated assessment.* https://www.ema.europa.eu/en/human-regulatory-overview/marketing-authorisation/accelerated-assessment (accessed August 15, 2024).

EMA. n.d.-b. *Accelerating Clinical Trials in the EU (ACT EU).* https://www.ema.europa.eu/en/human-regulatory-overview/research-development/clinical-trials-human-medicines/accelerating-clinical-trials-eu-act-eu (accessed August 1, 2024).

EMA. n.d.-c. *Applying for orphan designation.* https://www.ema.europa.eu/en/human-regulatory-overview/research-development/orphan-designation-research-development/applying-orphan-designation (accessed February 20, 2024).

EMA. n.d.-d. *Class waivers.* https://www.ema.europa.eu/en/human-regulatory-overview/research-development/paediatric-medicines-research-development/paediatric-investigation-plans/class-waivers (accessed August 6, 2024).

EMA. n.d.-e. *Class waivers.* https://www.ema.europa.eu/en/human-regulatory-overview/research-and-development/paediatric-medicines-research-and-development/paediatric-investigation-plans/class-waivers (accessed August 15, 2024).

EMA. n.d.-f. *Clinical efficacy and safety: General.* https://www.ema.europa.eu/en/human-regulatory-overview/research-and-development/scientific-guidelines/clinical-efficacy-safety-guidelines/clinical-efficacy-safety-general (accessed August 6, 2024).

EMA. n.d.-g. *Conditional marketing authorization.* https://www.ema.europa.eu/en/human-regulatory-overview/marketing-authorisation/conditional-marketing-authorisation (accessed February 20, 2024).

EMA. n.d.-h. *Data Analysis and Real World Interrogation Network (DARWIN EU).* https://www.ema.europa.eu/en/about-us/how-we-work/big-data/real-world-evidence/data-analysis-real-world-interrogation-network-darwin-eu (accessed August 6, 2024).

EMA. n.d.-i. *EU Innovation Network (EU-IN).* https://www.ema.europa.eu/en/committees/working-parties-other-groups/eu-innovation-network-eu (accessed July 10, 2024).

EMA. n.d.-j. *European Medicines Agency (EMA).* https://european-union.europa.eu/institutions-law-budget/institutions-and-bodies/search-all-eu-institutions-and-bodies/european-medicines-agency-ema_en#:~:text=The%20European%20Medicines%20Agency%20(EMA,European%20Economic%20Area%20(EEA (accessed August 15, 2024).

EMA. n.d.-k. *Exceptional circumstances.* https://www.ema.europa.eu/en/glossary/exceptional-circumstances (accessed March 10, 2024).

EMA. n.d.-l. *Getting involved.* https://www.ema.europa.eu/en/partners-networks/patients-and-consumers/getting-involved (accessed March 15, 2024).

EMA. n.d.-m. *Oprhan incentives.* https://www.ema.europa.eu/en/human-regulatory-overview/research-and-development/orphan-designation-research-and-development/orphan-incentives (accessed February 19, 2024).

EMA. n.d.-n. *Orphan designation: Overview.* https://www.ema.europa.eu/en/human-regulatory-overview/orphan-designation-overview (accessed June 25, 2024).

EMA. n.d.-o. *Paediatric investigation plans.* https://www.ema.europa.eu/en/human-regulatory-overview/research-development/paediatric-medicines-research-development/paediatric-investigation-plans (accessed August 15, 2024).

EMA. n.d.-p. *Patients' and Consumers' Working Party.* https://www.ema.europa.eu/en/committees/working-parties-other-groups/comp-working-parties-other-groups/patients-consumers-working-party (accessed August 6, 2024).

EMA. n.d.-q. *PRIME: Priority Medicines.* https://www.ema.europa.eu/en/human-regulatory-overview/research-development/prime-priority-medicines (accessed August 15, 2024).

EMA. n.d.-r. *Qualification of novel methodologies for medicine development.* https://www.ema.europa.eu/en/qualification-novel-methodologies-medicine-development (accessed August 6, 2024).

EMA. n.d.-s. *Scientific advice and protocol assistance.* https://www.ema.europa.eu/en/human-regulatory-overview/research-development/scientific-advice-protocol-assistance (accessed March 10, 2024).

EMA. n.d.-t. *Support to SMEs.* https://www.ema.europa.eu/en/about-us/support-smes (accessed August 7, 2024).
EMA. n.d.-u. *Supporting innovation.* https://www.ema.europa.eu/en/human-regulatory-overview/research-development/supporting-innovation (accessed July 10, 2024).
EMA. n.d.-v. *Who we are.* https://www.ema.europa.eu/en/about-us/who-we-are (accessed July 9, 2024).
EMA and FDA (U.S. Food and Drug Administration). 2021. *General principles: EMA-FDA parallel scientific advice.* https://www.ema.europa.eu/en/documents/other/general-principles-european-medicines-agency-food-and-drug-administration-parallel-scientific-advice_en.pdf (accessed August 1, 2024).
European Commission. 2022. *European Partnership on Rare Diseases.* https://cordis.europa.eu/programme/id/HORIZON_HORIZON-HLTH-2023-DISEASE-07-01 (accessed August 6, 2024).
European Commission. 2014. *Guideline on the format and content of applications for designation as orphan medicinal products and on the transfer of designations from one sponsor to another.* https://health.ec.europa.eu/system/files/2016-11/2014-03_guideline_rev4_final_0.pdf (accessed August 1, 2024).
European Joint Programme on Rare Diseases. n.d. *European Joint Programme on Rare Diseases.* https://www.ejprarediseases.org/ (accessed August 6, 2024).
European Union. 2022. *The EU Decentralised Clinical Trials project (EU DCT project).* https://www.hma.eu/fileadmin/dateien/HMA_joint/00-_About_HMA/03-Working_Groups/CTCG/2022_08_CTCG_EU_DCT_project.pdf (accessed August 1, 2024).
FDA. 1998. *Providing clinical evidence of effectiveness for human drug and biological product: Guidance for industry.* https://www.fda.gov/media/71655/download (accessed August 1, 2024).
FDA. 2009. *Formal meetings between the FDA and sponsors or applicants.* https://www.fda.gov/media/72253/download (accessed August 1, 2024).
FDA. 2010. *Guidance for the use of Bayesian statistics in medical device clinical trials: Guidance for industry and FDA staff.* https://www.fda.gov/media/71512/download (accessed August 1, 2024).
FDA. 2011. *E16 biomarkers related to drug or biotechnology product development: Context, structure, and format of qualification submissions.* https://www.fda.gov/media/81311/download (accessed August 1, 2024).
FDA. 2017. *Best practices for communication between IND sponsors and FDA during drug development guidance for industry and review staff: Good review practice.* https://www.fda.gov/media/94850/download (accessed August 1, 2024).
FDA. 2018a. *Biomarker qualification: Evidentiary framework: Guidance for industry and FDA staff.* https://www.fda.gov/media/122319/download (accessed August 1, 2024).
FDA. 2018b. *Biomarker qualification: Evidentiary framework: Guidance for industry and FDA staff.* https://www.fda.gov/media/122319/download (accessed August 1, 2024).
FDA. 2018c. *Breakthrough therapy.* https://www.fda.gov/patients/fast-track-breakthrough-therapy-accelerated-approval-priority-review/breakthrough-therapy (accessed August 6, 2024).
FDA. 2018d. *Clinical trial endpoints for the approval of cancer drugs and biologics.* https://www.fda.gov/media/71195/download (accessed August 1, 2024).
FDA. 2018e. *E17 general principles for planning and design of multiregional clinical trials.* https://www.fda.gov/media/99974/download (accessed August 1, 2024).
FDA. 2018f. *Fast track.* https://www.fda.gov/patients/fast-track-breakthrough-therapy-accelerated-approval-priority-review/fast-track (accessed August 7, 2024).
FDA. 2018g. *Meta-analyses of randomized controlled clinical trials to evaluate the safety of human drugs or biological products: Guidance for industry.* https://www.fda.gov/media/117976/download (accessed August 1, 2024).

FDA. 2018h. *Priority review.* https://www.fda.gov/patients/fast-track-breakthrough-therapy-accelerated-approval-priority-review/priority-review (accessed March 5, 2024).

FDA. 2018i. *Rare diseases: Early drug development and the role of pre-IND meetings.* https://www.fda.gov/media/117322/download (accessed August 1, 2024).

FDA. 2019a. *Adaptive designs for clinical trials of drugs and biologics: Guidance for industry.* https://www.fda.gov/media/78495/download (accessed August 1, 2024).

FDA. 2019b. *Demonstrating substantial evidence of effectiveness for human drug and biological products: Guidance for industry.* https://www.fda.gov/media/133660/download (accessed August 1, 2024).

FDA. 2019c. Rare diseases: Natural history studies for drug development: Guidance for industry. https://www.fda.gov/media/122425/download (accessed August 1, 2024).

FDA. 2019d. *Rare pediatric disease priority review vouchers guidance for industry.* https://www.fda.gov/media/90014/download (accessed August 1, 2024).

FDA. 2020a. *CURE ID app lets clinicians report novel uses of existing drugs.* https://www.fda.gov/drugs/science-and-research-drugs/cure-id-app-lets-clinicians-report-novel-uses-existing-drugs (accessed August 6, 2024).

FDA. 2020b. *Interacting with the FDA on complex innovative trial designs for drugs and biological products: Guidance for industry.* https://www.fda.gov/media/130897/download (accessed August 1, 2024).

FDA. 2020c. *Patient-focused drug development: Collecting comprehensive and representative input.* https://www.fda.gov/media/139088/download (accessed August 1, 2024).

FDA. 2020d. *Pediatric study plans: Content of and process for submitting initial pediatric study plans and amended initial pediatric study plans: Guidance for industry.* https://www.fda.gov/media/86340/download (accessed August 1, 2024).

FDA. 2020e. *Qualification process for drug development tools: Guidance for industry and FDA staff.* https://www.fda.gov/media/133511/download (accessed August 1, 2024).

FDA. 2022a. *About CDER small business and industry assistance (SBIA).* https://www.fda.gov/drugs/cder-small-business-industry-assistance-sbia/about-cder-small-business-and-industry-assistance-sbia (accessed August 6, 2024).

FDA. 2022b. *Externally-led patient-focused drug development meetings.* https://www.fda.gov/industry/prescription-drug-user-fee-amendments/externally-led-patient-focused-drug-development-meetings (accessed August 7, 2024).

FDA. 2022c. *General clinical pharmacology considerations for pediatric studies of drugs, including biological products.* https://www.fda.gov/media/90358/download (accessed August 1, 2024).

FDA. 2022d. *Master protocols: Efficient clinical trial design strategies to expedite development of oncology drugs and biologics: Guidance for industry.* https://www.fda.gov/media/120721/download (accessed August 1, 2024).

FDA. 2022e. *Multiple endpoints in clinical trials.* https://www.fda.gov/media/162416/download (accessed August 1, 2024).

FDA. 2022f. *Patient-focused drug development: Methods to identify what is important to patients: Guidance for industry, Food and Drug Administration staff, and other stakeholders.* https://www.fda.gov/media/131230/download (accessed August 1, 2024).

FDA. 2022g. *Patient-focused drug development: Selecting, developing, or modifying fit-for-purpose clinical outcome assessments.* https://www.fda.gov/media/159500/download (accessed August 1, 2024).

FDA. 2023a. *Benefit-risk assessment for new drug and biological products: Guidance for industry.* https://www.fda.gov/media/152544/download (accessed August 1, 2024).

FDA. 2023b. *Clinical outcome assessment (COA) qualification program.* https://www.fda.gov/drugs/drug-development-tool-ddt-qualification-programs/clinical-outcome-assessment-coa-qualification-program (accessed August 6, 2024).

FDA. 2023c. *Complex innovative trial design meeting program.* https://www.fda.gov/drugs/development-resources/complex-innovative-trial-design-meeting-program (accessed March 19, 2024).

FDA. 2023d. *Considerations for the design and conduct of externally controlled trials for drug and biological products: Guidance for industry.* https://www.fda.gov/media/164960/download (accessed August 1, 2024).

FDA. 2023e. *Considerations for the use of real-world data and real-world evidence to support regulatory decision-making for drug and biological products.* https://www.fda.gov/media/171667/download (accessed August 1, 2024).

FDA. 2023f. *Data standards for drug and biological product submissions containing real-world data.* https://www.fda.gov/media/153341/download (accessed August 1, 2024).

FDA. 2023g. *Decentralized clinical trials for drugs, biological products, and devices.* https://www.fda.gov/media/167696/download (accessed August 1, 2024).

FDA. 2023h. *Demonstrating substantial evidence of effectiveness with one adequate and well-controlled clinical investigation and confirmatory evidence: Guidance for industry.* https://www.fda.gov/media/172166/download (accessed August 1, 2024).

FDA. 2023i. *FDA-EMA Parallel Scientific Advice (PSA) program.* https://www.fda.gov/drugs/news-events-human-drugs/fda-ema-parallel-scientific-advice-psa-program-03162022 (accessed August 6, 2024).

FDA. 2023j. *Formal meetings between the FDA and sponsors or applicants of PDUFA products.* https://www.fda.gov/media/172311/download (accessed August 1, 2024).

FDA. 2023k. *Frequently asked questions (FAQ) about designating an orphan product.* https://www.fda.gov/industry/designating-orphan-product-drugs-and-biological-products/frequently-asked-questions-faq-about-designating-orphan-product (accessed March 19, 2024).

FDA. 2023l. *International agreements & information sharing.* https://www.fda.gov/drugs/cder-international-program/international-agreements-information-sharing (accessed August 6, 2024).

FDA. 2023m. *Orphan products grants program.* https://www.fda.gov/industry/medical-products-rare-diseases-and-conditions/orphan-products-grants-program (accessed August 6, 2024).

FDA. 2023n. *Patient-focused drug development: Incorporating clinical outcome assessments into endpoints for regulatory decision-making: Guidance for industry, Food and Drug Administration staff, and other stakeholders.* https://www.fda.gov/media/166830/download (accessed August 1, 2024).

FDA. 2023o. *Rare diseases: Considerations for the development of drugs and biological products: Guidance for industry.* https://www.fda.gov/media/119757/download (accessed August 1, 2024).

FDA. 2023p. *Real-world data: Assessing registries to support regulatory decision-making for drug and biological products: Guidance for industry.* https://www.fda.gov/media/154449/download (accessed August 1, 2024).

FDA. 2023q. *Support for clinical Trials Advancing Rare disease Therapeutics pilot program; program announcement.* https://www.federalregister.gov/documents/2023/10/02/2023-21235/support-for-clinical-trials-advancing-rare-disease-therapeutics-pilot-program-program-announcement (accessed August 1, 2024).

FDA. 2023r. *Using Bayesian statistical approaches to advance our ability to evaluate drug products.* https://www.fda.gov/drugs/cder-small-business-industry-assistance-sbia/using-bayesian-statistical-approaches-advance-our-ability-evaluate-drug-products (accessed August 1, 2024).

FDA. 2024a. *About the FDA patient representative program.* https://www.fda.gov/patients/learn-about-fda-patient-engagement/about-fda-patient-representative-program (accessed March 10, 2024).

FDA. 2024b. *Accelerated approval program.* https://www.fda.gov/drugs/nda-and-bla-approvals/accelerated-approval-program (accessed August 6, 2024).

FDA. 2024c. *Accelerating Rare disease Cures (ARC) program.* https://www.fda.gov/about-fda/center-drug-evaluation-and-research-cder/accelerating-rare-disease-cures-arc-program (accessed February 20, 2024).

FDA. 2024d. *Advancing real-world evidence program.* https://www.fda.gov/drugs/development-resources/advancing-real-world-evidence-program?utm_medium=email&utm_source=govdelivery#:~:text=As%20announced%20in%20the%20Federal%2cnew%20indications%20of%20approved%20medical (accessed August 7, 2024).

FDA. 2024e. *Biomarker qualification program.* https://www.fda.gov/drugs/drug-development-tool-ddt-qualification-programs/biomarker-qualification-program (accessed August 6, 2024).

FDA. 2024f. *CDER patient-focused drug development.* https://www.fda.gov/drugs/development-approval-process-drugs/cder-patient-focused-drug-development (accessed March 05, 2024).

FDA. 2024g. *CDER pilot grant program: Standard core clinical outcome assessments (COAs) and their related endpoints.* https://www.fda.gov/drugs/development-approval-process-drugs/cder-pilot-grant-program-standard-core-clinical-outcome-assessments-coas-and-their-related-endpoints (accessed August 7, 2024).

FDA. 2024h. *Clinical pharmacology considerations for the development of oligonucleotide therapeutics.* https://www.fda.gov/media/159414/download (accessed August 1, 2024).

FDA. 2024i. *Designating an orphan product: Drugs and biological products.* https://www.fda.gov/industry/medical-products-rare-diseases-and-conditions/designating-orphan-product-drugs-and-biological-products (accessed August 15, 2024).

FDA. 2024j. *FDA-led Patient-Focused Drug Development (PFDD) public meetings.* https://www.fda.gov/industry/prescription-drug-user-fee-amendments/fda-led-patient-focused-drug-development-pfdd-public-meetings (accessed August 7, 2024).

FDA. 2024k. *FDA Patient-Focused Drug Development guidance series for enhancing the incorporation of the patient's voice in medical product development and regulatory decision making.* https://www.fda.gov/drugs/development-approval-process-drugs/fda-patient-focused-drug-development-guidance-series-enhancing-incorporation-patients-voice-medical (accessed August 7, 2024).

FDA. 2024l. *FDA patient listening sessions.* https://www.fda.gov/patients/learn-about-fda-patient-engagement/fda-patient-listening-sessions (accessed August 1, 2024).

FDA. 2024m. *FDA patient listening sessions.* https://www.fda.gov/patients/learn-about-fda-patient-engagement/fda-patient-listening-sessions (accessed August 7, 2024).

FDA. 2024n. *Guidance documents for rare disease drug development.* https://www.fda.gov/drugs/guidances-drugs/guidance-documents-rare-disease-drug-development (accessed August 6, 2024).

FDA. 2024o. *LEADER 3D: Learning and Education to Advance and Empower Rare Disease Drug Developers: Public report of external stakeholder analysis.* https://www.fda.gov/media/176557/download?attachment= (accessed August 15, 2024).

FDA. 2024p. *Model-informed drug development paired meeting program.* https://www.fda.gov/drugs/development-resources/model-informed-drug-development-paired-meeting-program (accessed August 6, 2024).

FDA. 2024q. *Patient listening session summaries.* https://www.fda.gov/patients/learn-about-fda-patient-engagement/patient-listening-session-summaries#:~:text=Patient%20Listening%20Sessions%20can%20either,advocates%20participate%20in%20the%20session. (accessed August 7, 2024).

FDA. 2024r. *Project Orbis.* https://www.fda.gov/about-fda/oncology-center-excellence/project-orbis (accessed August 6, 2024).

FDA. 2024s. *Rare Disease Endpoint Advancement pilot program.* https://www.fda.gov/drugs/development-resources/rare-disease-endpoint-advancement-pilot-program (accessed August 6, 2024).

FDA. 2024t. *Rare pediatric disease designation and priority review voucher programs.* https://www.fda.gov/industry/medical-products-rare-diseases-and-conditions/rare-pediatric-disease-designation-and-priority-review-voucher-programs (accessed August 15, 2024).

FDA. 2024u. *Support for clinical Trials Advancing Rare disease Therapeutics (START) pilot program.* https://www.fda.gov/science-research/clinical-trials-and-human-subject-protection/support-clinical-trials-advancing-rare-disease-therapeutics-start-pilot-program (accessed August 6, 2024).

Flynn, R., K. Plueschke, C. Quinten, V. Strassmann, R. G. Duijnhoven, M. Gordillo-Maranon, M. Rueckbeil, C. Cohet, and X. Kurz. 2022. Marketing authorization applications made to the European Medicines Agency in 2018-2019: What was the contribution of real-world evidence? *Clinical Pharmacology & Therapeutics* 111(1):90-97.

GAO (U.S. Government Accountability Office). 2023. *Pediatric cancer studies: Early results of the Research to Accelerate Cures and Equity for Children Act.* https://www.gao.gov/products/gao-23-105947 (accessed August 1, 2024).

ICH (International Council for Harmonisation of Technical Requirements for Pharmaceuticals for Human Use). 1998. *Statistical principles for clinical trials E9.* https://database.ich.org/sites/default/files/E9_Guideline.pdf (accessed August 1, 2024).

ICH. 2001. *E10 choice of control group and related issues in clinical trials: Guidance for industry.* https://www.ema.europa.eu/en/documents/scientific-guideline/ich-e-10-choice-control-group-clinical-trials-step-5_en.pdf (accessed August 1, 2024).

ICH. 2019. *Final concept paper - E20: Adaptive clinical trials.* https://database.ich.org/sites/default/files/E20_FinalConceptPaper_2019_1107_0.pdf (accessed August 1, 2024).

ICH. 2021. *General considerations for clinical studies E8(R1).* https://database.ich.org/sites/default/files/ICH_E8-R1_Guideline_Step4_2021_1006.pdf (accessed August 1, 2024).

Ionan, A. C., J. Clark, J. Travis, A. Amatya, J. Scott, J. P. Smith, S. Chattopadhyay, M. J. Salerno, and M. Rothmann. 2023. Bayesian methods in human drug and biological products development in CDER and CBER. *Therapeutic Innovation & Regulatory Science* 57(3):436-444.

Lee, K. J., R. Bent, and J. Vaillancourt. 2023. Selected FDA programs on rare disease: Processes to Evaluate the Safety and Efficacy of Drugs for Rare Diseases or Conditions in the United States and the European Union (Meeting 1 - Virtual).

Michaeli, T., H. Jürges, and D. T. Michaeli. 2023. FDA approval, clinical trial evidence, efficacy, epidemiology, and price for non-orphan and ultra-rare, rare, and common orphan cancer drug indications: Cross sectional analysis. *BMJ* 381:e073242.

Thirstrup, S. 2023. Orphan medicines in EU: Processes to Evaluate the Safety and Efficacy of Drugs for Rare Diseases or Conditions in the United States and the European Union (Meeting 2 - Hybrid).

Thor, S., T. Vetter, A. Marcal, and S. Kweder. 2023. EMA-FDA parallel scientific advice: Optimizing development of medicines in the global age. *Therapeutic Innovation & Regulatory Science 2023 57(4)* CC BY 4.0.

Ungstrup, E., and D. Vanags. 2023. *Aligning global drug development for pediatric populations.* https://www.pharmalex.com/thought-leadership/blogs/aligning-global-drug-development-for-pediatric-populations/ (accessed August 15, 2024).